*HERE'S AMERICA'S FAVORITE DIET GUIDE*

# CALORIES AND CARBOHYDRATES

*THE BOOK THAT MAKES IT FUN TO LOSE THOSE EXTRA POUNDS*

Whether you aim to lose five pounds or fifty, the only safe, healthy way is to eat an adequate, well-balanced diet, choosing your calories from many different kinds of foods in order to ensure that you're getting sufficient vitamins, minerals, and other nutrients. CALORIES AND CARBOHYDRATES contains the most accurate and dependable caloric and carbohydrate counts for practically everything you will eat and drink—thousands and thousands of brand names and basic foods, including alcoholic beverages and take-out foods such as your favorites from McDONALD'S or BURGER KING.

**So diet—and enjoy it!**

# SIGNET Books for Your Reference Shelf

# Barbara Kraus

# CALORIES
## and
# CARBOHYDRATES

## FOURTH REVISED EDITION

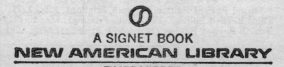

A SIGNET BOOK
**NEW AMERICAN LIBRARY**
TIMES MIRROR

*For Vito Squicciarini*

SIGNET TRADEMARK REG. U.S. PAT. OFF. AND FOREIGN COUNTRIES
REGISTERED TRADEMARK—MARCA REGISTRADA
HECHO EN CHICAGO, U.S.A.

SIGNET, SIGNET CLASSICS, MENTOR, PLUME, MERIDIAN, AND NAL BOOKS
are published by The New American Library, Inc.,
1633 Broadway, New York, New York 10019

First Signet Printing, August, 1973
Second Revised Edition (Seventh Printing), July, 1975
Third Revised Edition (Fourteenth Printing), March, 1979
Fourth Revised Edition (Nineteenth Printing), May, 1981

22 23 24 25 26 27

PRINTED IN THE UNITED STATES OF AMERICA

# Contents

# Introduction

This dictionary of foods lists several thousand brand-name products and basic foods with their caloric and carbohydrate content. The calorie yield of your diet versus the amount of energy you expend is the key to whether you maintain your ideal weight, gain too many pounds or lose weight.

Because of the relationship of weight to health, many individuals are "counting calories" at every meal. Interest has also been directed to the carbohydrate content of the diet in relation to weight control. Comprehensive information on these values in basic foods and brand-name products is not readily available in any one source. Nor is the information regularly reported in portions that are usually eaten or bought at the grocery store. To compound the problem, hundreds of new food items appear in our stores every year.

## *Arrangement of This Book*

Foods are listed alphabetically by brand name or by the name of the food. The singular form is used for the entries, that is, blackberry instead of blackberries. Most items are listed individually though a few are grouped (see p. xiii) for example, all candies are listed together so that if you are looking for *Mars* bar, you look first under Candy, then under *M* in alphabetical order. But, if you are looking for a breakfast food such as Oatmeal, you will find it under *O* in the main alphabet. Many cross references are included to assist in finding items called by different names.

Under the main headings, it was often not possible nor even desirable to follow an alphabetical arrangement. For basic foods such as apricots, for example, the first entries are for the fresh product weighed with seeds as it is purchased in the store, then the fruit in small portions as they may be eaten or measured. These entries are followed by the processed products, canned (although it may actually be a bottle or jar), dehydrated, dried and frozen. This basic plan, with adaptations where necessary, was followed for fruits, vegetables and meats.

In almost all entries where data were available the U.S. Department of Agriculture figures are shown first. The Department values represent averages from several manufacturers and are shown for comparison with the values from individual companies or for use where particular brands are not available.

All brand-name products have been italicized and company names appear in parentheses.


## Portions Used

The portion column is a most important one to read and note. Common household measures are used insofar as possible. For some items, the amounts given are those commonly purchased in the store, such as 1 pound of meat. These quantities can be divided into the number of servings used in the home and the nutritive values available to each person served can then be readily determined. Of course, any ingredients added to preparing such products must also be taken into account.

The smaller portions given are for foods as served or measured in moderate amounts, such as ½ cup of juice reconstituted, or 4 ounces of meat. Be sure to adjust the calories and carbohydrates to the actual portions you use. For example, if you serve 1 cup of juice instead of ½ cup, multiply the calories and carbohydrates shown for the smaller amount by 2.

Don't fool yourself about the size of portions you use. If you are serious about controlling the calories and carbohydrates in your diet, weigh your foods until you can accurately gauge the weight visually. Remember, the calories and carbohydrates go up with any increase in the weight of foods. Remember, too, that 4 ounces by weight may be very different from 4 fluid ounces or ½ cup. Ounces in the table are always ounces by weight unless specified as fluid ounces, or fractions of a cup or other volumetric measure. Foods that are fluffy in texture, such as flaked coconut and bean sprouts, vary greatly in weight per cup depending on how tightly they are packed into the cup. Such foods as canned green beans also vary when weighed with or without liquid, for example, canned green beans with liquid weigh 4.2 ounces for ½ cup, but drained beans weigh 2.5 ounces for the same ½ cup. Check the weights of your serving portions regularly. Bear in mind that you can cut calories and carbohydrates by cutting the serving size.

It was impossible to convert all the portions to a uniform basis. Some sources were only able to report data in terms of weights with no information on cup or other volumetric measures. I have shown small portions in quantities that might reasonably be expected to be served or measured in the home or institution. Package sizes are useful to show the composition of products as they are purchased and may be divided into the number of serving portions prepared from the entire product, taking into account any added ingredients.

You will find in the portion column the phrases "weighed with bone," or "weighed with skin and seeds" or other inedible parts. These descriptions apply to the products as you purchase them in the markets but the caloric values and the carbohydrate content as shown are for the amount of edible food after you discard the bone, skin, seed or other inedible part. The weight given in the "measure or quantity" column is to the nearest gram or fraction of an ounce.

Data on the composition of foods are constantly changing for many reasons. Better sampling and analytical methods, improvements in marketing procedures and changes in formulas of mixed products, all may alter values for carbohydrates and other nutrients as well as caloric values. Weights of packaged foods are frequently changed. It is essential to read label information to be informed about these matters and to make intelligent use of food tables.

I will be constantly revising and updating this book along with my individual calorie and carbohydrate annual guides (*The Barbara Kraus 1981 Calorie and Carbohydrate Guides to Brand Names and Basic Foods*) to help keep you as up-to-date as possible.

## Calories

What is a calorie? It is not a nutrient nor is it a good guide to the nutritive value of a food. It is more like a yardstick to measure the energy that a food will yield in the body. You need energy for your body functions as well as for exercise.

If your diet contains more calories than your body uses for these purposes, the extra "energy" will be stored as fat.

If your plan is to cut down on calories, the easiest way to do so is to consult the calorie column of this counter and keep an accurate count of your total intake of food and beverages for a period of seven days. If you have not gained or lost weight during that week divide that number by seven and you'll have your maintenance diet expressed in calories. To lose weight, you must reduce your daily or weekly intake of calories below this maintenance level. (To gain, increase the intake.)

One pound of fat is equal to 3,500 calories. Add this number of calories to those you need to balance your energy requirements and you will gain one pound; subtract it, and you will lose a pound.

## Carbohydrates

The carbohydrate column shows the amount of this nutrient in grams for the quantities of foods indicated in the portion column. Some dietitians are giving special attention to this nutrient at present in connection with weight control. Carbohydrates include sugars, starches, acids and other nutrients. The values in this book are total carbohydrates, by difference, the basis on which calories from carbohydrates are calculated in the U.S. diet.

## Other Nutrients

Do not forget that other nutrients are extremely important in diet planning—protein, fat, minerals and vitamins. Calories yielded by alcohol must also be taken into consideration. From a nutrition viewpoint, perhaps the best advice that can be given to the dieter is to eat a varied diet with all classes of foods represented. Meat, fish, chicken, fats and oils, milk, vegetables, fruits and grain products are all important sources of essential nutrients and some foods from each of these classes of foods should be included in the diet every day. With the great abundance and variety of foods on the grocer's shelves, there is no reason why the dieter should not enjoy a tasty, nutritious and attractive diet. Just eat in moderation and there is no need to eliminate any one food altogether, except in special conditions under a doctor's directions. Choose wisely and eat well.

## Sources of Data

Values in this dictionary are based on publications issued by the U.S. Department of Agriculture and on data submitted by manufacturers and processors. The U.S. Department of Agriculture issues basic tables on food composition for use in the United States. The commercial products from U.S.D.A. publications represent average values obtained on products of more than one company. The figures designated "home recipe" are based on recipes on file with the Department of Agriculture. Data on commercial products listed by brand name in this publication are based on values supplied by manufacturers and processors for their own individual products. Very few supermarket brand names, such as Pathmark or private labels were included in this book inasmuch as they are not usually analyzed under these trade names. Every care has been taken to interpret the data and the descriptions supplied by the companies as fully and accurately as possible. Many values have been recalculated to different portions from those submitted in order to bring about greater uniformity among similar items.

Calories in these different sources are not always on a strictly uniform basis. In the Department of Agriculture, calories are calculated using specific factors, which make allowances for losses in digestion and metabolism. The technical explanation of these factors is given in Handbook 74 of the United States Department of Agriculture. Most manufacturers use average factors of 4, 9 and 4 for calories yielded by each gram of protein, fat and carbohydrate respectively; a factor of 7 is used as an average value to calculate the calories from one gram of alcohol. These differences in procedure will give somewhat different results for products of similar composition. Some manufacturers have adopted the values from U.S. Department of Agriculture publications as representative of their own products. In these cases, it will be apparent in the table that the data from the companies match exactly those from U.S.D.A. publications.

Analyses of foods to provide information on nutritive values are extremely expensive to conduct. Many small companies have not been able to afford to have their products analyzed and thus were unable to provide data for this book or were able to provide only the calories or only the carbohydrates. Other companies have simply never gotten around to having the analysis done. New requirements for labeling nutritive values of products may provide information on additional items in the future. Therefore, wherever data for carbohydrates were unavailable, blank spaces were left which may be filled in by the reader at a later time.

Bear in mind that small differences in calorie values on similar products of the same weight are not important in diet planning. They may be due to different methods of calculating the calories or to small differences in the nutritive values of the samples analyzed because no two foods ever have exactly the same composition. Some differences may also be due to the way the food was measured as noted in the case of green beans earlier.

Carbohydrates in this book are usually total carbohydrates by difference. A few manufacturers reported only "available carbohydrates." These values were omitted.

## Foods Listed by Groups

Certain foods are reported together rather than as individual items in the main alphabet. For example: Baby Food; Bread; Cake; Cake Icing; Cake Icing Mix; Cake Mix; Candy; Cheese; Cookie; Cookie Mix; Cracker; Gravy; Pie; Pie Filling; Salad Dressing; Sauce and Soft Drinks.

BARBARA KRAUS

# Abbreviations and Symbols

(USDA) = United States Department
    of Agriculture
(HEW/FAO) = Health, Education
    and Welfare/Food
    and Agriculture
    Organization
* = prepared as package directs[1]
< = less than
& = and
″ = inch
canned = bottles or jars
    as well as cans
dia. = diameter
fl. = fluid

liq. = liquid
lb. = pound
med. = medium
oz. = ounce
pkg. = package
pt. = pint
qt. = quart
sq. = square
T. = tablespoon
Tr. = trace
tsp. = teaspoon
wt. = weight

italics or name in parentheses = registered trademark, ®
Blank spaces indicate that no data are available.

# Equivalents

*By Weight*
1 pound = 16 ounces
1 ounce = 28.35 grams
3.52 ounces = 100 grams

*By Volume*
1 quart = 4 cups
1 cup = 8 fluid ounces
1 cup = ½ pint
1 cup = 16 tablespoons
2 tablespoons = 1 fluid ounce
1 tablespoon = 3 teaspoons

[1]If the package directions call for whole or skim milk, the data given here are for whole milk, unless otherwise stated.

| Food and Description | Measure or Quantity | Calories | Carbohydrates (grams) |
|---|---|---|---|
| | A | | |
| **ABALONE** (USDA): | | | |
| Raw, meat only | 4 oz. | 111 | 3.9 |
| Canned | 4 oz. | 91 | 2.6 |
| **ABISANTE LIQUEUR** | | | |
| (Leroux) 100 proof | 1 fl. oz. | 87 | 1.0 |
| *AC'CENT* | ¼ tsp. (1 gram) | 3 | 0. |
| **ACEROLA**, fresh (USDA) | ½ lb. (weighed with seeds) | 52 | 12.6 |
| **ALBACORE**, raw, meat only (USDA) | 4 oz. | 201 | 0. |
| **ALCOHOLIC BEVERAGES** (See individual listings) | | | |
| **ALE** (See **BEER**) | | | |
| **ALEWIFE** (USDA): | | | |
| Raw, meat only | 4 oz. | 144 | 0. |
| Canned, solids & liq. | 4 oz. | 160 | 0. |
| **ALEXANDER COCKTAIL** MIX (Holland House) | .6-oz. pkg. | 69 | 16.0 |
| **ALLSPICE** (French's) | 1 tsp. | 6 | 1.3 |
| **ALMOND:** | | | |
| In shell: | | | |
| (USDA) | 10 nuts (25 grams) | 60 | 2.0 |
| (USDA) | 1 cup (2.8 oz.) | 187 | 6.1 |

(USDA): United States Department of Agriculture
(HEW/FAO): Health, Education and Welfare/Food and Agriculture Organization
* Prepared as Package Directs

| Food and Description | Measure or Quantity | Calories | Carbohydrates (grams) |
|---|---|---|---|
| Shelled: | | | |
| (USDA) whole | ½ cup (2.5 oz.) | 425 | 13.8 |
| (USDA) whole | 1 oz. | 170 | 5.5 |
| (USDA) whole | 13-15 almonds (.6 oz.) | 105 | 3.4 |
| (USDA) chopped | 1 cup (4.5 oz.) | 777 | 25.4 |
| (Blue Diamond) | ½ cup | 504 | 19.4 |
| Blanched (Blue Diamond) salted | ½ cup | 492 | 15.3 |
| Chocolate-covered (See CANDY) | | | |
| Flavored (Blue Diamond) | 1 oz. | 180 | 9.5 |
| Roasted: | | | |
| (USDA) salted | ½ cup (2.8 oz.) | 492 | 15.3 |
| (Blue Diamond) diced | 1 oz. | 176 | 5.5 |
| (Flavor House) dry roasted | 1 oz. | 178 | 5.5 |
| (Planters) dry roasted | 1 oz. | 170 | 6.0 |
| **ALMOND EXTRACT:** | | | |
| (Durkee) | 1 tsp. | 13 | |
| (Ehlers) | 1 tsp. | 12 | |
| (French's) | 1 tsp. | 12 | |
| (Virginia Dare) | 1 tsp. (4 grams) | 10 | 0. |
| **ALMOND MEAL,** partially defatted (USDA) | 1 oz. | 116 | 8.2 |
| **ALPHA-BITS,** oat cereal (Post) | 1 cup (1 oz.) | 173 | 23.8 |
| **A.M.** fruit juice drink (Mott's) | 6 fl. oz. | 90 | 22.0 |
| **AMARANTH,** raw (USDA): | | | |
| Untrimmed | 1 lb. (weighed untrimmed) | 103 | 18.6 |
| Trimmed | 4 oz. | 41 | 7.4 |
| **AMARETTO DELIGHT COCKTAIL** (Mr. Boston) 12½% alcohol | 3 fl. oz. | 204 | 27.6 |

| Food and Description | Measure or Quantity | Calories | Carbo-hydrates (grams) |
|---|---|---|---|
| *AMARETTO DI SARONNO* | 1 fl. oz. | 82 | 9.0 |
| **AMARETTO SOUR COCKTAIL** (Mr. Boston) 12½% alcohol | 3 fl. oz. | 123 | 15.6 |
| **ANCHOVY, PICKLED,** canned (USDA) not heavily salted, drained | 2-oz. can | 79 | .1 |
| **ANGEL FOOD CAKE** (See CAKE, Angel Food) | | | |
| **ANGEL FOOD CAKE MIX** (See CAKE MIX, Angel Food) | | | |
| **ANISE EXTRACT:** | | | |
| (Durkee) | 1 tsp. | 16 | |
| (Ehlers) | 1 tsp. | 26 | |
| (French's) | 1 tsp. | 26 | |
| (Virginia Dare) | 1 tsp. (4 grams) | 22 | 0. |
| **ANISE SEED,** dried (HEW/FAO) | ½ oz. | 58 | 6.3 |
| **ANISETTE LIQUEUR,** red or white: | | | |
| (Dekuyper) | 1 fl. oz. (1.2 oz.) | 95 | 11.4 |
| (Mr. Boston) | 1 fl. oz. | 88 | 10.8 |
| **APPLE,** any variety: Fresh (USDA): | | | |
| Eaten with skin | 1 lb. (weighed with skin & core) | 242 | 60.5 |
| Eaten with skin | 1 med., 2½" dia. (about 4 per lb.) | 66 | 15.3 |

(USDA): United States Department of Agriculture
(HEW/FAO): Health, Education and Welfare/Food and Agriculture Organization
* Prepared as Package Directs

| Food and Description | Measure or Quantity | Calories | Carbohydrates (grams) |
|---|---|---|---|
| Eaten without skin | 1 lb. (weighed with skin & core) | 211 | 55.0 |
| Eaten without skin | 1 med., 2½″ dia. (about 4 per lb.) | 53 | 13.9 |
| Pared, diced or sliced | 1 cup (3.9 oz.) | 59 | 15.5 |
| Pared, quartered | 1 cup (4.4 oz.) | 68 | 17.6 |
| Dehydrated (USDA): | | | |
| Uncooked | 1 oz. | 100 | 26.1 |
| Cooked, sweetened | ½ cup (4.5 oz.) | 97 | 25.0 |
| Dried: | | | |
| (USDA) uncooked | 1 cup (3 oz.) | 234 | 61.0 |
| (USDA) cooked, unsweetened | ½ cup (4.5 oz.) | 99 | 25.9 |
| (USDA) cooked, sweetened | ½ cup (4.9 oz.) | 157 | 40.9 |
| (Del Monte) uncooked | 1 cup (2 oz.) | 151 | 37.2 |
| (Sun-Maid) | 2-oz. serving | 150 | 40.0 |
| Frozen, sweetened, slices, not thawed (USDA) | 10-oz. pkg. | 264 | 68.9 |
| **APPLE BROWN BETTY,** home recipe (USDA) | 1 cup (7.6 oz.) | 325 | 63.9 |
| **APPLE BUTTER:** | | | |
| (USDA) | 1 T. (.6 oz.) | 33 | 8.2 |
| (Smucker's) cider or spiced | 1 T. (.6 oz.) | 38 | 9.0 |
| **APPLE CIDER:** | | | |
| (USDA) | ½ cup (4.4 oz.) | 58 | 14.8 |
| (Mott's) sweet | ½ cup | 59 | 14.6 |
| *Mix, *Country Time* | 8 fl. oz. | 98 | 24.5 |
| **APPLE-CRANBERRY JUICE,** canned (Lincoln) | 6 fl. oz. | 104 | 26.0 |
| **APPLE DRINK,** canned: | | | |
| (Ann Page) | 6 fl. oz. (6.3 oz.) | 80 | 20.0 |
| (Hi-C) | 6 fl. oz. | 92 | 23.0 |
| **APPLE, ESCALLOPED,** frozen (Stouffer's) | ⅓ of 12-oz. pkg. | 138 | 27.8 |

| Food and Description | Measure or Quantity | Calories | Carbohydrates (grams) |
|---|---|---|---|
| **APPLE FRITTERS,** frozen (Mrs. Paul's) | 2-oz. fritter | 117 | 16.1 |
| **APPLE JACKS,** cereal (Kellogg's) | 1 cup (1 oz.) | 110 | 26.0 |
| **APPLE JELLY:** | | | |
| Sweetened: | | | |
| (Smucker's) | 1 T. (.7 oz.) | 57 | 14.0 |
| (White House) | 1 T. (.7 oz.) | 46 | 13.0 |
| Dietetic or low calorie: | | | |
| (Dia-Mel) | 1 T. (.5 oz.) | 6 | 0. |
| (Diet Delight) | 1 T. (.6 oz.) | 14 | 3.5 |
| (Featherweight) | 1 T. | 16 | 3.0 |
| (Slenderella) | 1 T. (.6 oz.) | 24 | 6.0 |
| (Tillie Lewis) *Tasti Diet* | 1 T. (.5 oz.) | 11 | 2.6 |
| **APPLE JUICE:** | | | |
| Canned: | | | |
| (USDA) | ½ cup (4.4 oz.) | 58 | 14.8 |
| (Ann Page) | ½ cup (4.4 oz.) | 79 | 20.0 |
| (Lincoln) cocktail | ½ cup (4.4 oz.) | 65 | 16.7 |
| (Minute Maid) | 6 fl. oz. | 100 | 24.0 |
| (Mott's) regular or McIntosh | ½ cup (4.4 oz.) | 59 | 14.6 |
| *Frozen (Minute Maid) | 6-fl.-oz. serving | 100 | 24.0 |
| **APPLE PIE** (See PIE, Apple) | | | |
| **APPLE PIE FILLING** (See PIE FILLING, Apple) | | | |
| **APPLESAUCE,** canned: | | | |
| Sweetened: | | | |
| (USDA) | ½ cup (4.5 oz.) | 116 | 30.5 |
| (Del Monte) | ½ cup (4.6 oz.) | 97 | 23.7 |

(USDA): United States Department of Agriculture
(HEW/FAO): Health, Education and Welfare/Food and Agriculture Organization
* Prepared as Package Directs

| Food and Description | Measure or Quantity | Calories | Carbo- hydrates (grams) |
|---|---|---|---|
| (Mott's) natural style | ½ cup | 107 | 26.2 |
| (Stokely-Van Camp) | ½ cup (4.5 oz.) | 90 | 22.5 |
| Unsweetened, dietetic or low calorie: | | | |
| (USDA) | ½ cup (4.3 oz.) | 50 | 13.2 |
| (Diet Delight) | ½ cup (4.3 oz.) | 54 | 13.3 |
| (Featherweight) | ½ cup | 50 | 12.0 |
| (Mott's) natural style | 4-oz. serving | 45 | 11.0 |
| (Tillie Lewis) *Tasti Diet* | ½ cup (4.1 oz.) | 61 | 15.2 |
| **APPLE SPREAD,** low sugar (Smucker's) | 1 T. | 24 | 6.0 |
| **APPLE TURNOVER,** chilled (Pillsbury) | 1 turnover | 170 | 26.0 |
| **APRICOT:** | | | |
| Fresh (USDA): | | | |
| Whole | 1 lb. (weighed with pits) | 217 | 54.6 |
| Whole | 3 apricots (about 12 per lb.) | 55 | 13.7 |
| Halves | 1 cup (5.5 oz.) | 79 | 19.8 |
| Canned, regular pack, solids & liq.: | | | |
| (USDA) juice pack | 4 oz. | 61 | 15.4 |
| (USDA) light syrup | 4 oz. | 75 | 19.1 |
| (USDA) heavy syrup, halves | ½ cup (4.6 oz.) | 111 | 28.4 |
| (USDA) heavy syrup, halves | 3 med. halves with 1¾-T. syrup (3.0 oz.) | 73 | 18.7 |
| (USDA) extra heavy syrup | 4 oz. | 115 | 29.5 |
| (Del Monte): | | | |
| halves, unpeeled | ½ cup | 101 | 24.4 |
| whole, peeled | ½ cup | 104 | 25.0 |
| (Libby's) heavy syrup, halves | ½ cup | 110 | 26.8 |
| (Stokely-Van Camp) | ½ cup (4.6 oz.) | 110 | 27.0 |

| Food and Description | Measure or Quantity | Calories | Carbo-hydrates (grams) |
|---|---|---|---|
| Canned, unsweetened or dietetic: | | | |
| (USDA) water pack, halves, solids & liq. | ½ cup (4.3 oz.) | 46 | 11.8 |
| (Del Monte) *Lite*, un-peeled, extra light syrup, solids & liq. | ½ cup (4.3 oz.) | 64 | 15.1 |
| (Diet Delight) juice pack, solids & liq. | ½ cup (4.4 oz.) | 64 | 15.0 |
| (Diet Delight) water pack, solids & liq. | ½ cup | 35 | 9.0 |
| (Featherweight) juice pack, solids & liq. | ½ cup | 50 | 12.0 |
| (Featherweight) water pack, solids & liq. | ½ cup | 30 | 9.0 |
| (Tillie Lewis) *Tasti Diet*, unpeeled, solids & liq. | ½ cup (4.3 oz.) | 60 | 15.0 |
| Dehydrated: | | | |
| (USDA) uncooked, sulfured | 4 oz. | 376 | 95.9 |
| (USDA) cooked, sugar added, solids & liq. | 4 oz. | 135 | 34.6 |
| Dried: | | | |
| (USDA) | | | |
| Uncooked | 1 cup (4.6 oz.) | 338 | 86.5 |
| Uncooked | 10 large halves (¼ cup or 1.7 oz.) | 125 | 31.9 |
| Cooked, sweetened | ½ cup with liq. (4.7 oz.) | 164 | 42.4 |
| Cooked, unsweetened | ½ cup with liq. (4.4 oz.) | 106 | 27.0 |
| (Del Monte) | ½ cup (2.3 oz.) | 145 | 39.9 |
| (Sun-Maid) | ¼ cup (2 oz.) | 140 | 35.0 |
| Frozen, unthawed, sweet-ened (USDA) | 10-oz. pkg. | 278 | 71.2 |

(USDA): United States Department of Agriculture
(HEW/FAO): Health, Education and Welfare/Food and Agriculture Organization
* Prepared as Package Directs

| Food and Description | Measure or Quantity | Calories | Carbohydrates (grams) |
|---|---|---|---|
| **APRICOT BRANDY** (See BRANDY, FLAVORED) | | | |
| **APRICOT, CANDIED** (USDA) | 1 oz. | 96 | 24.5 |
| **APRICOT LIQUEUR** (Dekuyper) 60 proof | 1 fl. oz. | 82 | 8.3 |
| **APRICOT NECTAR,** canned, sweetened: | | | |
| (USDA) | ½ cup (4.4 oz.) | 71 | 18.3 |
| (Del Monte) | ½ cup (4.4 oz.) | 75 | 18.0 |
| **APRICOT & PINEAPPLE PRESERVE:** | | | |
| Sweetened (Smucker's) | 1 T. (.7 oz.) | 53 | 13.5 |
| Low calorie or dietetic: | | | |
| (Diet Delight) | 1 T. (.6 oz.) | 13 | 3.4 |
| (Featherweight) artificially sweetened | 1 T. | 8 | 2.0 |
| (Tillie Lewis) *Tasti Diet* | 1 T. (.5 oz.) | 12 | 2.8 |
| **APRICOT PRESERVE:** | | | |
| Sweetened (Smucker's) | 1 T. (.7 oz.) | 53 | 13.5 |
| Low calorie or dietetic: | | | |
| (Dia-Mel) | 1 T. | 6 | 0. |
| (Featherweight) | 1 T. | 16 | 4.0 |
| **APRICOT SOUR COCKTAIL:** | | | |
| (Holland House) liquid mix | 2 fl. oz. | 86 | 24.0 |
| (National Distillers) *Duet,* 12½% alcohol | 2 fl. oz. | 48 | 1.6 |
| (Party Tyme) dry mix | ½ oz. pkg. | 50 | 11.6 |
| (Party Tyme) liquid mix | 2 fl. oz. | 58 | 14.0 |
| (Party Tyme) 12½% alcohol | 2 fl. oz. | 66 | 5.7 |
| **APRICOT SPREAD,** low sugar (Smucker's) | 1 T. | 24 | 6.0 |
| **APRICOT SYRUP,** sweetened (Smucker's) | 1 T. (.6 oz.) | 50 | 13.0 |

| Food and Description | Measure or Quantity | Calories | Carbohydrates (grams) |
|---|---|---|---|
| **AQUAVIT** (Leroux) 90 proof | 1 fl. oz. | 75 | Tr. |
| **ARTICHOKE,** Globe or French (See also **JERUSALEM ARTICHOKE**): | | | |
| Raw, whole (USDA) | 1 lb. (weighed untrimmed) | 85 | 19.2 |
| Boiled, without salt, drained (USDA) | 4 oz. | 50 | 11.2 |
| Canned (Cara Mia) marinated, drained | 6-oz. jar | 175 | 12.6 |
| Frozen: | | | |
| (Birds Eye) deluxe hearts | ⅓ of 9-oz. pkg. | 34 | 5.5 |
| (Cara Mia) | ⅓ of 9-oz. pkg. | 35 | 7.5 |
| **ASPARAGUS:** | | | |
| Raw (USDA) whole spears | 1 lb. (weighed untrimmed) | 66 | 12.7 |
| Boiled (USDA) without salt, drained: | | | |
| Whole spears | 4 spears (½" at base, 2.1 oz.) | 12 | 2.2 |
| Cut spears, 1½"-2" pieces | 1 cup (5.1 oz.) | 29 | 5.2 |
| Canned, regular pack: | | | |
| (USDA) green spears, solids & liq. | 1 cup (8.6 oz.) | 44 | 7.1 |
| (USDA) green spears, drained | 1 cup (8.3 oz.) | 49 | 8.0 |
| (USDA) green spears only | 4 med. spears (2.8 oz.) | 17 | 2.7 |
| (USDA) green, liquid only | 2 T. liquid | 3 | .7 |
| (USDA) white spears, solids & liq. | 1 cup (8.6 oz.) | 44 | 8.1 |

(USDA): United States Department of Agriculture
(HEW/FAO): Health, Education and Welfare/Food and Agriculture Organization
* Prepared as Package Directs

| Food and Description | Measure or Quantity | Calories | Carbohydrates (grams) |
|---|---|---|---|
| (USDA) white, spears only | 4 med. spears (2.8 oz.) | 18 | 2.9 |
| (USDA) white, liquid only | 2 T. liquid | 3 | .8 |
| (Del Monte): | | | |
| Green, spears, solids & liq. | 1 cup (8.6 oz.) | 47 | 6.4 |
| Green, spears, drained solids | 1 cup (8.5 oz.) | 65 | 7.5 |
| White, spears, solids & liq. | 1 cup (8.6 oz.) | 48 | 7.3 |
| White, spears, drained solids | 1 cup (8.5 oz.) | 55 | 8.0 |
| (Green Giant) green, cut spears, solids & liq. | ½ of 10½-oz. can | 22 | 2.5 |
| (Kounty Kist) green, cut spears, solids & liq. | ⅓ of 14-oz. can | 19 | 2.3 |
| (Kounty Kist) green, spears, solids & liq. | ½ of 15-oz. can | 31 | 3.6 |
| (Le Sueur) green, spears, solids & liq. | ¼ of 19-oz. can | 20 | 2.3 |
| (Lindy) green, cut spears, solids & liq. | ⅓ of 10½-oz. can | 14 | 1.7 |
| (Stokely-Van Camp) green, spears, solids & liq. | 1 cup (8.4 oz.) | 45 | 6.0 |
| (Stokely-Van Camp) green, cut spears, solids & liq. | 1 cup (8.4 oz.) | 46 | 6.0 |
| Canned, dietetic pack: | | | |
| (USDA) green, spears, solids & liq. | 4 oz. | 18 | 3.1 |
| (USDA) green, spears, drained solids | 4 oz. | 23 | 3.5 |
| (USDA) green, liquid only | 4-oz. liquid | 10 | 2.3 |
| (USDA) white, spears, solids & liq. | 4 oz. | 18 | 3.4 |
| (Diet Delight) solids & liq. | ½ cup (4.2 oz.) | 18 | 2.3 |

| Food and Description | Measure or Quantity | Calories | Carbo-hydrates (grams) |
|---|---|---|---|
| (Tillie Lewis) *Tasti Diet*, cut spears, solids & liq. | ½ cup | 18 | 4.0 |
| Frozen: | | | |
| (USDA) cuts & tips, unthawed | 4 oz. | 26 | 4.1 |
| (USDA) cuts & tips, boiled, drained | ½ cup (3.2 oz.) | 20 | 3.2 |
| (USDA) spears, unthawed | 4 oz. | 27 | 4.4 |
| (USDA) spears, boiled, drained | 4 oz. | 26 | 4.3 |
| (Birds Eye) cuts, 5-minute style | ⅛ of 10-oz. pkg. | 25 | 3.0 |
| (Birds Eye) spears, regular or jumbo | ⅛ of 10-oz. pkg. | 28 | 3.4 |
| (Green Giant) cut spears, in butter sauce | ⅛ of 9-oz. pkg. | 41 | 2.6 |
| (McKenzie) cuts & tips | 3.3-oz. serving | 30 | 3.8 |
| (McKenzie) spears | 4-oz. serving | 29 | 8.0 |
| (Seabrook Farms) cuts & tips | 3.3-oz. serving | 30 | 3.8 |
| (Seabrook Farms) spears | ⅓ of 12-oz. pkg. | 29 | 8.0 |
| (Stouffer's) souffle | ⅓ of 12-oz. pkg. | 118 | 8.0 |
| **ASPARAGUS SOUP,** cream of, canned: | | | |
| (USDA): | | | |
| Condensed | 8 oz. (by weight) | 123 | 19.1 |
| Prepared with equal volume water | 1 cup (8.5 oz.) | 65 | 10.1 |
| Prepared with equal volume milk | 1 cup (8.5 oz.) | 144 | 16.3 |
| *(Campbell) condensed | 8-oz. serving | 80 | 9.6 |
| *AUNT JEMIMA SYRUP* | ¼ cup | 212 | 54.0 |

(USDA): United States Department of Agriculture
(HEW/FAO): Health, Education and Welfare/Food and Agriculture Organization
* Prepared as Package Directs

| *Food and Description* | *Measure or Quantity* | *Calories* | *Carbo-hydrates (grams)* |
|---|---|---|---|
| **AVOCADO,** peeled, pitted, all commercial varieties (USDA): | | | |
| Whole | 1 fruit (10.7 oz., weighed with seed & skin) | 378 | 14.3 |
| Cubed | 1 cup (5.3 oz.) | 251 | 9.5 |
| Puree | 1 cup (8.1 oz.) | 384 | 14.5 |
| ****AWAKE*** (Birds Eye) | 6 fl. oz. | 88 | 21.2 |
| ***AYDS,*** all flavors | 1 piece (7 grams) | 25 | 5.0 |

# B

| *Food and Description* | *Measure or Quantity* | *Calories* | *Carbo-hydrates (grams)* |
|---|---|---|---|
| **BABY FOOD:** | | | |
| *Advance* (Similac) | 1 fl. oz. | 16 | 1.5 |
| Apple & apricot: | | | |
| Junior (Beech-Nut) | 7¾-oz. serving | 93 | 24.4 |
| Strained (Beech-Nut) | 4¾-oz. serving | 57 | 14.0 |
| Apple Betty: | | | |
| Junior (Beech-Nut) | 7¾-oz. serving | 118 | 27.7 |
| Strained (Beech-Nut) | 4¾-oz. serving | 73 | 17.0 |
| Apple-Blueberry: | | | |
| Junior (Beech-Nut) | 7½-oz. serving | 121 | 28.6 |
| Strained (Beech-Nut) | 4½-oz. serving | 72 | 16.6 |
| Apple-cherry juice: | | | |
| Strained: | | | |
| (Beech-Nut) | 4⅕ fl. oz. (4.4 oz.) | 56 | 14.0 |
| (Gerber) | 4.2-fl.-oz. can | 62 | 14.7 |
| Apple dessert: | | | |
| Junior (Gerber) Dutch | 7¾-oz. serving | 151 | 35.4 |
| Strained (Gerber) Dutch | 4¾-oz. serving | 97 | 21.3 |
| Apple grape juice: | | | |
| Strained: | | | |
| (Beech-Nut) | 4⅕ fl. oz. | 56 | 13.9 |
| (Gerber) | 4.2-oz. can | 56 | 13.6 |
| Apple juice: | | | |
| Strained: | | | |
| (Beech-Nut) | 4⅕ fl. oz. | 54 | 13.6 |

| *Food and Description* | *Measure or Quantity* | *Calories* | *Carbohydrates (grams)* |
|---|---|---|---|
| (Gerber) | 4.2-oz. can | 58 | 14.2 |
| Apple peach juice: | | | |
| Strained: | | | |
| (Beech-Nut) | 4⅕ fl. oz. | 59 | 14.6 |
| (Gerber) | 4.2-fl. oz. can | 55 | 13.1 |
| Apple plum juice, strained (Gerber) | 4.2-fl.-oz. can | 60 | 14.7 |
| Apple raspberry: | | | |
| Junior (Gerber) | 7¾-oz. serving | 138 | 33.0 |
| Strained (Gerber) | 4¾-oz. serving | 87 | 20.5 |
| Applesauce: | | | |
| Junior: | | | |
| (Beech-Nut) | 7¾-oz. serving | 97 | 24.1 |
| (Gerber) | 7½-oz. jar | 102 | 24.2 |
| Strained: | | | |
| (Beech-Nut) | 4¾-oz. serving | 60 | 14.8 |
| (Gerber) | 4½-oz. jar | 65 | 15.4 |
| Applesauce & apricots: | | | |
| Junior (Gerber) | 7½-oz. serving | 109 | 25.6 |
| Strained (Gerber) | 4½-oz. serving | 75 | 17.9 |
| Applesauce & cherries: | | | |
| Junior (Beech-Nut) | 7¾-oz. serving | 115 | 28.4 |
| Strained (Beech-Nut) | 4¾-oz. serving | 71 | 17.4 |
| Applesauce & pineapple: | | | |
| Junior (Gerber) | 7½-oz. serving | 99 | 23.4 |
| Strained (Gerber) | 4½-oz. jar | 69 | 16.6 |
| Applesauce & raspberries: | | | |
| Junior (Beech-Nut) | 7¾-oz. serving | 102 | 24.6 |
| Strained (Beech-Nut) | 4¾-oz. serving | 61 | 15.1 |
| Apricot with tapioca: | | | |
| Junior (Gerber) | 7½-oz. serving | 103 | 23.9 |
| Strained (Gerber) | 4½-oz. serving | 56 | 12.8 |
| Apricot with tapioca & apple juice: | | | |
| Junior (Beech-Nut) | 7¾-oz. serving | 117 | 28.8 |
| Strained (Beech-Nut) | 4¾-oz. serving | 72 | 17.6 |
| Banana & apple juice, junior (Beech-Nut) | 7¾-oz. serving | 146 | 35.2 |

(USDA): United States Department of Agriculture
(HEW/FAO): Health, Education and Welfare/Food and Agriculture Organization
* Prepared as Package Directs

| Food and Description | Measure or Quantity | Calories | Carbo-hydrates (grams) |
|---|---|---|---|
| Banana & pineapple, strained (Beech-Nut) | 4¾-oz. serving | 67 | 16.3 |
| Banana & pineapple with tapioca: | | | |
| Junior: | | | |
| (Beech-Nut) | 7¾-oz. serving | 103 | 26.0 |
| (Gerber) | 7½-oz. serving | 109 | 25.6 |
| Strained (Gerber) | 4½-oz. serving | 71 | 16.6 |
| Banana with tapioca: | | | |
| Junior: | | | |
| (Beech-Nut) | 7¾-oz. serving | 72 | 27.5 |
| (Gerber) | 7½-oz. serving | 114 | 25.6 |
| Strained: | | | |
| (Beech-Nut) | 4¾-oz. serving | 72 | 16.9 |
| (Gerber) | 4½-oz. serving | 66 | 15.4 |
| Bean, green: | | | |
| Junior (Beech-Nut) | 7¼-oz. serving | 62 | 13.0 |
| Strained: | | | |
| (Beech-Nut) | 4½-oz. serving | 38 | 8.1 |
| (Gerber) | 4½-oz. serving | 33 | 6.3 |
| Bean, green, creamed Junior (Gerber) | 7½-oz. serving | 91 | 18.3 |
| Bean, green, with potatoes & ham, casserole, toddler (Gerber) | 6¼-oz. serving | 129 | 13.7 |
| Beef: | | | |
| Junior (Gerber) | 3½-oz. serving | 94 | .3 |
| Strained (Gerber) | 3½-oz. serving | 90 | Tr. |
| Beef & beef broth: | | | |
| Junior (Beech-Nut) | 7½-oz. serving | 235 | .4 |
| Strained (Beech-Nut) | 4½-oz. serving | 152 | .3 |
| Beef & beef broth: | | | |
| Junior (Beech-Nut) | 3½-oz. serving | 88 | .7 |
| Strained (Beech-Nut) | 4½-oz. serving | 132 | 8.0 |
| Beef with beef heart, strained (Gerber) | 4½-oz. serving | 118 | 10.2 |
| Beef dinner, high meat: | | | |
| Junior: | | | |
| (Beech-Nut) with vegetables & cereal | 4½-oz. serving | 132 | 8.0 |
| (Gerber) with vegetables | 4½-oz. serving | 118 | 10.2 |

| Food and Description | Measure or Quantity | Calories | Carbohydrates (grams) |
|---|---|---|---|
| Strained: | | | |
| (Beech-Nut) with vegetables & cereal | 4½-oz. serving | 132 | 8.1 |
| (Gerber) with vegetables | 4½-oz. serving | 100 | 7.7 |
| Beef dinner & egg noodles: | | | |
| Junior: | | | |
| (Beech-Nut) | 7½-oz. serving | 122 | 17.0 |
| (Gerber) with vegetables | 7½-oz. serving | 130 | 19.4 |
| Strained: | | | |
| (Beech-Nut) | 4½-oz. serving | 72 | 9.9 |
| (Gerber) with vegetables | 4½-oz. serving | 78 | 11.6 |
| Beef & rice with tomato sauce, Toddler (Gerber) | 6¼-oz. serving | 133 | 16.9 |
| Beef lasagna, Toddler (Gerber) | 6¼-oz. serving | 114 | 16.3 |
| Beef liver, Strained (Gerber) | 3½-oz. serving | 97 | 2.4 |
| Beef stew, Toddler (Gerber) | 6¼-oz. serving | 116 | 12.3 |
| Beet, strained (Gerber) | 4½-oz. serving | 46 | 9.5 |
| Carrot: | | | |
| Junior: | | | |
| (Beech-Nut) | 7½-oz. serving | 67 | 13.8 |
| (Gerber) | 7½-oz. serving | 58 | 12.0 |
| Strained: | | | |
| (Beech-Nut) | 4½-oz. serving | 40 | 8.3 |
| (Gerber) | 4½-oz. serving | 33 | 6.8 |
| Cereal, dry: | | | |
| Barley: | | | |
| (Beech-Nut) | ½-oz. serving | 55 | 9.9 |
| (Gerber) | 6 T. (½ oz.) | 53 | 10.4 |
| High-protein: | | | |
| (Beech-Nut) | ½-oz. serving | 52 | 5.2 |
| (Gerber) | 6 T. (½ oz.) | 53 | 5.9 |

(USDA): United States Department of Agriculture
(HEW/FAO): Health, Education and Welfare/Food and Agriculture Organization
* Prepared as Package Directs

| Food and Description | Measure or Quantity | Calories | Carbo-hydrates (grams) |
|---|---|---|---|
| High protein with apple & orange (Gerber) | 6 T. (½ oz.) | 54 | 7.8 |
| Mixed: | | | |
|   (Beech-Nut) | ½-oz. serving | 54 | 9.6 |
|   (Gerber) | 6 T. (½ oz.) | 54 | 9.8 |
| Mixed with banana (Gerber) | 6 T. (½ oz.) | 55 | 10.7 |
| Mixed, & honey (Beech-Nut) | ½-oz. serving | 55 | 9.9 |
| Oatmeal: | | | |
|   (Beech-Nut) | ½-oz. serving | 51 | 9.6 |
|   (Gerber) | 6 T. (½ oz.) | 56 | 9.3 |
| Oatmeal, with banana (Gerber) | 6 T. (½ oz.) | 56 | 10.1 |
| Oatmeal & honey (Beech-Nut) | ½ oz. | 57 | 9.9 |
| Rice: | | | |
|   (Beech-Nut) | ½-oz. serving | 54 | 11.3 |
|   (Gerber) | 6 T. (½ oz.) | 54 | 10.8 |
| Rice with banana (Gerber) | 6 T. (½ oz.) | 56 | 10.7 |
| Rice & honey (Beech-Nut) | ½-oz. serving | 54 | 11.3 |
| Wheat & honey (Beech-Nut) | ½-oz. serving | 52 | 1.1 |
| Cereal or Mixed Cereal: | | | |
| With applesauce & banana: | | | |
|   Junior (Gerber) | 7½-oz. serving | 140 | 29.8 |
|   Strained: | | | |
|     (Beech-Nut) | 4½-oz. serving | 86 | 18.9 |
|     (Gerber) | 4½-oz. serving | 82 | 16.6 |
| & egg yolk: | | | |
|   Junior (Gerber) | 7½-oz. serving | 114 | 15.6 |
|   Strained (Gerber) | 4½-oz. serving | 68 | 9.3 |
| & egg yolk & bacon: | | | |
|   Junior (Beech-Nut) | 7½-oz. serving | 180 | 14.9 |
|   Strained (Beech-Nut) | 4½-oz. serving | 113 | 8.9 |
| High protein with applesauce & bananas, strained (Gerber) | 4¾-oz. serving | 115 | 20.2 |

| Food and Description | Measure or Quantity | Calories | Carbo-hydrates (grams) |
|---|---|---|---|
| Oatmeal with applesauce & banana: | | | |
| Junior (Gerber) | 7½-oz. serving | 121 | 23.4 |
| Strained: | | | |
| (Beech-Nut) | 4¾-oz. serving | 83 | 17.1 |
| (Gerber) | 4½-oz. serving | 74 | 14.1 |
| Rice, with applesauce & bananas, strained: | | | |
| (Beech-Nut) | 4¾-oz. serving | 96 | 21.4 |
| (Gerber) | 4¾-oz. serving | 93 | 20.2 |
| Rice with mixed fruit, junior (Gerber) | 7¾-oz. serving | 166 | 37.4 |
| Cheese, cottage: | | | |
| With pineapple: | | | |
| Junior (Gerber) | 7¾-oz. serving | 203 | 40.3 |
| Strained (Gerber) | 4¾-oz. serving | 120 | 23.4 |
| With pineapple juice: | | | |
| Junior (Beech-Nut) | 7¾-oz. serving | 149 | 28.4 |
| Strained (Beech-Nut) | 4¾-oz. serving | 91 | 17.4 |
| Cherry-vanilla pudding: | | | |
| Junior (Gerber) | 7¾-oz. serving | 171 | 41.2 |
| Strained (Gerber) | 4¾-oz. serving | 100 | 23.6 |
| Chicken: | | | |
| Junior (Gerber) | 3½-oz. serving | 125 | .3 |
| Strained (Gerber) | 3½-oz. serving | 131 | .2 |
| Chicken & chicken broth: | | | |
| Junior (Beech-Nut) | 7½-oz. serving | 181 | 12.8 |
| Strained (Beech-Nut) | 4½-oz. serving | 128 | .3 |
| Chicken dinner, high meat: | | | |
| Junior (Beech-Nut) with vegetables & cereal | 4½-oz. serving | 90 | 8.9 |
| Strained (Beech-Nut) with vegetables & cereal | 4½-oz. serving | 90 | 8.8 |
| Chicken dinner & noodle: | | | |
| Junior: | | | |
| (Beech-Nut) | 7½-oz. serving | 86 | 16.6 |
| (Gerber) | 7½-oz. serving | 111 | 16.4 |

(USDA): United States Department of Agriculture
(HEW/FAO): Health, Education and Welfare/Food and Agriculture Organization
\* Prepared as Package Directs

| *Food and Description* | *Measure or Quantity* | *Calories* | *Carbo-hydrates (grams)* |
|---|---|---|---|
| Strained: | | | |
| (Beech-Nut) | 4½-oz. serving | 59 | 10.5 |
| (Gerber) | 4½-oz. serving | 73 | 10.9 |
| Chicken dinner & vegetables: | | | |
| Junior (Gerber) | 4½-oz. serving | 132 | 8.4 |
| Strained (Gerber) | 4½-oz. serving | 127 | 6.6 |
| Chicken soup, cream of, strained (Gerber) | 4½-oz. serving | 73 | 9.1 |
| Chicken stew, toddler (Gerber) | 6-oz. serving | 143 | 10.4 |
| Chicken sticks, junior (Gerber) | 2½-oz. serving | 130 | 1.0 |
| Cookie (See also **COOKIE**) animal-shaped (Gerber) | 6.5-gram cookie | 28 | 4.2 |
| Cookie, Arrowroot (Gerber) | 5.5-gram cookie | 25 | 4.0 |
| Corn, creamed: | | | |
| Junior: | | | |
| (Beech-Nut) | 7½-oz. serving | 142 | 30.9 |
| (Gerber) | 7½-oz. serving | 146 | 29.8 |
| Strained: | | | |
| (Beech-Nut) | 4½-oz. serving | 85 | 18.5 |
| (Gerber) | 4½-oz. serving | 87 | 17.8 |
| Custard: | | | |
| Chocolate, strained (Gerber) | 4½-oz. serving | 115 | 21.2 |
| Vanilla: | | | |
| Junior (Gerber) | 7¾-oz. serving | 206 | 35.4 |
| Strained (Gerber) | 4½-oz. serving | 118 | 20.2 |
| Egg yolk, strained: | | | |
| (Beech-Nut) | 3⅓-oz. serving | 185 | .4 |
| (Gerber) | 3⅓-oz. serving | 184 | 1.0 |
| Fruit dessert: | | | |
| Junior: | | | |
| (Beech-Nut) | 7¾-oz. serving | 114 | 28.2 |
| (Gerber) | 7¾-oz. serving | 153 | 37.1 |
| Strained: | | | |
| (Beech-Nut) | 4½-oz. serving | 66 | 16.4 |
| (Gerber) | 4¾-oz. serving | 95 | 22.7 |
| Fruit dessert, tropical & apple juice, junior (Beech-Nut) | 7¾-oz. serving | 82 | 20.3 |

| Food and Description | Measure or Quantity | Calories | Carbohydrates (grams) |
|---|---|---|---|
| Fruit juice, mixed, strained: | | | |
| (Beech-Nut) | 4⅛ fl. oz. | 58 | 14.6 |
| (Gerber) | 1 can (4.2 fl. oz.) | 69 | 16.3 |
| Fruit, mixed with yogurt, strained (Beech-Nut) | 4¾-oz. serving | 76 | 17.3 |
| Grits with egg yolk, strained (Gerber) | 4½-oz. serving | 78 | 10.4 |
| Ham: | | | |
| Junior (Gerber) | 3½-oz. serving | 111 | .5 |
| Strained (Gerber) | 3½-oz. serving | 106 | .8 |
| Ham dinner, high meat (Beech-Nut): | | | |
| Junior, with vegetables & cereal | 4½-oz. serving | 126 | 7.9 |
| Strained, with vegetables & cereal | 4½-oz. serving | 126 | 7.7 |
| Ham dinner with vegetables (Gerber): | | | |
| Junior | 4½-oz. serving | 114 | 9.7 |
| Strained | 4½-oz. serving | 94 | 7.0 |
| Ham & ham broth, strained (Beech-Nut) | 4½-oz. serving | 143 | .3 |
| Hawaiian Delight, junior (Gerber) | 7¾-oz. serving | 206 | 46.0 |
| *Isomil* (Similac), ready-to-feed | 1 fl. oz. | 20 | 1.9 |
| Lamb (Gerber): | | | |
| Junior | 3½-oz. serving | 98 | .5 |
| Strained | 3½-oz. serving | 96 | .2 |
| Lamb & lamb broth (Beech-Nut): | | | |
| Junior | 7½-oz. serving | 265 | .4 |
| Strained | 4½-oz. serving | 157 | .2 |
| Macaroni & cheese (Gerber): | | | |
| Junior | 7½-oz. serving | 132 | 17.5 |
| Strained | 4½-oz. serving | 81 | 10.4 |

(USDA): United States Department of Agriculture
(HEW/FAO): Health, Education and Welfare/Food and Agriculture Organization
* Prepared as Package Directs

| Food and Description | Measure or Quantity | Calories | Carbo-hydrates (grams) |
|---|---|---|---|
| Macaroni with tomato & beef: | | | |
| Junior (Gerber) | 7½-oz. serving | 115 | 19.8 |
| Strained: | | | |
| (Beech-Nut) | 4½-oz. serving | 81 | 10.7 |
| (Gerber) | 4½-oz. serving | 72 | 11.6 |
| MBF (Gerber): | | | |
| Concentrate | 15-fl.-oz. can | 599 | 57.0 |
| *Diluted, 1 to 1 | 1 fl. oz. (2 T.) | 21 | 1.9 |
| Meat sticks, junior (Gerber) | 2½-oz. serving | 97 | .7 |
| Orange apple, banana juice, strained (Gerber) | 1 can (4.2 fl. oz.) | 70 | 16.3 |
| Orange-apple juice, strained (Beech-Nut) | 4⅙ fl. oz. | 55 | 13.2 |
| Orange-apple juice, strained (Gerber) | 1 can (4.2 fl. oz.) | 63 | 14.3 |
| Orange-apricot juice, strained (Gerber) | 1 can (4.2 oz.) | 66 | 15.0 |
| Orange-banana juice, strained (Beech-Nut) | 4⅛ fl. oz. | 58 | 13.9 |
| Orange juice, strained: | | | |
| (Beech-Nut) | 4⅛ fl. oz. | 56 | 13.2 |
| (Gerber) | 1 can (4.2 fl. oz.) | 60 | 13.0 |
| Orange-pineapple dessert, strained (Beech-Nut) | 4¾-oz. serving | 67 | 16.5 |
| Orange-pineapple juice, strained: | | | |
| (Beech-Nut) | 4⅛ fl. oz. | 57 | 13.7 |
| (Gerber) | 1 can (4.2 fl. oz.) | 69 | 16.1 |
| Orange pudding, strained (Gerber) | 4¾-oz. serving | 113 | 24.0 |
| Pea: | | | |
| Junior (Beech-Nut) | 7¼-oz. serving | 114 | 19.1 |
| Strained: | | | |
| (Beech-Nut) | 4½-oz. serving | 67 | 11.2 |
| (Gerber) | 4½-oz. serving | 54 | 8.4 |
| Peach: | | | |
| Junior: | | | |
| (Beech-Nut) | 7¾-oz. serving | 97 | 22.9 |
| (Gerber) | 7½-oz. serving | 103 | 23.4 |
| Strained: | | | |
| (Beech-Nut) | 4¾-oz. serving | 59 | 14.0 |

| Food and Description | Measure or Quantity | Calories | Carbohydrates (grams) |
|---|---|---|---|
| (Gerber) | 4½-oz. serving | 63 | 14.1 |
| Peach apple with yogurt, strained (Beech-Nut) | 4¾-oz. serving | 71 | 15.9 |
| Peach cobbler (Gerber): | | | |
| Junior | 7¾-oz. serving | 161 | 37.2 |
| Strained | 4¾-oz. serving | 99 | 22.7 |
| Peach melba (Beech-Nut): | | | |
| Junior | 7¾-oz. serving | 107 | 25.9 |
| Strained | 4¾-oz. serving | 66 | 15.9 |
| Pear: | | | |
| Junior: | | | |
| (Beech-Nut) | 7½-oz. serving | 106 | 26.2 |
| (Gerber) | 7½-oz. serving | 110 | 25.6 |
| Strained: | | | |
| (Beech-Nut) | 4½-oz. serving | 64 | 15.7 |
| (Gerber) | 4½-oz. serving | 66 | 15.4 |
| Pear & pineapple: | | | |
| Junior: | | | |
| (Beech-Nut) | 7½-oz. serving | 121 | 29.6 |
| (Gerber) | 7½-oz. serving | 111 | 25.6 |
| Strained | | | |
| (Beech-Nut) | 4½-oz. serving | 73 | 17.8 |
| (Gerber) | 4½-oz. serving | 65 | 14.8 |
| Pineapple dessert, strained (Beech-Nut) | 4¾-oz. serving | 66 | 16.2 |
| Plum with tapioca (Gerber): | | | |
| Junior | 7½-oz. serving | 135 | 31.9 |
| Strained | 4½-oz. serving | 82 | 19.2 |
| Plum with tapioca and apple juice (Beech-Nut): | | | |
| Junior | 7¾-oz. serving | 120 | 29.3 |
| Strained | 4¾-oz. serving | 73 | 17.9 |
| Pork, strained (Gerber) | 3½-oz. serving | 115 | .5 |
| Pretzel (Gerber) | 6-gram pretzel | 23 | 4.8 |
| Prune-orange juice, strained: | | | |
| (Beech-Nut) | 4⅛ fl. oz. | 66 | 15.7 |
| (Gerber) | 1 can (4.2 fl. oz.) | 76 | 17.8 |

(USDA): United States Department of Agriculture
(HEW/FAO): Health, Education and Welfare/Food and Agriculture Organization
* Prepared as Package Directs

| Food and Description | Measure or Quantity | Calories | Carbo-hydrates (grams) |
|---|---|---|---|
| Prune with tapioca: | | | |
| Junior: | | | |
| (Beech-Nut) | 7¾-oz. serving | 174 | 40.5 |
| (Gerber) | 7¾-oz. serving | 179 | 41.8 |
| Strained: | | | |
| (Beech-Nut) | 4¾-oz. serving | 107 | 24.8 |
| (Gerber) | 4¾-oz. serving | 104 | 24.3 |
| Raspberry dessert with yogurt (Gerber): | | | |
| Junior | 7½-oz. serving | 162 | 33.2 |
| Strained | 4½-oz. serving | 97 | 20.0 |
| *Similac, powder & powder with iron | 1 fl. oz. | 20 | 2.0 |
| *Similac, ready-to-feed or concentrated liquid, with & without added iron | 1 fl. oz. | 20 | 2.0 |
| Spaghetti & meatballs, toddler (Gerber) | 6¼-oz. serving | 131 | 20.2 |
| Spaghetti with tomato sauce & beef, junior: | | | |
| (Beech-Nut) | 7½-oz. serving | 131 | 19.4 |
| (Gerber) | 7½-oz. serving | 140 | 22.4 |
| Spinach, creamed (Gerber): | | | |
| Junior | 7½-oz. serving | 101 | 12.8 |
| Strained | 4½-oz. serving | 68 | 8.6 |
| Split pea & ham, junior: | | | |
| (Beech-Nut) | 7½-oz. serving | 149 | 23.4 |
| (Gerber) | 7½-oz. serving | 147 | 23.2 |
| Squash: | | | |
| Junior: | | | |
| (Beech-Nut) | 7½-oz. serving | 57 | 11.7 |
| (Gerber) | 7½-oz. serving | 59 | 11.5 |
| Strained: | | | |
| (Beech-Nut) | 4½-oz. serving | 34 | 7.0 |
| (Gerber) | 4½-oz. serving | 33 | 6.8 |
| Sweet potato: | | | |
| Junior: | | | |
| (Beech-Nut) | 7¾-oz. serving | 118 | 27.5 |
| (Gerber) | 7¾-oz. serving | 132 | 29.8 |
| Strained | | | |
| (Beech-Nut) | 4½-oz. serving | 68 | 15.9 |
| (Gerber) | 4¾-oz. serving | 80 | 18.2 |
| Teething biscuit (Gerber) | 11-gram biscuit | 42 | 8.3 |

| Food and Description | Measure or Quantity | Calories | Carbo-hydrates (grams) |
|---|---|---|---|
| Turkey (Gerber): | | | |
| Junior | 3½-oz. serving | 130 | Tr. |
| Strained | 3½-oz. serving | 121 | .3 |
| Turkey dinner, high meat: | | | |
| Junior: | | | |
| (Beech-Nut) with vegetables & cereal | 4½-oz. serving | 112 | 8.9 |
| (Gerber) with vegetables | 4½-oz. serving | 95 | 9.3 |
| Strained: | | | |
| (Beech-Nut) with vegetables & cereal | 4½-oz. serving | 104 | 7.8 |
| (Gerber) with vegetables | 4½-oz. serving | 133 | 8.6 |
| Turkey dinner & rice (Beech-Nut): | | | |
| Junior | 7½-oz. serving | 83 | 16.0 |
| Strained | 4½-oz. serving | 59 | 12.0 |
| Turkey & rice with vegetables (Gerber): | | | |
| Junior | 7½-oz. serving | 130 | 17.9 |
| Strained | 4½-oz. serving | 66 | 9.3 |
| Turkey sticks, junior (Gerber) | 2½-oz. serving | 153 | 1.1 |
| Turkey & turkey broth, strained (Beech-Nut) | 4½-oz. serving | 140 | .2 |
| Veal (Gerber): | | | |
| Junior | 3½-oz. serving | 95 | .1 |
| Strained | 3½-oz. serving | 89 | .3 |
| Veal dinner, high meat: | | | |
| Junior: | | | |
| (Beech-Nut) with vegetables & cereal | 4½-oz. serving | 108 | 8.1 |
| (Gerber) with vegetables | 4½-oz. serving | 106 | 11.4 |
| Strained: | | | |
| (Beech-Nut) with vegetables & cereal | 4½-oz. serving | 126 | 7.0 |

(USDA): United States Department of Agriculture
(HEW/FAO): Health, Education and Welfare/Food and Agriculture Organization
* Prepared as Package Directs

| Food and Description | Measure or Quantity | Calories | Carbohydrates (grams) |
|---|---|---|---|
| (Gerber) with vegetables | 4½-oz. serving | 104 | 9.3 |
| Veal & veal broth, strained (Beech-Nut) | 4½-oz. serving | 143 | .2 |
| Vegetables & bacon: | | | |
| Junior: | | | |
| (Beech-Nut) | 7½-oz. serving | 137 | 18.9 |
| (Gerber) | 7½-oz. serving | 181 | 18.8 |
| Strained: | | | |
| (Beech-Nut) | 4½-oz. serving | 83 | 9.9 |
| (Gerber) | 4½-oz. serving | 98 | 11.4 |
| Vegetables & beef: | | | |
| Junior: | | | |
| (Beech-Nut) | 7½-oz. serving | 123 | 18.1 |
| (Gerber) | 7½-oz. serving | 138 | 20.7 |
| Strained: | | | |
| (Beech-Nut) | 4½-oz. serving | 79 | 10.9 |
| (Gerber) | 4½-oz. serving | 59 | 7.5 |
| Vegetable & chicken: | | | |
| Junior: | | | |
| (Beech-Nut) | 7½-oz. serving | 89 | 15.9 |
| (Gerber) | 7½-oz. serving | 121 | 19.2 |
| Strained: | | | |
| (Beech-Nut) | 4½-oz. serving | 58 | 9.9 |
| (Gerber) | 4½-oz. serving | 55 | 8.3 |
| Vegetable dinner, mixed, strained (Beech-Nut) | 4½-oz. serving | 55 | 12.0 |
| Vegetables, garden, strained: | | | |
| (Beech-Nut) | 4½-oz. serving | 66 | 12.5 |
| (Gerber) | 4½-oz. serving | 37 | 5.8 |
| Vegetables & ham: | | | |
| Junior (Gerber) | 7½-oz. serving | 121 | 17.3 |
| Strained: | | | |
| (Beech-Nut) | 4½-oz. serving | 75 | 10.9 |
| (Gerber) | 4½-oz. serving | 66 | 9.0 |
| Vegetable & lamb (Gerber): | | | |
| Junior | 7½-oz. serving | 141 | 17.9 |
| Strained | 4½-oz. serving | 86 | 10.5 |
| Vegetables & lamb with rice & barley (Beech-Nut): | | | |
| Junior | 7½-oz. serving | 86 | 17.0 |

| Food and Description | Measure or Quantity | Calories | Carbo-hydrates (grams) |
|---|---|---|---|
| Strained | 4½-oz. serving | 74 | 10.0 |
| Vegetables & liver, junior (Gerber) | 7½-oz. serving | 95 | 16.6 |
| Vegetables & liver with rice & barley (Beech-Nut): | | | |
| Junior | 7½-oz. serving | 91 | 16.8 |
| Strained | 4½-oz. serving | 57 | 9.8 |
| Vegetables, mixed (Gerber): | | | |
| Junior | 7½-oz. serving | 85 | 16.8 |
| Strained | 4½-oz. serving | 53 | 10.1 |
| Vegetables & turkey (Gerber): | | | |
| Junior | 7½-oz. serving | 107 | 16.8 |
| Strained | 4½-oz. serving | 65 | 9.6 |
| Toddler, casserole | 6¼-oz. serving | 148 | 15.4 |
| Zwieback (Nabisco) (See also ZWIEBACK) | ¼-oz. piece | 30 | 5.0 |
| | | | |
| BACON, cured: | | | |
| Raw (USDA): | | | |
| slab | 1 oz. (weighed with rind) | 177 | .3 |
| Sliced | 1 oz. | 189 | .3 |
| Broiled or fried crisp: (USDA): | | | |
| Medium slice | 1 slice (7.5 grams) | 43 | .2 |
| Thick slice | 1 slice (12 grams) | 72 | .4 |
| Thin slice | 1 slice (5 grams) | 30 | .2 |
| (Lazy Maple) | 3-4 slices (.8 oz.) | 140 | 0. |
| (Oscar Mayer): | | | |
| Medium slice, drained | 1 slice (6 grams) | 36 | .1 |
| Thick slice, drained | 1 slice (11 grams) | 66 | .2 |
| Swift Premium | 3-4 slices (.8 oz.) | 137 | .7 |
| Canned (USDA) | 1 oz. | 194 | .3 |
| | | | |
| BACON BITS: | | | |
| (Ann Page) imitation | 1 tsp. (1.8 grams) | 8 | .5 |
| (Durkee) imitation | 1 tsp. (2 grams) | 8 | .5 |

(USDA): United States Department of Agriculture
(HEW/FAO): Health, Education and Welfare/Food and Agriculture Organization
* Prepared as Package Directs

| Food and Description | Measure or Quantity | Calories | Carbo-hydrates (grams) |
|---|---|---|---|
| (French's) imitation, crumbles | 1 tsp. (2 grams) | 6 | <.5 |
| (Hormel) | 1 tsp. (3 grams) | 11 | .1 |
| **BACON, CANADIAN:** | | | |
| Unheated (Oscar Mayer) | 1-oz. slice | 38 | .2 |
| Broiled or fried (USDA) drained | 1 oz. | 79 | Tr. |
| **BAC ONION** (Lawry's) | 1 tsp. (4 grams) | 14 | 2.1 |
| **BACO NOIR BURGUNDY WINE** (Great Western) 12.5% alcohol | 3 fl. oz. | 69 | 2.1 |
| **BACON, SIMULATED,** cooked, *Sizzlean* (Swift) | 1 strip (.4 oz.) | 50 | 0. |
| **BAC*Os** (General Mills) | 1 T. | 40 | 2.0 |
| **BAGEL** (USDA): | | | |
| Egg | 3″ dia. (1.9 oz.) | 162 | 28.3 |
| Water | 3″ dia. (1.9 oz.) | 163 | 30.5 |
| **BAKING POWDER:** | | | |
| Phosphate (USDA) | 1 tsp. (3.8 grams) | 5 | 1.1 |
| SAS (USDA) | 1 tsp. (3 grams) | 4 | .9 |
| Tartrate (USDA) | 1 tsp. (2.8 grams) | 2 | .5 |
| (Calumet) | 1 tsp. (3.6 grams) | 2 | 1.0 |
| **BALSAMPEAR,** fresh (HEW/FAO): | | | |
| Whole | 1 lb. (weighed with cavity contents) | 69 | 16.3 |
| Flesh only | 4 oz. | 22 | 5.1 |
| **BAMBOO SHOOT:** | | | |
| Raw (USDA) trimmed | 4 oz. | 31 | 5.9 |
| Canned: | | | |
| (Chun King) drained | ½ of 8½-oz. can | 20 | 3.0 |
| (La Choy) drained | 8-oz. can | 24 | 3.7 |

| Food and Description | Measure or Quantity | Calories | Carbo-hydrates (grams) |
|---|---|---|---|
| **BANANA (USDA):** | | | |
| Common yellow: | | | |
| Fresh: | | | |
| Whole | 1 lb. (weighed with skin) | 262 | 68.5 |
| Small size | 4.9-oz. banana (7¾" x 1¹¹/₃₂") | 81 | 21.1 |
| Medium size | 6.2-oz. banana (8¾" x 1¹³/₃₂") | 101 | 26.4 |
| Large size | 7-oz. banana (9¾" x 1⁷/₁₆") | 116 | 30.2 |
| Mashed | 1 cup (about 2 med.) | 191 | 50.0 |
| Sliced | 1 cup (1¼ med.) | 128 | 33.3 |
| Dehydrated flakes | ½ cup (1.8 oz.) | 170 | 44.3 |
| Red, fresh, whole | 1 lb. (weighed with skin) | 278 | 72.2 |
| **BANANA, BAKING (See PLANTAIN)** | | | |
| **BANANA EXTRACT,** imitation (Durkee) | 1 tsp. | 20 | DNA |
| **BANANA ICE CREAM** (Breyer's) red raspberry & strawberry twirl | ¼ pt. | 150 | 21.0 |
| **BANANA PIE (See PIE, Banana)** | | | |
| **BANANA PUDDING (See PUDDING or PIE FILLING, Banana)** | | | |
| **BARBADOS CHERRY (See ACEROLA)** | | | |

(USDA): United States Department of Agriculture
(HEW/FAO): Health, Education and Welfare/Food and Agriculture Organization
* Prepared as Package Directs

| Food and Description | Measure or Quantity | Calories | Carbo-hydrates (grams) |
|---|---|---|---|
| **BARBECUE SEASONING** (French's) | 1 tsp. (2.5 grams) | 6 | 1.0 |
| **BARDOLINO WINE,** Italian red (Antinori) 12% alcohol | 3 fl. oz. | 84 | 6.3 |
| **BARLEY,** pearled, dry: Light: | | | |
| (USDA) | ¼ cup (1.8 oz.) | 174 | 39.4 |
| (Quaker-Scotch) | ¼ cup (1.7 oz.) | 172 | 36.3 |
| Pot or Scotch (USDA) | 2 oz. | 197 | 43.8 |
| **BASIL:** Fresh (HEW/FAO) sweet, leaves | ½ oz. | 6 | 1.0 |
| Dried (French's) leaves | 1 tsp. (1.1 grams) | 3 | .7 |
| **BASS** (USDA): Black Sea: Raw, whole | 1 lb. (weighed whole) | 165 | 0. |
| Baked, stuffed, home recipe | 4 oz. | 294 | 12.9 |
| Smallmouth & largemouth, raw: Whole | 1 lb. (weighed whole) | 146 | 0. |
| Meat only | 4 oz. | 118 | 0. |
| Striped: Raw, whole | 1 lb. (weighed whole) | 205 | 0. |
| Raw, meat only | 4 oz. | 119 | 0. |
| Oven-fried | 4 oz. | 222 | 7.6 |
| White, raw, meat only | 4 oz. | 111 | 0. |
| **BAY LEAF** (French's) | 1 tsp. (1.3 grams) | 5 | 1.0 |
| **B AND B LIQUEUR** (Julius Wile) 86 proof | 1 fl. oz. | 94 | 5.7 |
| **B.B.Q. SAUCE & BEEF,** frozen (Banquet) sliced, cooking bag | 5-oz. bag | 126 | 12.5 |

| Food and Description | Measure or Quantity | Calories | Carbo-hydrates (grams) |
|---|---|---|---|
| **BEAN, BAKED,** canned: | | | |
| (USDA): | | | |
|   With pork & molasses sauce | 1 cup (9 oz.) | 383 | 53.8 |
|   With pork & tomato sauce | 1 cup (9 oz.) | 311 | 48.5 |
|   With tomato sauce | 1 cup (9 oz.) | 306 | 58.7 |
| (Ann Page): | | | |
|   With pork & molasses sauce. Boston style | ½ of 16-oz. can | 287 | 49.8 |
|   With pork & tomato sauce | ½ of 16-oz. can | 235 | 41.6 |
|   Vegetarian in tomato sauce | ½ of 16-oz. can | 236 | 44.1 |
| (B & M): | | | |
|   Pea bean with pork in brown sugar sauce | 8-oz. can | 336 | 51.2 |
|   Red kidney in brown sugar sauce | ½ of 16-oz. can | 360 | 49.6 |
|   Yellow eye bean in brown sugar sauce | ½ of 16-oz. can | 360 | 50.4 |
| (Campbell): | | | |
|   Home style | ½ of 16-oz. can | 300 | 52.0 |
|   Old fashioned in molasses & brown sugar sauce | ½ of 16-oz. can | 290 | 49.0 |
|   With pork & tomato sauce | 8-oz. can | 260 | 43.0 |
| (Libby's) *Deep Brown:* | | | |
|   With pork in molasses sauce | ½ of 14-oz. can | 228 | 40.6 |
|   With pork in tomato sauce | ½ of 14-oz. can | 220 | 40.2 |
|   Vegetarian in tomato sauce | ½ of 14-oz. can | 214 | 40.8 |
| (Morton House) with tomato sauce | ½ of 16-oz. can | 270 | 45.0 |
| (Sultana) with pork in tomato sauce | ½ of 16-oz. can | 232 | 41.8 |

(USDA): United States Department of Agriculture
(HEW/FAO): Health, Education and Welfare/Food and Agriculture Organization
* Prepared as Package Directs

| Food and Description | Measure or Quantity | Calories | Carbo-hydrates (grams) |
|---|---|---|---|
| (Van Camp) vegetarian style | 1 cup | 260 | 48.0 |
| **BEAN, BARBECUE** (Campbell) | ½ of 15¾-oz. can | 277 | 45.4 |
| **BEAN, BAYO,** black or brown, dry (USDA) | 4 oz. | 384 | 69.4 |
| **BEAN, BLACK,** dry (USDA) | 4 oz. | 384 | 69.4 |
| **BEAN, BROWN,** dry (USDA) | 4 oz. | 384 | 69.4 |
| **BEAN, CALICO,** dry (USDA) | 4 oz. | 396 | 72.2 |
| **BEAN, CHILI** (See CHILI) | | | |
| **BEAN & FRANKFURTER,** canned: | | | |
| (USDA) | 1 cup (9 oz.) | 367 | 32.1 |
| (Campbell) in tomato & molasses sauce | 8-oz. can | 370 | 16.0 |
| **BEAN & FRANKFURTER DINNER,** frozen: | | | |
| (Banquet) | 10¾-oz. dinner | 591 | 63.1 |
| (Morton) | 10¾-oz. dinner | 528 | 79.4 |
| (Swanson) | 11¼-oz. dinner | 550 | 75.0 |
| **BEAN, GREEN or SNAP:** Fresh (USDA): | | | |
| Whole | 1 lb. (weighed untrimmed) | 128 | 28.3 |
| French style | ½ cup (1.4 oz.) | 13 | 2.8 |
| Boiled, drained, whole (USDA) | ½ cup (2.2 oz.) | 16 | 3.3 |
| Boiled, drained, 1½ to 2" pieces (USDA) | ½ cup (2.4 oz.) | 17 | 3.7 |
| Canned, regular pack: (USDA): | | | |
| Solids & liq. | ½ cup (4.2 oz.) | 22 | 5.0 |
| Whole, drained solids | 4 oz. | 27 | 5.9 |
| Cut, drained solids | ½ cup (2.5 oz.) | 17 | 3.6 |

| Food and Description | Measure or Quantity | Calories | Carbo-hydrates (grams) |
|---|---|---|---|
| Drained liquid (Comstock) cut or French style, solids & liq. | 4 oz. | 11 | 2.7 |
|  | ½ cup | 23 | 4.0 |
| (Del Monte): |  |  |  |
| Cut, solids & liq. | ½ cup | 21 | 3.8 |
| Cut, drained solids | ½ cup | 30 | 5.3 |
| French-style, solids & liq. | ½ cup | 18 | 3.4 |
| French-style, drained solids | ½ cup | 27 | 4.9 |
| Seasoned, solids & liq. | ½ cup | 22 | 4.1 |
| Seasoned, drained solids | ½ cup | 30 | 5.5 |
| Whole, solids & liq. | ½ cup | 17 | 2.9 |
| Whole, drained solids | ½ cup | 26 | 4.3 |
| (Green Giant) whole, cut or French-style, solids & liq. | ½ of 8-oz. can | 15 | 2.6 |
| (Kounty Kist) cut, French style or whole, solids & liq. | ¼ of 16-oz. can | 15 | 2.7 |
| (Libby's) cut, Blue Lake, solids & liq. | ¼ of 16-oz. can | 21 | 4.1 |
| (Libby's) French-style, Blue Lake, solids & liq. | ¼ of 16-oz. can | 21 | 4.0 |
| (Lindy) cut, French-style or whole, solids & liq. | ¼ of 16-oz. can | 15 | 2.7 |
| (Stokely-Van Camp) cut, sliced or whole, solids & liq. | ½ cup (4.2 oz.) | 20 | 4.0 |
| Canned dietetic pack: |  |  |  |
| (USDA) solids & liq. | 4 oz. | 18 | 4.1 |
| (USDA) drained solids | 4 oz. | 25 | 5.4 |
| (Blue Boy) solids & liq. | 4-oz. serving | 22 | 4.7 |

(USDA): United States Department of Agriculture
(HEW/FAO): Health, Education and Welfare/Food and Agriculture Organization
* Prepared as Package Directs

| Food and Description | Measure or Quantity | Calories | Carbohydrates (grams) |
|---|---|---|---|
| (Diet Delight) solids & liq. | ½ cup (4.2 oz.) | 17 | 3.4 |
| (Featherweight) cut, solids & liq. | ½ cup | 20 | 5.0 |
| (Tillie Lewis) *Tasti Diet* | ½ cup | 20 | 4.0 |
| Frozen: | | | |
| (USDA): | | | |
| Cut or French-style, unthawed | 10-oz. pkg. | 74 | 17.0 |
| Cut or French-style, boiled, drained | ½ cup (2.8 oz.) | 20 | 4.6 |
| (Birds Eye): | | | |
| Cut, 5-minute style | ⅓ of 9-oz. pkg. | 25 | 5.0 |
| French, 5-minute style | ⅓ of 9-oz. pkg. | 30 | 6.0 |
| French-style, with sliced mushrooms | ⅓ of 9-oz. pkg. | 32 | 6.1 |
| With pearl onions | ⅓ of 9-oz. pkg. | 32 | 6.2 |
| Whole, deluxe | ⅓ of 9-oz. pkg. | 26 | 5.0 |
| (Green Giant): | | | |
| Cut or French-style, in butter sauce | ⅓ of 9-oz. pkg. | 31 | 3.0 |
| With onions & bacon bits | ⅓ of 9-oz. pkg. | 32 | 3.6 |
| (McKenzie) French or whole | ⅓ of 9-oz. pkg. | 29 | 5.8 |
| (Seabrook Farms) French-style or whole | ⅓ of 9-oz. pkg. | 29 | 5.8 |
| BEAN, GREEN, & MUSHROOM CASSEROLE, frozen (Stouffer's) | ½ of 9½-oz. pkg. | 143 | 11.9 |
| BEAN, ITALIAN: | | | |
| Canned (Del Monte): | | | |
| Solids & liq. | 1 cup | 57 | 10.9 |
| Drained solids | ½ cup | 43 | 8.2 |
| Frozen: | | | |
| (Bird's Eye) 5-minute style | ⅓ of 9-oz. pkg. | 30 | 6.0 |
| (McKenzie) | ⅓ of 9-oz. pkg. | 37 | 7.1 |
| (Seabrook Farms) | ⅓ of 9-oz. pkg. | 37 | 7.1 |

| Food and Description | Measure or Quantity | Calories | Carbo-hydrates (grams) |
|---|---|---|---|
| **BEAN, KIDNEY or RED:** | | | |
| Dry (USDA) | 1 lb. | 1556 | 280.8 |
| Dry (USDA) | ½ cup (3.3 oz.) | 319 | 57.6 |
| Cooked (USDA) | ½ cup (3.3 oz.) | 109 | 19.8 |
| Canned, regular pack: | | | |
| (USDA) solids & liq. | ½ cup (4.5 oz.) | 115 | 21.0 |
| (Ann Page) | ¼ of 15½-oz. can | 104 | 19.3 |
| (Ann Page) in chili gravy | ½ of 15-oz. can | 208 | 33.7 |
| (Blue Boy) solids & liq. | 4-oz. serving | 115 | 17.8 |
| (Van Camp) red | 1 cup | 230 | 43.0 |
| (Van Camp) New Orleans style | 1 cup | 210 | 38.0 |
| **BEAN, LIMA:** | | | |
| Raw (USDA): | | | |
| Young, whole | 1 lb. (weighed in pod) | 223 | 40.1 |
| Mature, dry | ½ cup (3.4 oz.) | 331 | 61.4 |
| Young, without shell | 1 lb. (weighed shelled) | 558 | 100.2 |
| Boiled, drained (USDA) mature | ½ cup (3.4 oz.) | 131 | 24.3 |
| Canned, regular pack: | | | |
| (USDA) solids & liq. | ½ cup (4.4 oz.) | 88 | 16.6 |
| (USDA) drained solids | ½ cup (3 oz.) | 81 | 15.5 |
| (Del Monte) solids & liq. | ½ cup | 76 | 14.1 |
| (Del Monte) drained solids | ½ cup | 108 | 19.7 |
| (Libby's) solids & liq. | ½ cup (4.3 oz.) | 91 | 16.0 |
| (Stokely-Van Camp) solids & liq. | ½ cup (4.4 oz.) | 90 | 16.5 |
| (Sultana) baby, solids & liq. | ¼ of 15-oz. can | 93 | 17.0 |
| (Sultana) butter bean, solids & liq. | ¼ of 15-oz. can | 82 | 14.6 |

(USDA): United States Department of Agriculture
(HEW/FAO): Health, Education and Welfare/Food and Agriculture
Organization
* Prepared as Package Directs

| Food and Description | Measure or Quantity | Calories | Carbo-hydrates (grams) |
|---|---|---|---|
| Canned, dietetic pack: | | | |
| (USDA) solids & liq., low sodium | 4-oz. serving | 79 | 14.6 |
| (USDA) drained solids, low sodium | 4-oz. serving | 108 | 20.1 |
| (Featherweight) solids & liq. | ½ cup | 73 | 16.0 |
| Frozen: | | | |
| (USDA): | | | |
| Baby, unthawed | 4-oz. serving | 138 | 26.1 |
| Fordhooks, unthawed | 4-oz. serving | 112 | 21.7 |
| Boiled, drained solids | ½ cup (3.1 oz.) | 106 | 20.0 |
| Boiled, Fordhooks, drained | ½ cup (3 oz.) | 83 | 16.0 |
| (Birds Eye): | | | |
| Baby butter | ⅓ of 10-oz. pkg. | 140 | 26.0 |
| Baby, 5-minute style | ⅓ of pkg. | 120 | 22.0 |
| Fordhooks, 5-minute style | ⅓ pkg. | 100 | 18.0 |
| Tiny, deluxe | ⅓ of 10-oz. pkg. | 111 | 20.0 |
| (Green Giant): | | | |
| Baby | ¼ of 16-oz. pkg. | 124 | 22.4 |
| Baby, in butter sauce | ⅓ of 10-oz. pkg. | 107 | 15.7 |
| Speckled butter bean, Southern recipe | ⅓ of 10-oz. pkg. | 105 | 13.2 |
| (Kounty Kist) baby | ⅙ of 20-oz. pkg. | 154 | 27.5 |
| (McKenzie & Seabrook Farms): | | | |
| Baby | ⅓ of 10-oz. pkg. | 126 | 23.6 |
| Baby butterbean | ⅓ of 10-oz. pkg. | 139 | 26.1 |
| Fordhook | ⅓ of 10-oz. pkg. | 98 | 17.9 |
| Speckled butterbean | ⅓ of 10-oz. pkg. | 126 | 23.4 |
| **BEAN, MUNG, dry (USDA)** | ½ cup (3.7 oz.) | 357 | 63.3 |
| **BEAN, PINTO, dry (USDA)** | ½ cup (3.4 oz.) | 335 | 61.2 |
| **BEAN, RED (See BEAN, KIDNEY or BEAN, RED MEXICAN)** | | | |
| **BEAN, RED MEXICAN:** Dry (USDA) | 4-oz. serving | 396 | 72.2 |

| Food and Description | Measure or Quantity | Calories | Carbo-hydrates (grams) |
|---|---|---|---|
| **BEAN, REFRIED,** canned (Ortega) | ½ cup (4.8 oz.) | 170 | 25.0 |
| **BEAN SALAD,** canned: | | | |
| (Green Giant) | ¼ of 17-oz. can | 92 | 19.9 |
| (Nalley's) | 4½-oz. serving | 155 | 29.4 |
| **BEAN SOUP,** canned: | | | |
| (USDA) condensed, with pork | 8 oz. (by wt.) | 304 | 39.3 |
| *(USDA) condensed, with pork, prepared with equal volume water | 1 cup (8.8 oz.) | 168 | 21.8 |
| *(Ann Page) with bacon | 1 cup | 141 | 19.0 |
| (Campbell): | | | |
| *Chunky* with ham | 11-oz. can | 300 | 35.0 |
| *Condensed, with bacon | 10-oz. serving | 100 | 12.0 |
| *Soup For One,* old fashioned | 7¾-oz. can | 210 | 28.0 |
| **BEAN SOUP, BLACK,** canned: | | | |
| *(Campbell) condensed | 11-oz. serving | 130 | 21.0 |
| (Crosse & Blackwell) with sherry | ½ of 13-oz. can | 80 | 18.0 |
| **BEAN SOUP, NAVY** (USDA) dehydrated | 1 oz. | 93 | 17.8 |
| **BEAN SPROUT:** | | | |
| Mung (USDA): | | | |
| Raw | ½ lb. | 80 | 15.0 |
| Raw | ½ cup (1.6 oz.) | 19 | 3.5 |
| Boiled, drained | ½ cup (2.2 oz.) | 17 | 3.2 |
| Soy (USDA): | | | |
| Raw | ½ lb. | 104 | 12.0 |
| Raw | ½ cup (1.9 oz.) | 25 | 2.9 |
| Boiled, drained | 4 oz. | 43 | 4.2 |

(USDA): United States Department of Agriculture
(HEW/FAO): Health, Education and Welfare/Food and Agriculture
            Organization
* Prepared as Package Directs

| Food and Description | Measure or Quantity | Calories | Carbo-hydrates (grams) |
|---|---|---|---|
| Canned: | | | |
| (Chun King) drained | ¼ of 16-oz. can | 20 | 2.0 |
| (La Choy) drained | 1 cup (4.5 oz.) | 13 | 1.3 |
| **BEAN, WAX (See BEAN, YELLOW)** | | | |
| **BEAN, WHITE (USDA):** | | | |
| Raw: | | | |
| Great Northern | ½ cup (3.1 oz.) | 303 | 54.6 |
| Navy or pea | ½ cup | 354 | 63.8 |
| White | 1 oz. | 96 | 17.4 |
| Cooked: | | | |
| Great Northern | ½ cup (3 oz.) | 100 | 18.0 |
| Navy or pea | ½ cup (3.4 oz.) | 113 | 20.4 |
| All other white | 4-oz. serving | 134 | 24.0 |
| **BEAN, YELLOW or WAX:** | | | |
| Raw, whole (USDA) | 1 lb. (weighed untrimmed) | 108 | 24.0 |
| Boiled, drained (USDA) 1″ pieces | ½ cup (2.9 oz.) | 18 | 3.7 |
| Canned, regular pack: | | | |
| (USDA): | | | |
| Solids & liq. | ½ cup (4.2 oz.) | 23 | 5.0 |
| Drained solids | ½ cup (2.2 oz.) | 15 | 3.2 |
| Drained liquid | 4-oz. serving | 12 | 2.8 |
| (Comstock) solids & liq. | ½ cup | 23 | 4.5 |
| (Del Monte): | | | |
| Cut, solids & liq. | ½ cup (4 oz.) | 19 | 3.4 |
| Cut, drained solids | ½ cup | 25 | 4.5 |
| French-style, solids & liq. | ½ cup (4 oz.) | 19 | 3.6 |
| (Libby's) solids & liq. | ½ of 8-oz. can | 23 | 4.4 |
| (Stokely-Van Camp) cut, solids & liq. | ½ cup (4.3 oz.) | 23 | 4.0 |
| Canned, dietetic pack: | | | |
| (USDA) solids & liq. | 4-oz. serving | 17 | 3.9 |
| (USDA) drained solids | 4-oz. serving | 24 | 5.3 |
| (Blue Boy) solids & liq. | 4-oz. serving | 28 | 4.7 |
| (Featherweight) cut, solids & liq. | ½ cup | 20 | 5.0 |

| Food and Description | Measure or Quantity | Calories | Carbo- hydrates (grams) |
|---|---|---|---|
| Frozen: | | | |
| (USDA) cut, unthawed | 4-oz. serving | 32 | 7.4 |
| (USDA) boiled, drained | 4-oz. serving | 31 | 7.0 |
| (Birds Eye) cut, 5-minute style | ⅓ of 9-oz. pkg. | 30 | 4.0 |
| **BEAUJOLAIS WINE**, French Burgundy (Barton & Guestier) St. Louis, 12% alcohol | 3 fl. oz. | 60 | .1 |
| **BEAUNE WINE:** | | | |
| *Clos de Feves*, French Burgundy (Chanson) 12% alcohol | 3 fl. oz. | 84 | 6.3 |
| *St. Vincent*, French Burgundy (Chanson) 12% alcohol | 3 fl. oz. | 84 | 6.3 |
| **BEAVER**, roasted (USDA) | 4-oz. serving | 281 | 0. |
| **BEECHNUT (USDA):** | | | |
| Whole | 4 oz. (weighed in shell) | 393 | 14.0 |
| Shelled | 4 oz. (weighed shelled) | 644 | 23.0 |

**BEEF.** Values for beef cuts are given below for "lean and fat" and for "lean only." Beef purchased by the consumer at the retail store usually is trimmed to about one-half inch layer of fat. This is the meat described as "lean and fat." If all the fat that can be cut off with a knife is removed, the

---

(USDA): United States Department of Agriculture
(HEW/FAO): Health, Education and Welfare/Food and Agriculture Organization
* Prepared as Package Directs

| Food and Description | Measure or Quantity | Calories | Carbo-hydrates (grams) |
|---|---|---|---|
| remainder is the "lean only." These cuts still contain flecks of fat known as "marbling" distributed through the meat. Cooked meats are medium done. | | | |
| Choice grade cuts (USDA): | | | |
| Brisket: | | | |
| Raw | 1 lb. (weighed with bone) | 1284 | 0. |
| Braised: | | | |
| Lean & fat | 4 oz. | 467 | 0. |
| Lean only | 4 oz. | 252 | 0. |
| Chuck: | | | |
| Raw | 1 lb (weighed with bone) | 984 | 0. |
| Braised or pot-roasted: | | | |
| Lean & fat | 4 oz. | 371 | 0. |
| Lean only | 4 oz. | 243 | 0. |
| Dried (See BEEF CHIPPED) | | | |
| Fat, separable, cooked | 1 oz. | 207 | 0. |
| Filet mignon. There are no data available on its composition. For dietary estimates, the data for sirloin steak, lean only, afford the closest approximation. | | | |
| Flank: | | | |
| Raw | 1 lb. | 653 | 0. |
| Braised | 4 oz. | 222 | 0. |
| Foreshank: | | | |
| Raw | 1 lb. (weighed with bone) | 531 | 0. |
| Simmered: | | | |
| Lean & fat | 4 oz. | 310 | 0. |
| Lean only | 4 oz. | 209 | 0. |
| Ground: | | | |
| Lean: | | | |
| Raw | 1 lb. | 812 | 0. |
| Raw | 1 cup (8 oz.) | 405 | 0. |
| Broiled | 4 oz. | 248 | 0. |

| Food and Description | Measure or Quantity | Calories | Carbohydrates (grams) |
|---|---|---|---|
| Regular: | | | |
| Raw | 1 lb. | 1216 | 0. |
| Raw | 1 cup (8 oz.) | 606 | 0. |
| Broiled | 4 oz. | 324 | 0. |
| Heel of round: | | | |
| Raw | 1 lb. | 966 | 0. |
| Roasted: | | | |
| Lean & fat | 4 oz. | 296 | 0. |
| Lean only | 4 oz. | 204 | 0. |
| Hindshank: | | | |
| Raw | 1 lb. (weighed with bone) | 604 | 0. |
| Simmered: | | | |
| Lean & fat | 4 oz. | 409 | 0. |
| Lean only | 4 oz. | 209 | 0. |
| Neck: | | | |
| Raw | 1 lb. (weighed with bone) | 820 | 0. |
| Pot-roasted: | | | |
| Lean & fat | 4 oz. | 332 | 0. |
| Lean only | 4 oz. | 222 | 0. |
| Plate: | | | |
| Raw | 1 lb. (weighed with bone) | 1615 | 0. |
| Simmered: | | | |
| Lean & fat | 4 oz. | 538 | 0. |
| Lean only | 4 oz. | 252 | 0. |
| Rib roast: | | | |
| Raw | 1 lb. (weighed with bone) | 1673 | 0. |
| Lean & fat | | | |
| Lean only | 4 oz. | 499 | 0. |
| Round: | 4 oz. | 273 | 0. |
| Raw | | | |
| Roasted: | 1 lb. (weighed with bone) | 863 | 0. |
| Broiled: | | | |
| Lean & fat | 4 oz. | 296 | 0. |

(USDA): United States Department of Agriculture
(HEW/FAO): Health, Education and Welfare/Food and Agriculture Organization
* Prepared as Package Directs

| Food and Description | Measure or Quantity | Calories | Carbo-hydrates (grams) |
|---|---|---|---|
|    Lean only | 4 oz. | 214 | 0. |
| Rump: | | | |
|   Raw | 1 lb. (weighed with bone) | 1167 | 0. |
|   Roasted: | | | |
|     Lean & fat | 4 oz. | 393 | 0. |
|     Lean only | 4 oz. | 236 | 0. |
| Steak, club: | | | |
|   Raw | 1 lb. (weighed without bone) | 1724 | 0. |
|   Broiled: | | | |
|     Lean & fat | 4 oz. | 515 | 0. |
|     Lean only | 4 oz. | 277 | 0. |
|     One 8-oz. steak (weighed without bone before cooking) will give you: | | | |
|     Lean & fat | 5.9 oz. | 754 | 0. |
|     Lean only | 3.4 oz. | 234 | 0. |
| Steak, porterhouse: | | | |
|   Raw | 1 lb. (weighed with bone) | 1603 | 0. |
|   Broiled: | | | |
|     Lean & fat | 4 oz. | 527 | 0. |
|     Lean only | 4 oz. | 254 | 0. |
|     One 16-oz. steak (weighed with bone before cooking) will give you: | | | |
|     Lean & fat | 10.2 oz. | 1339 | 0. |
|     Lean only | 5.9 oz. | 372 | 0. |
| Steak, ribeye broiled: | | | |
|     One 10-oz. steak (weighed before cooking without bone) will give you: | | | |
|     Lean & fat | 7.3 oz. | 911 | 0. |
|     Lean only | 3.8 oz. | 258 | 0. |
| Steak, sirloin, double-bone: | | | |
|   Raw | 1 lb. (weighed with bone) | 1240 | 0. |
|   Broiled: | | | |
|     Lean & fat | 4 oz. | 463 | 0. |
|     Lean only | 4 oz. | 245 | 0. |

| Food and Description | Measure or Quantity | Calories | Carbo-hydrates (grams) |
|---|---|---|---|
| One 16-oz. steak (weighed before cooking with bone) will give you: | | | |
| Lean & fat | 8.9 oz. | 1028 | 0. |
| Lean only | 5.9 oz. | 359 | 0. |
| One 12-oz. steak (weighed before cooking with bone) will give you: | | | |
| Lean & fat | 6.6 oz. | 767 | 0. |
| Lean only | 4.4 oz. | 268 | 0. |
| Steak, sirloin, hipbone: | | | |
| Raw | 1 lb. (weighed with bone) | 1585 | 0. |
| Broiled: | | | |
| Lean & fat | 4 oz. | 552 | 0. |
| Lean only | 4 oz. | 272 | 0. |
| Steak, sirloin, wedge & round-bone: | | | |
| Raw | 1 lb. (weighed with bone) | 1316 | 0. |
| Broiled: | | | |
| Lean & fat | 4 oz. | 439 | 0. |
| Lean only | 4 oz. | 235 | 0. |
| Steak, T-bone: | | | |
| Raw | 1 lb. (weighed with bone) | 1596 | 0. |
| Broiled: | | | |
| Lean & fat | 4 oz. | 536 | 0. |
| Lean only | 4 oz. | 253 | 0. |
| One 16-oz. steak (weighed before cooking with bone) will give you: | | | |
| Broiled: | | | |
| Lean & fat | 4 oz. | 463 | 0. |
| Lean only | 4 oz. | 245 | 0. |

(USDA): United States Department of Agriculture
(HEW/FAO): Health, Education and Welfare/Food and Agriculture Organization
* Prepared as Package Directs

| Food and Description | Measure or Quantity | Calories | Carbo-hydrates (grams) |
|---|---|---|---|
| **BEEFAMATO COCKTAIL** | | | |
| (Mott's) | ½ cup | 49 | 10.7 |
| **BEEF BOUILLON,** cubes or powder: | | | |
| (Herb-Ox) | 1 cube (4 grams) | 6 | .5 |
| (Herb-Ox) | 1 packet (4 grams) | 8 | .8 |
| (Maggi) | 1 cube (3.5 grams) | 6 | 0. |
| *MBT* | 1 packet (5.5 grams) | 14 | 2.0 |
| **BEEF BROTH (See BEEF SOUP)** | | | |
| **BEEF, CHIPPED:** | | | |
| Uncooked (USDA) | ½ cup (2.9 oz.) | 166 | 0. |
| Cooked, creamed, home recipe (USDA) | ½ cup (4.3 oz.) | 188 | 8.7 |
| Frozen (Banquet) creamed | 5-oz. bag | 124 | 10.5 |
| Frozen (Stouffer's) creamed | ½ of 11-oz. pkg. | 231 | 10.0 |
| **BEEF, CORNED (See CORNED BEEF)** | | | |
| **BEEF DINNER or ENTREE,** frozen: | | | |
| (Banquet) | 11-oz. dinner | 312 | 20.9 |
| (Banquet) chopped | 11-oz. dinner | 443 | 32.8 |
| (Morton): | | | |
| Chopped sirloin, *Steak House* | 9½-oz. dinner | 748 | 43.2 |
| Rib eye, *Steak House* | 9-oz. dinner | 816 | 38.4 |
| Sirloin strip, *Steak House* | 9½-oz. dinner | 896 | 43.2 |
| Sliced, *Country Table* | 14-oz. dinner | 512 | 55.7 |
| Tenderloin, *Steak House* | 9½-oz. dinner | 896 | 43.2 |
| (Swanson): | | | |
| Chopped, *Hungry Man* | 18-oz. dinner | 730 | 70.0 |
| Sliced, with gravy & whipped potatoes | 8-oz. entree | 190 | 23.0 |
| Sliced, *Hungry Man* | 12¼-oz. entree | 330 | 23.0 |

| Food and Description | Measure or Quantity | Calories | Carbo-hydrates (grams) |
|---|---|---|---|
| Sliced, *Hungry Man* | 17-oz. dinner | 540 | 51.0 |
| 3-course | 15-oz. dinner | 490 | 58.0 |
| TV dinner | 11½-oz. dinner | 370 | 34.0 |
| (Weight Watchers) beef-steak with peppers & mushrooms | 10-oz. meal | 387 | 11.1 |
| (Weight Watchers) sirloin, 3-compartment | 16-oz. meal | 516 | 10.0 |
| **BEEF, DRIED,** canned: | | | |
| (Hormel) creamed, *Short Orders* | 7½-oz. can | 160 | 9.0 |
| (Swift) | 1-oz. serving | 35 | 0. |
| **BEEF GOULASH:** | | | |
| Canned, regular pack: | | | |
| (Bounty) | 7½-oz. can | 203 | 16.3 |
| (Hormel) *Short Orders* | 7½-oz. can | 230 | 16.0 |
| **BEEF GROUND** (See BEEF, Ground) | | | |
| **BEEF, GROUND, SEASON-ING MIX:** | | | |
| (Durkee) | 1.1-oz. pkg. | 91 | 18.0 |
| *(Durkee) | 1 cup | 654 | 9.0 |
| (Durkee) with onion | 1.1-oz. pkg. | 102 | 13.0 |
| *(Durkee) with onion | 1 cup | 659 | 6.5 |
| (French's) with onion | 1⅛-oz. pkg. | 100 | 24.0 |
| **BEEF HASH, ROAST,** frozen (Stouffer's) | ½ of 11½-oz. pkg. | 262 | 10.9 |
| **BEEF PEPPER ORIENTAL,** frozen (Chun King): | | | |
| Dinner | 11-oz. dinner | 310 | 43.0 |
| Pouch | 12-oz. pouch | 160 | 20.0 |

(USDA): United States Department of Agriculture
(HEW/FAO): Health, Education and Welfare/Food and Agriculture
        Organization
* Prepared as Package Directs

| Food and Description | Measure or Quantity | Calories | Carbo-hydrates (grams) |
|---|---|---|---|
| **BEEF PIE:** | | | |
| Home recipe, baked (USDA) | 4¼" pie (8 oz. before baking) | 558 | 42.7 |
| Frozen: | | | |
| (Banquet) | 8-oz. pie | 409 | 40.9 |
| (Morton) | 8-oz. pie | 316 | 31.8 |
| (Stouffer's) | 10-oz. pie | 552 | 37.8 |
| (Swanson) | 8-oz. pie | 430 | 43.0 |
| (Swanson) *Hungry Man* | 16-oz. pie | 770 | 65.0 |
| (Swanson) steak burger, *Hungry Man* | 16-oz. pie | 830 | 69.0 |
| **BEEF, POTTED** (USDA) | 1-oz. serving | 70 | 0. |
| **BEEF PUFFS,** frozen (Durkee) | 1 piece | 47 | 3.0 |
| **BEEF ROAST,** canned (USDA) | 4-oz. serving | 254 | 0. |
| **BEEF SHORT RIBS,** frozen (Stouffer's) boneless, with vegetable gravy | ½ of 11½-oz. pkg. | 347 | 2.0 |
| **BEEF SOUP:** | | | |
| Canned, regular pack: (USDA): | | | |
| Bouillon, condensed | 8 oz. (by weight) | 59 | 5.0 |
| *Bouillon, condensed, prepared with equal volume water | 1 cup (8.5 oz.) | 31 | 2.6 |
| Consomme, condensed | 8 oz. (by weight) | 59 | 5.0 |
| *Consomme, condensed, prepared with equal volume water | 1 cup (8.5 oz.) | 31 | 2.6 |
| & noodle, condensed | 8 oz. (by weight) | 129 | 13.2 |
| *& noodle, condensed, prepared with equal volume water | 1 cup (8.5 oz.) | 67 | 7.0 |
| *(Ann Page) & vegetable | 1 cup | 71 | 9.5 |
| (Campbell): | | | |
| *Broth, condensed | 10-oz. serving | 30 | 2.0 |

| Food and Description | Measure or Quantity | Calories | Carbo-hydrates (grams) |
|---|---|---|---|
| *Broth, & barley, condensed | 11-oz. serving | 90 | 13.0 |
| *Broth, & noodles, condensed | 10-oz. serving | 80 | 10.0 |
| *Chunky* | 10¾-oz. can | 220 | 22.0 |
| *Chunky, & noodles* | 10¾-oz. can | 280 | 24.0 |
| *Chunky, sirloin burger* | 10¾-oz. can | 230 | 24.0 |
| *Condensed | 11-oz. serving | 110 | 15.0 |
| *Consomme, condensed, gelatin added | 11-oz. serving | 45 | 4.0 |
| *& noodle, condensed | 10-oz. serving | 90 | 9.0 |
| (College Inn) broth | 1 cup | 18 | 1.0 |
| (Swanson) broth | ½ of 13¾-oz. can | 20 | 1.0 |
| Canned. dietetic pack (Dia-Mel) & noodle | 8-oz. serving | 70 | 5.0 |
| Mix: | | | |
| *(USDA) | 1 cup (8.1 oz.) | 64 | 11.0 |
| *(Lipton) & noodle, *Cup-a-Soup* | 6 fl. oz. | 35 | 6.0 |
| *(Nestle) & noodle, *Souptime* | 6 fl. oz. | 30 | 4.0 |
| (Weight Watchers) broth | .2-oz. packet | 10 | 1.0 |
| **BEEF STEW:** | | | |
| Home recipe (USDA) | 1 cup | 218 | 15.2 |
| Canned. regular pack: | | | |
| (USDA) | 15-oz. can | 336 | 30.2 |
| *Dinty Moore* | 7½-oz. serving | 184 | 12.8 |
| (Libby's) | 8-oz. serving | 233 | 33.8 |
| (Morton House) | ⅓ of 24-oz. can | 240 | 17.0 |
| (Nalley's) | 7½-oz. serving | 226 | 17.0 |
| (Swanson) | ½ of 15¼-oz. can | 192 | 18.2 |
| Canned. dietetic or low calorie: | | | |
| (Dia-Mel) | 8-oz. can | 200 | 19.0 |
| (Featherweight) | 7¼-oz. can | 210 | 24.0 |
| Frozen: | | | |
| (Banquet) buffet | 2-lb. pkg. | 700 | 90.9 |

(USDA): United States Department of Agriculture
(HEW/FAO): Health, Education and Welfare/Food and Agriculture Organization
* Prepared as Package Directs

| Food and Description | Measure or Quantity | Calories | Carbo-hydrates (grams) |
|---|---|---|---|
| (Green Giant) & biscuits, Bake n' Serve | 14-oz. pkg. | 368 | 40.6 |
| (Green Giant) boil-in-bag | 9-oz. pkg. | 165 | 20.2 |
| (Stouffer's) | 10-oz. serving | 305 | 15.9 |
| **BEEF STEW SEASONING MIX:** | | | |
| (Durkee) | 1.8-oz. pkg. | 99 | 22.0 |
| *(Durkee) | 1 cup | 379 | 16.8 |
| (French's) | 1⅞-oz. pkg. | 150 | 36.0 |
| **BEEF STIX,** packaged | | | |
| (Vienna) | 1-oz. serving | 163 | 1.4 |
| **BEEF STOCK BASE** | | | |
| (French's) | 1 tsp. (4 grams) | 8 | 2.0 |
| **BEEF STROGANOFF,** frozen (Stouffer's) with parsley noodles | 9¾-oz. serving | 390 | 30.7 |
| **BEER,** canned: | | | |
| Regular: | | | |
| Black Horse Ale, 5% alcohol | 12 fl. oz. | 162 | 13.8 |
| Black Label | 12 fl. oz. | 140 | 11.3 |
| Buckeye, 4.6% alcohol | 12 fl. oz. | 144 | 11.0 |
| Budweiser, 4.9% alcohol | 12 fl. oz. | 156 | 12.3 |
| Budweiser, 3.9% alcohol | 12 fl. oz. | 137 | 11.9 |
| Busch Bavarian, 4.9% alcohol | 12 fl. oz. | 156 | 12.3 |
| Busch Bavarian, 3.9% alcohol | 12 fl. oz. | 137 | 11.9 |
| Eastside Lager | 12 fl. oz. | 145 | DNA |
| Heidelberg, 4.6% alcohol | 12 fl. oz. | 133 | 10.7 |
| Knickerbocker, 4.6% alcohol | 12 fl. oz. | 160 | 13.7 |
| Meister Brau Premium, 4.6% alcohol | 12 fl. oz. | 144 | 11.0 |
| Meister Brau Premium, Draft, 4.6% alcohol | 12 fl. oz. | 144 | 11.0 |
| Michelob, 4.9% alcohol | 12 fl. oz. | 160 | 12.8 |
| Pabst Blue Ribbon | 12 fl. oz. | 150 | DNA |

| Food and Description | Measure or Quantity | Calories | Carbo- hydrates (grams) |
|---|---|---|---|
| *Rheingold*, 4.6% alcohol | 12 fl. oz. | 160 | 13.7 |
| *Schmidt*, regular or extra special, 4.8% alcohol | 12 fl. oz. | 165 | 14.9 |
| *Schmidt*, 3.2 low gravity | 12 fl. oz. | 142 | 13.6 |
| *Stroh Bohemian*, 3.2 low gravity | 12 fl. oz. | 126 | 11.6 |
| *Tuborg USA*, 4.8% alcohol | 12 fl. oz. | 140 | 12.1 |
| Low carbohydrate: | | | |
| *Gablinger's*, 4.5% alcohol | 12 fl. oz. | 99 | .2 |
| *Meister Brau Lite*, 4.6% alcohol | 12 fl. oz. | 96 | 1.4 |
| *Stroh Light* | 12 fl. oz. | 115 | 7.1 |
| **BEER, NEAR:** | | | |
| *Goetz Pale*, 0.2% alcohol | 12 fl. oz. | 78 | 3.9 |
| *Kingsbury*, 0.5% alcohol | 12 fl. oz. | 45 | 10.7 |
| **BEET:** | | | |
| Raw (USDA) | 1 lb. (weighed with skins, without tops) | 137 | 31.4 |
| Raw (USDA) diced | ½ cup (2.4 oz.) | 29 | 6.6 |
| Boiled (USDA) drained: | | | |
| Whole | 2 beets (2″ dia., 3.5 oz.) | 32 | 7.2 |
| Diced | ½ cup (3 oz.) | 27 | 6.1 |
| Sliced | ½ cup (3.6 oz.) | 33 | 7.3 |
| Canned, regular pack: | | | |
| (USDA) solids & liq. | ½ cup (4.3 oz.) | 42 | 9.7 |
| (USDA) whole, drained solids | ½ cup (2.8 oz.) | 30 | 7.0 |
| (USDA) diced, drained solids | ½ cup (2.9 oz.) | 30 | 7.2 |
| (USDA) sliced, drained solids | ½ cup (3.1 oz.) | 33 | 7.7 |
| (Del Monte): | | | |
| Pickled, sliced, solids & liq. | ½ cup | 77 | 18.1 |

(USDA): United States Department of Agriculture
(HEW/FAO): Health, Education and Welfare/Food and Agriculture Organization
* Prepared as Package Directs

| Food and Description | Measure or Quantity | Calories | Carbohydrates (grams) |
|---|---|---|---|
| Pickled, sliced, drained solids | ½ cup | 81 | 18.9 |
| Sliced, solids & liq. | ½ cup | 29 | 7.0 |
| Sliced, drained solids | ½ cup | 36 | 3.6 |
| Whole, tiny, solids & liq. | ½ cup | 42 | 9.1 |
| (Libby's): | | | |
| Harvard, diced, solids & liq. | ½ cup (4.2 oz.) | 87 | 20.8 |
| Pickled, sliced, solids & liq. | ¼ of 16-oz. jar | 78 | 18.5 |
| (Stokely-Van Camp): | | | |
| Cut, solids & liq. | ½ cup | 45 | 9.5 |
| Diced, solids & liq. | ½ cup | 35 | 7.5 |
| Harvard, solids & liq. | ½ cup (4.5 oz.) | 80 | 18.0 |
| Pickled, solids & liq. | ½ cup (4.3 oz.) | 95 | 22.5 |
| Whole, solids & liq. | ½ cup (4.3 oz.) | 45 | 10.0 |
| Canned, dietetic pack: | | | |
| (USDA) solids & liq. | 4-oz. serving | 36 | 8.8 |
| (USDA) drained solids | 4-oz. serving | 42 | 9.9 |
| (Blue Boy) whole, solids & liq. | ¼ of 16-oz. can | 39 | 9.2 |
| (Comstock) water packed | ½ cup | 30 | 6.5 |
| (Featherweight) sliced, solids & liq. | ½ cup | 40 | 10.0 |
| (Tillie Lewis) Tasti Diet | ½ cup | 35 | 8.0 |
| **BEET GREENS** (USDA): | | | |
| Raw, whole | 1 lb. (weighed untrimmed) | 61 | 11.7 |
| Boiled, leaves & stems, drained | ½ cup (2.6 oz.) | 13 | 2.4 |
| **BENEDICTINE LIQUEUR** (Julius Wile) 86 proof | 1 fl. oz. | 112 | 10.3 |
| **BIG H,** burger sauce (Hellmann's) | 1 T. | 71 | 1.6 |
| **BIG MAC** (See McDONALD'S) | | | |
| **BIG WHEEL** (Hostess) | 1.3-oz. cake | 170 | 21.1 |

| Food and Description | Measure or Quantity | Calories | Carbo- hydrates (grams) |
|---|---|---|---|
| **BISCUIT**, home recipe (USDA) baking powder | 1-oz. biscuit (2" dia.) | 103 | 12.8 |
| **BISCUIT DOUGH,** refrigerated (Pillsbury): | | | |
| *Ballard,* oven-ready | 1 biscuit | 60 | 11.0 |
| Buttermilk | 1 biscuit | 105 | 10.5 |
| Buttermilk extra light | 1 biscuit | 60 | 10.5 |
| Cornbread | 1 biscuit | 95 | 12.5 |
| Country-style | 1 biscuit | 55 | 10.5 |
| *1869 Brand* baking powder | 1 biscuit | 105 | 13.0 |
| *1869 Brand* prebaked | 1 biscuit | 100 | 12.0 |
| *Hungry Jack,* buttermilk or regular | 1 biscuit | 90 | 11.5 |
| *Hungry Jack,* buttermilk, extra light | 1 biscuit | 60 | 10.5 |
| **BISCUIT MIX** (USDA): | | | |
| Dry, with enriched flour | 1 oz. | 120 | 19.5 |
| *Baked from mix, with added milk | 1-oz. biscuit | 91 | 14.6 |
| ***BI-SICLE*** (Popsicle Industries) | 2½ fl. oz. | 112 | 21.4 |
| **BITTERS** (Angostura) | 1 tsp. | 14 | DNA |
| **BLACKBERRY:** Fresh (USDA) includes boysenberry, dewberry, youngsberry: | | | |
| With hulls | 1 lb. (weighed untrimmed) | 250 | 55.6 |
| Hulled | ½ cup (2.6 oz.) | 41 | 9.4 |
| Canned, regular pack (USDA) solids & liq.: | | | |
| Juice pack | 4-oz. serving | 61 | 13.7 |
| Light syrup | 4-oz. serving | 82 | 19.6 |

(USDA): United States Department of Agriculture
(HEW/FAO): Health, Education and Welfare/Food and Agriculture
          Organization
* Prepared as Package Directs

| Food and Description | Measure or Quantity | Calories | Carbo-hydrates (grams) |
|---|---|---|---|
| Heavy syrup | ½ cup (4.6 oz.) | 118 | 28.9 |
| Extra heavy syrup | 4-oz. serving | 125 | 30.7 |
| Frozen (USDA): | | | |
| Sweetened, unthawed | 4-oz. serving | 109 | 27.7 |
| Unsweetened, unthawed | 4-oz. serving | 55 | 12.9 |

**BLACKBERRY BRANDY**
**(See BRANDY, FLAVORED)**

**BLACKBERRY JELLY:**

| | | | |
|---|---|---|---|
| Sweetened (Smucker's) | 1 T. (.7 oz.) | 53 | 13.5 |
| Dietetic or low calorie: | | | |
| (Featherweight) | 1 T. | 16 | 4.0 |
| (Slenderella) | 1 T. | 24 | 6.0 |

**BLACKBERRY LIQUEUR:**

| | | | |
|---|---|---|---|
| (Bols) 60 proof | 1 fl. oz. | 96 | 8.9 |
| (Hiram Walker) 60 proof | 1 fl. oz. | 100 | 12.8 |

**BLACKBERRY PRESERVE or JAM:**

| | | | |
|---|---|---|---|
| Sweetened (Smucker's) | 1 T. (.7 oz.) | 53 | 13.5 |
| Dietetic or low calorie: | | | |
| (Dia-Mel) | 1 T. | 6 | 0. |
| (Diet Delight) | 1 T. (.6 oz.) | 13 | 3.3 |
| (Featherweight) | 1 T. | 16 | 4.0 |

**BLACKBERRY SOUR COCKTAIL, liquid mix**

| | | | |
|---|---|---|---|
| (Holland House) | 1½ fl. oz. | 75 | 18.0 |

**BLACKBERRY SPREAD, low sugar (Smucker's)**

| | | | |
|---|---|---|---|
| | 1 T. | 24 | 6.0 |

**BLACKBERRY SYRUP**

| | | | |
|---|---|---|---|
| (Smucker's) | 1 T. (.6 oz.) | 50 | 13.0 |

**BLACKBERRY WINE (Mogen David) 12% alcohol**

| | | | |
|---|---|---|---|
| | 3 fl. oz. | 135 | 18.7 |

**BLACK-EYED PEA (See also COWPEA):**

| | | | |
|---|---|---|---|
| Boiled (USDA) drained | ½ cup (3 oz.) | 111 | 20.1 |

| Food and Description | Measure or Quantity | Calories | Carbohydrates (grams) |
|---|---|---|---|
| Canned (Sultana) with pork | ½ of 15-oz. can | 204 | 33.9 |
| Frozen: | | | |
| (Birds Eye) | ⅓ of 10-oz. pkg. | 130 | 23.0 |
| (Green Giant) Southern recipe | ⅓ of 10-oz. pkg. | 106 | 12.7 |
| (McKenzie) | ⅓ of 10-oz. pkg. | 130 | 22.7 |
| (Seabrook Farms) | ⅓ of 10-oz. pkg. | 130 | 22.7 |
| **BLACK RUSSIAN COCK-TAIL,** liquid mix (Holland House) | 1½ fl. oz. | 138 | 34.5 |
| **BLANCMANGE (See VANILLA PUDDING)** | | | |
| **BLOOD PUDDING** or **SAUSAGE** (USDA) | 1 oz. | 112 | .1 |
| **BLOODY MARY MIX:** | | | |
| Dry (Holland House) | 1 serving (.5 oz.) | 56 | 14.0 |
| Liquid (Sacramento) | 5½-fl.-oz. can | 39 | 9.1 |
| **BLUEBERRY:** | | | |
| Fresh (USDA): | | | |
| Whole | 1 lb. (weighed untrimmed) | 259 | 63.8 |
| Trimmed | ½ cup (2.6 oz.) | 45 | 11.2 |
| Canned, regular pack (USDA) solids & liq., syrup pack, extra heavy | ½ cup (4.4 oz.) | 126 | 32.5 |
| Canned, dietetic or low calorie: | | | |
| (USDA) water pack, solids & liq. | ½ cup (4.3 oz.) | 47 | 11.9 |
| (Featherweight) water pack, solids & liq. | ½ cup | 41 | 10.7 |
| Frozen (USDA): | | | |
| Sweetened, solids & liq. | ½ cup (4 oz.) | 120 | 30.2 |
| Unsweetened, solids & liq. | ½ cup (2.9 oz.) | 45 | 11.2 |

(USDA): United States Department of Agriculture
(HEW/FAO): Health, Education and Welfare/Food and Agriculture Organization
* Prepared as Package Directs

| Food and Description | Measure or Quantity | Calories | Carbo-hydrates (grams) |
|---|---|---|---|
| **BLUEBERRY PIE** (See PIE, Blueberry) | | | |
| **BLUEBERRY PRESERVE or JAM:** | | | |
| Sweetened (Smucker's) | 1 T. | 53 | 13.5 |
| Dietetic (Dia-Mel) | 1 T. | 6 | 0. |
| **BLUEBERRY SYRUP:** | | | |
| Sweetened (Smucker's) | 1 T. (.6 oz.) | 50 | 13.0 |
| Dietetic (Featherweight) | 1 T. | 14 | 3.0 |
| **BLUEBERRY TURNOVER,** refrigerated (Pillsbury) | 1 turnover (3.3 oz.) | 170 | 23.0 |
| **BLUEFISH** (USDA): | | | |
| Raw: | | | |
| Whole | 1 lb. (weighed whole) | 271 | 0. |
| Meat only | 4 oz. | 133 | 0. |
| Baked or broiled | 4.4-oz. piece (3½" x 3" x ½") | 199 | 0. |
| Fried | 5.3-oz. piece (3½" x 3" x ½") | 308 | 7.0 |
| **BODY BUDDIES,** cereal (General Mills): | | | |
| Brown sugar & honey | 1 cup (1 oz.) | 110 | 25.0 |
| Natural Fruit Flavor | ¾ cup (1 oz.) | 110 | 25.0 |
| **BOLOGNA:** | | | |
| (Eckrich): | | | |
| Beef | 1-oz. serving | 95 | 1.5 |
| Garlic | 1-oz. serving | 95 | 1.5 |
| Ring | 1-oz. serving | 100 | 1.5 |
| Ring, pickled | 1-oz. serving | 95 | 1.5 |
| Sliced | 1-oz. serving | 95 | 1.5 |
| Sliced, thick | 1.7-oz. slice | 160 | 3.0 |
| Sliced, thick | 1.8-oz. slice | 170 | 3.0 |
| (Hormel): | | | |
| Beef | 1-oz. serving | 86 | .3 |
| Coarse ground | 1-oz. serving | 76 | .9 |

| Food and Description | Measure or Quantity | Calories | Carbo-hydrates (grams) |
|---|---|---|---|
| Fine ground | 1-oz. serving | 82 | .6 |
| Meat | 1-oz. serving | 85 | .2 |
| (Oscar Mayer): | | | |
| Beef | .5-oz. slice | 45 | .4 |
| Beef | .8-oz. slice | 72 | .7 |
| Beef, thick slice | 1.3-oz. slice | 118 | 1.1 |
| Beef Lebanon | .8-oz. slice | 51 | .4 |
| Garlic beef | .8-oz. slice | 73 | .4 |
| German brand | .8-oz. slice | 55 | .3 |
| Meat, round | .8-oz. slice | 73 | .7 |
| Meat, square | 1-oz. slice | 91 | .8 |
| Meat, thick, round | 1.3-oz. slice | 118 | 1.1 |
| Meat, thin, round | .5-oz. slice | 45 | .4 |
| Ring, Wisconsin-made, coarse ground | 1-oz. serving | 81 | .4 |
| Ring, Wisconsin-made, fine ground | 1-oz. serving | 87 | .7 |
| (Swift) | 1-oz. slice | 95 | 1.5 |
| (Vienna) beef | 1-oz. serving | 84 | .7 |
| **BOLOGNA & CHEESE,** packaged (Oscar Mayer) | .8-oz. slice | 72 | .6 |
| **BONITO:** | | | |
| Raw (USDA): | | | |
| Whole | 1 lb. (weighed whole) | 442 | 0. |
| Meat only | 4 oz. | 191 | 0. |
| Canned (Star-Kist): | | | |
| Chunk, in oil | 6½-oz. can | 604 | 0. |
| Solid, in oil | 7-oz. can | 650 | 0. |
| *BOO\*BERRY,* cereal | 1 cup (1 oz.) | 110 | 24.0 |
| **BORDEAUX WINE** (See also individual regional, vineyard, or brand names or **CLARET WINE**) Rouge (Cruse) 10½% alcohol | 3 fl. oz. | 63 | DNA |

(USDA): United States Department of Agriculture
(HEW/FAO): Health, Education and Welfare/Food and Agriculture Organization
* Prepared as Package Directs

| Food and Description | Measure or Quantity | Calories | Carbo-hydrates (grams) |
|---|---|---|---|
| **BOSCO** (Best Foods) | 1 T. (.7 oz.) | 56 | 13.3 |
| **BOUILLON CUBE** (See individual flavors) | | | |
| **BOURBON WHISKY,** unflavored (See **DISTILLED LIQUEUR**) | | | |
| **BOYSENBERRY:** Fresh (See **BLACKBERRY**) Frozen, sweetened (USDA) | 10-oz. pkg. | 273 | 69.3 |
| **BOYSENBERRY JELLY,** sweetened (Smucker's) | 1 T. | 53 | 13.5 |
| **BOYSENBERRY PRESERVE** or **JAM:** Sweetened (Smucker's) | 1 T. (.7 oz.) | 53 | 13.5 |
| Dietetic or low calorie (Slenderella) | 1 T. (.6 oz.) | 24 | 6.0 |
| **BOYSENBERRY SPREAD,** low sugar (Smucker's) | 1 T. | 24 | 6.0 |
| **BOYSENBERRY SYRUP,** sweetened (Smucker's) | 1 T. | 50 | 13.0 |
| **BRAINS,** all animals, raw (USDA) | 1 oz. | 60 | 17.5 |
| **BRAN,** crude (USDA) | 1 oz. | 60 | 17.5 |
| **BRAN BREAKFAST CEREAL:** (Kellogg's): | | | |
| *All-Bran* | ⅓ cup (1 oz.) | 70 | 22.0 |
| *Bran-Buds* | ⅓ cup (1 oz.) | 70 | 22.0 |
| *Cracklin' Bran* | ⅓ cup (1 oz.) | 110 | 19.0 |
| 40% bran flakes | ⅔ cup (1 oz.) | 90 | 23.0 |
| With raisins | ¾ cup (1.3 oz.) | 120 | 29.0 |
| (Nabisco) 100% bran | ½ cup (1 oz.) | 70 | 21.0 |
| (Post) 40% bran flakes | ⅔ cup (1 oz.) | 107 | 22.6 |

| Food and Description | Measure or Quantity | Calories | Carbo-hydrates (grams) |
|---|---|---|---|
| (Post) with raisins | ½ cup (1 oz.) | 102 | 21.4 |
| (Quaker) *Corn Bran* | ⅔ cup (1 oz.) | 109 | 23.3 |
| (Ralston Purina): | | | |
| Bran Chex | ⅔ cup (1 oz.) | 110 | 20.0 |
| Raisin | ½ cup (1 oz.) | 100 | 22.0 |
| *Shoprite,* 40% bran | ⅝ cup | 104 | 21.9 |
| *Shoprite,* raisin | ⅝ cup | 101 | 22.0 |
| (Van Brode) 40% bran | ⅝ cup | 104 | 21.9 |
| (Van Brode) raisin | ⅝ cup | 101 | 22.0 |

**BRANDY, unflavored (See DISTILLED LIQUOR)**

**BRANDY EXTRACT:**

| | | | |
|---|---|---|---|
| (Ehlers) pure | 1 tsp. | 16 | |
| (French's) imitation | 1 tsp. | 16 | |

**BRANDY, FLAVORED:**

| | | | |
|---|---|---|---|
| Apricot: | | | |
| (Leroux) | 1 fl. oz. | 92 | 8.6 |
| (Mr. Boston) | 1 fl. oz. | 94 | 8.9 |
| Blackberry: | | | |
| (Bols) | 1 fl. oz. | 100 | 7.4 |
| (Leroux) | 1 fl. oz. | 91 | 8.3 |
| (Mr. Boston) | 1 fl. oz. | 92 | 8.6 |
| Cherry: | | | |
| (Bols) | 1 fl. oz. | 100 | 7.4 |
| (Leroux) | 1 fl. oz. | 91 | 8.3 |
| (Mr. Boston) | 1 fl. oz. | 87 | 8.4 |
| Coffee: | | | |
| (Leroux) coffee & brandy | 1 fl. oz. | 91 | 8.3 |
| (Mr. Boston) | 1 fl. oz. | 100 | 10.6 |
| Ginger: | | | |
| (Garnier) | 1 fl. oz. | 74 | 4.0 |
| (Leroux) | 1 fl. oz. | 76 | 4.4 |
| (Leroux) sharp | 1 fl. oz. | 77 | 4.7 |
| (Mr. Boston) | 1 fl. oz. | 72 | 3.5 |
| Peach: | | | |
| (Hiram Walker) | 1 fl. oz. | 87 | 7.2 |

(USDA): United States Department of Agriculture
(HEW/FAO): Health, Education and Welfare/Food and Agriculture Organization
* Prepared as Package Directs

| Food and Description | Measure or Quantity | Calories | Carbo- hydrates (grams) |
|---|---|---|---|
| (Leroux) | 1 fl. oz. | 93 | 8.9 |
| (Mr. Boston) | 1 fl. oz. | 94 | 8.9 |
| **BRAUNSCHWEIGER:** | | | |
| (Oscar Mayer): | | | |
| Tube | 1-oz. serving | 94 | .7 |
| Tube, German brand | 1-oz. serving | 95 | .6 |
| (Swift) 8-oz. chub | 1-oz. serving | 109 | 1.4 |
| **BRAZIL NUT** (USDA): | | | |
| Whole, in shell | 1 cup (4.3 oz.) | 383 | 6.4 |
| Shelled | ½ cup (2.5 oz.) | 458 | 7.6 |
| Shelled | 4 nuts (.6 oz.) | 114 | 1.9 |
| **BREAD** (listed by type or brand name): | | | |
| *American Granary* (Arnold) | .9-oz. slice | 70 | 12.5 |
| Boston Brown (USDA) | 1.7-oz. slice (3" x ¾") | 101 | 21.9 |
| Bran, *Ideal Flatbread* | .2-oz. slice | 19 | 4.1 |
| *Bran'nola* (Arnold) | 1.2-oz. slice | 90 | 15.5 |
| Cinnamon raisin (Thomas') | .8-oz. slice | 60 | 11.7 |
| Cracked-wheat: | | | |
| (USDA) 20 slices to 1 lb. | .8-oz. slice | 60 | 12.0 |
| (Wonder) | 1-oz. slice | 75 | 13.5 |
| Date nut loaf (Thomas') cake | 1.1-oz. slice | 93 | 18.4 |
| Date nut roll (Dromedary) | .5-oz. slice | 80 | 13.0 |
| French: | | | |
| (USDA) 20 slices to 1 lb. | .8-oz. slice | 67 | 12.7 |
| (Arnold) *Francisco* | 1-oz. serving | 80 | 14.5 |
| (Arnold) *Francisco,* Vienna | .8-oz. slice | 80 | 14.5 |
| (Pepperidge Farm) | ⅐ of 14-oz. loaf | 150 | 27.0 |
| (Wonder) | 1-oz. slice | 75 | 13.5 |
| *Glutogen* Gluten (Thomas') | 1-oz. slice | 32 | 5.9 |
| *Hillbilly* (Wonder) | 1-oz. slice | 70 | 12.5 |
| *Hollywood* (Wonder) dark or light | 18-gram slice | 45 | 7.5 |
| *Hollywood* (Wonder) dark or light | 20-gram slice | 49 | 8.8 |
| Honey bran (Pepperidge Farm) | 1 slice | 95 | 17.5 |

| Food and Description | Measure or Quantity | Calories | Carbo-hydrates (grams) |
|---|---|---|---|
| *Honey Wheatberry* (Arnold) | 1.2-oz. slice | 90 | 16.0 |
| Italian: | | | |
|     (USDA) 20 slices to 1 lb. | .8-oz. slice | 63 | 13.0 |
|     (Pepperidge Farm) | ⅛ of 1-lb. loaf | 150 | 28.0 |
| Low sodium (Wonder) | 1-oz. slice | 70 | 13.5 |
| *Naturel* (Arnold) | .9-oz. slice | 65 | 12.0 |
| *Profile* (Wonder) dark or | | | |
|     light | 1-oz. slice | 75 | 12.5 |
| *Protogen* protein (Thomas') | .7-oz. slice | 45 | 8.3 |
| *Protogen* protein (Thomas') | | | |
|     frozen | .9-oz. slice | 55 | 10.2 |
| Pumpernickel: | | | |
|     (Arnold) | 1.1-oz. slice | 75 | 14.0 |
|     (Levy's) | 1-oz. slice | 70 | 14.0 |
|     (Pepperidge Farm) | 1 slice | 80 | 15.0 |
| Raisin: | | | |
|     Cinnamon (See Cinnamon | | | |
|       raisin) | | | |
|     (Arnold) tea | .9-oz. slice | 70 | 13.0 |
|     (Sun-Maid) | 1-oz. slice | 80 | 14.5 |
| *Roman Meal* | 1-oz. slice | 70 | 13.5 |
| Rye: | | | |
|     (Arnold) Jewish | 1.1-oz. slice | 75 | 14.0 |
|     (Arnold) melba thin | .7-oz. slice | 50 | 9.5 |
|     (Levy's) Real, with or | | | |
|       without seeds | 1-oz. slice | 70 | 13.0 |
|     (Pepperidge Farm) family | 1 slice | 85 | 15.0 |
|     *Wasa:* | | | |
|       Golden | .4-oz. slice | 40 | 8.6 |
|       Hearty | .5-oz. slice | 53 | 11.4 |
|       Lite | .3-oz. slice | 30 | 6.3 |
|       Seasoned | 1 slice | 34 | 7.1 |
|     (Wonder) | 1-oz. slice | 75 | 13.5 |
| Salt rising (USDA) | .9-oz. slice | 67 | 13.0 |
| Sesame, *Wasa* | 14-gram slice | 60 | 9.0 |
| Sourdough, *DiCarlo* | 1-oz. slice | 70 | 13.5 |
| Sourdough toast, *Wasa* | 12-gram slice | 46 | 9.5 |
| Sport, *Wasa* | .4-oz. slice | 43 | 9.1 |

| Food and Description | Measure or Quantity | Calories | Carbo-hydrates (grams) |
|---|---|---|---|
| Toaster cake (See **TOASTER CAKE**) | | | |
| Ultra thin, *Ideal Flatbread* | .1-oz. slice | 12 | 2.5 |
| Wheat: | | | |
| *Fresh Horizons* | 1-oz. slice | 54 | 9.6 |
| *Home Pride* | 1-oz. slice | 75 | 13.1 |
| (Pepperidge Farm) | 1 slice | 85 | 17.5 |
| (Wonder) | 1-oz. slice | 75 | 13.5 |
| (Wonder) 100% whole wheat | 1-oz. slice | 70 | 11.9 |
| Wheatberry, *Home Pride* | 1-oz. slice | 70 | 12.5 |
| Wheat germ (Pepperidge Farm) | 1 slice | 65 | 12.0 |
| White: | | | |
| (USDA): | | | |
| Prepared with 1-4% non-fat dry milk | .8-oz. slice | 62 | 11.6 |
| Prepared with 5-6% non-fat dry milk | .8-oz. slice | 63 | 11.5 |
| (Arnold): | | | |
| *Brick Oven* | .8-oz. slice | 65 | 11.0 |
| *Brick Oven* | 1.1-oz. slice | 85 | 14.5 |
| *Hearthstone,* 2-lb. loaf | 1.1-oz. slice | 85 | 15.0 |
| Country | 1.2-oz. slice | 95 | 17.0 |
| Melba thin | .5-oz. slice | 40 | 7.0 |
| *Fresh Horizons* | 1-oz. slice | 54 | 9.6 |
| *Home Pride* | 1-oz. slice | 75 | 13.0 |
| (Levy's) no salt added | .9-oz. slice | 80 | 14.0 |
| (Pepperidge Farm): | | | |
| Large loaf | 1 slice | 75 | 13.0 |
| Sandwich | 1 slice | 65 | 11.5 |
| Sliced | .8-oz. slice | 55 | 10.5 |
| Toasting | 1.2-oz. slice | 85 | 15.5 |
| Very thin slice | 1 slice | 40 | 7.5 |
| (Wonder) regular and with buttermilk | 1-oz. slice | 75 | 13.5 |
| Whole-wheat: | | | |
| (USDA): | | | |
| Prepared with 2% non-fat dry milk | .9-oz. slice | 61 | 11.9 |
| Prepared with 2% non-fat dry milk | .8-oz. slice | 56 | 11.0 |
| Prepared with water | .9-oz. slice | 60 | 12.3 |

| Food and Description | Measure or Quantity | Calories | Carbo-hydrates (grams) |
|---|---|---|---|
| (Arnold): | | | |
|   *Brick Oven* | .8-oz. slice | 60 | 9.5 |
|   *Brick Oven* | 1.1-oz. slice | 80 | 13.0 |
|   Melba thin | .5-oz. slice | 40 | 6.5 |
|   Stone ground, 100% | .8-oz. slice | 55 | 9.5 |
| (Pepperidge Farm) thin sliced | 1 slice | 70 | 12.0 |
| (Thomas') | .8-oz. slice | 56 | 10.1 |
| **BREAD, CANNED** (B&M): | | | |
|   Brown, plain | 1-oz. slice | 52 | 11.4 |
|   Brown, with raisins | 1-oz. slice | 52 | 11.1 |
| **BREAD CRUMBS:** | | | |
|   (Contadina) seasoned | ½ cup (2.1 oz.) | 228 | 44.3 |
|   (4C) plain | 2-oz. serving | 203 | 42.6 |
|   (4C) seasoned | 2-oz. serving | 192 | 38.6 |
| ***BREAD DOUGH,** frozen (Rich's): | | | |
|   French | 1⁄20 of loaf | 59 | 11.0 |
|   Italian | 1⁄20 of loaf | 60 | 11.0 |
|   Raisin | 1⁄20 of loaf | 66 | 12.3 |
| ***BREAD MIX** (Pillsbury): | | | |
|   Applesauce | 1⁄16 of loaf | 120 | 21.0 |
|   Apricot nut, banana, blueberry nut | 1⁄16 of loaf | 110 | 20.0 |
|   Cranberry | 1⁄16 of loaf | 120 | 22.0 |
|   Date | 1⁄12 of loaf | 120 | 23.0 |
| **BREAD PUDDING** with raisins, home recipe (USDA) | 1 cup (9.3 oz.) | 496 | 75.3 |
| **BREADFRUIT,** fresh (USDA): | | | |
|   Whole | 1 lb. (weighed untrimmed) | 360 | 91.5 |
|   Peeled & trimmed | 4 oz. | 117 | 29.7 |

(USDA): United States Department of Agriculture
(HEW/FAO): Health, Education and Welfare/Food and Agriculture Organization
* Prepared as Package Directs

| Food and Description | Measure or Quantity | Calories | Carbo-hydrates (grams) |
|---|---|---|---|
| **BREAKFAST BAR** | | | |
| (Carnation): | | | |
| Almond crunch | 1 piece | 210 | 20.0 |
| Chocolate chip | 1 piece | 200 | 20.0 |
| Chocolate crunch | 1 piece | 200 | 22.0 |
| Peanut butter crunch | 1 piece | 200 | 22.0 |
| **BREAKFAST DRINK**, instant: | | | |
| (Ann Page) grape or orange flavor | 2 tsps. (.6 oz.) | 63 | 15.9 |
| (Pillsbury): | | | |
| Chocolate or chocolate malt | 1 pouch | 130 | 26.0 |
| Strawberry or vanilla | 1 pouch | 130 | 27.0 |
| **BREAKFAST SQUARES** | | | |
| (General Mills) all flavors | 1 bar | 145 | 22.5 |
| ***BRIGHT & EARLY*** | 6 fl. oz. (6.6 oz.) | 90 | 21.6 |
| **BROCCOLI:** | | | |
| Raw (USDA): | | | |
| Whole | 1 lb. (weighed untrimmed) | 89 | 16.3 |
| Large leaves removed | 1 lb. (weighed partially trimmed) | 113 | 20.9 |
| Boiled (USDA): | | | |
| ½" pieces, drained | ½ cup (2.8 oz.) | 20 | 3.5 |
| Whole, drained | 1 med. stalk (6.3 oz.) | 47 | 8.1 |
| Frozen: | | | |
| (Birds Eye): | | | |
| In cheese sauce | ⅓ of 10-oz. pkg. | 110 | 8.0 |
| Chopped, spears or baby deluxe spears | ⅓ of 10-oz. pkg. | 25 | 4.0 |
| In Hollandaise sauce | ⅓ of 10-oz. pkg. | 100 | 2.9 |
| (Green Giant): | | | |
| Cuts in cheese sauce, Bake 'N Serve | ⅓ of 10-oz. pkg. | 91 | 5.6 |
| Spears in butter sauce | ½ of 10-oz. pkg. | 43 | 3.7 |
| (Kounty Kist) cut | ¼ of 18-oz. pkg. | 34 | 3.8 |

| Food and Description | Measure or Quantity | Calories | Carbohydrates (grams) |
|---|---|---|---|
| (Mrs. Paul's) & cheese, batter fried | ⅓ of 7¾-oz. pkg. | 161 | 18.6 |
| (McKenzie or Seabrook Farms): | | | |
| Chopped | ⅓ of 10-oz. pkg. | 30 | 4.1 |
| Spears | ⅓ of 10-oz. pkg. | 31 | 4.5 |
| (Stouffer's) au gratin | ⅓ of 10-oz. pkg. | 113 | 4.6 |

**BROWNIE (See COOKIE)**

**BRUSSELS SPROUTS:**

| | | | |
|---|---|---|---|
| Raw (USDA) | 1 lb. | 188 | 34.6 |
| Boiled (USDA) drained, 1¼"-1½" dia. | 1 cup (7-8 sprouts, 5.5 oz.) | 56 | 9.9 |
| Frozen: | | | |
| (USDA) Boiled, drained | 4-oz. serving | 37 | 7.4 |
| (Birds Eye) | ⅓ of 10-oz. pkg. | 30 | 5.0 |
| (Birds Eye) baby sprouts | ⅓ of 10-oz. pkg. | 42 | 5.8 |
| (Green Giant) | ¼ of 16-oz. pkg. | 47 | 7.3 |
| (Green Giant) in butter sauce | ⅓ of 10-oz. pkg. | 53 | 5.0 |
| (Green Giant) halves in cheese sauce | ⅓ of 10-oz. pkg. | 61 | 6.6 |
| (Kounty Kist) | ⅙ of 20-oz. pkg. | 47 | 7.3 |
| (Stouffer's) au gratin | ⅓ of 10⅞-oz. pkg. | 124 | 10.6 |

**BUCKWHEAT:**

| | | | |
|---|---|---|---|
| Flour (See FLOUR) | | | |
| Groats (Pocono): | | | |
| Brown, whole | 1 oz. | 104 | 19.4 |
| White, whole | 1 oz. | 102 | 20.1 |

**BUC*WHEATS, cereal**

| | | | |
|---|---|---|---|
| (General Mills) | ¾ cup (1 oz.) | 110 | 23.0 |

(USDA): United States Department of Agriculture
(HEW/FAO): Health, Education and Welfare/Food and Agriculture Organization
* Prepared as Package Directs

| Food and Description | Measure or Quantity | Calories | Carbo-hydrates (grams) |
|---|---|---|---|
| **BULGAR** (from hard red winter wheat) (USDA): | | | |
| Dry | | | |
| Canned: | 1 lb. | 1605 | 343.4 |
| Unseasoned | 4-oz. serving | 191 | 39.7 |
| Seasoned | 4-oz. serving | 206 | 37.2 |
| **BULLOCK'S HEART** (See CUSTARD APPLE) | | | |
| **BUN** (See ROLL) | | | |
| ***BURGER KING:*** | | | |
| Apple pie | 3-oz. pie | 240 | 32.0 |
| Cheeseburger | 1 burger | 350 | 30.0 |
| Cheeseburger, double meat | 1 burger | 530 | 32.0 |
| French fries | 1 regular order | 210 | 25.0 |
| Hamburger | 1 burger | 290 | 29.0 |
| Hamburger, double meat | 1 burger | 420 | 30.0 |
| Onion rings | 1 regular order | 270 | 29.0 |
| Shake: | | | |
| Chocolate | 1 shake | 340 | 57.0 |
| Vanilla | 1 shake | 340 | 52.0 |
| Steak sandwich | 1 sandwich | 540 | 58.0 |
| *Whaler* | 1 sandwich | 550 | 44.0 |
| *Whaler* with cheese | 1 sandwich | 650 | 45.0 |
| *Whopper:* | | | |
| Regular | 1 burger | 630 | 50.0 |
| With cheese | 1 burger | 740 | 52.0 |
| Double meat | 1 burger | 850 | 52.0 |
| Double meat with cheese | 1 burger | 950 | 54.0 |
| Junior | 1 burger | 370 | 31.0 |
| Junior with cheese | 1 burger | 420 | 22.0 |
| Junior, double meat | 1 burger | 490 | 33.0 |
| Junior, double meat with cheese | 1 burger | 550 | 34.0 |
| **BURGUNDY WINE** (See also individual regional, vineyard, grape or brand names): | | | |
| (Gallo) 13% alcohol | 3 fl. oz. | 52 | .9 |
| (Gallo) hearty, 14% alcohol | 3 fl. oz. | 48 | 1.2 |
| (Gold Seal) 12% alcohol | 3 fl. oz. | 82 | .4 |

| Food and Description | Measure or Quantity | Calories | Carbohydrates (grams) |
|---|---|---|---|
| (Great Western) 12% alcohol | 3 fl. oz. | 70 | 2.3 |
| (Inglenook) Navalle, 12% alcohol | 3 fl. oz. | 64 | 1.7 |
| (Inglenook) Vintage, 12% alcohol | 3 fl. oz. (2.9 oz.) | 59 | .3 |
| (Italian Swiss Colony) 13% alcohol | 3 fl. oz. | 61 | .9 |
| (Italian Swiss Colony) Gold Medal. 12.3% alcohol | 3 fl. oz. | 63 | .7 |
| (Louis M. Martini) 12½% alcohol | 3 fl. oz. | 90 | .2 |
| (Taylor) 12.5% alcohol | 3 fl. oz. | 75 | 3.3 |

**BURGUNDY WINE, SPARKLING:**

| | | | |
|---|---|---|---|
| (Barton & Guestier) French red. 12% alcohol | 3 fl. oz. | 69 | 2.2 |
| (Chanson) French red | 3 fl. oz. | 72 | 3.6 |
| (Gold Seal) 12% alcohol | 3 fl. oz. | 87 | 2.6 |
| (Great Western) 12% alcohol | 3 fl. oz. | 82 | 5.1 |
| (Lejon) 12% alcohol | 3 fl. oz. | 67 | 2.3 |
| (Taylor) 12.5% alcohol | 3 fl. oz. | 78 | 4.2 |

**BUTTER, salted or unsalted:**

| | | | |
|---|---|---|---|
| (USDA) | ¼ lb. (1 stick, ½ cup) | 812 | .5 |
| (USDA) | 1 T. (⅛ stick, .5 oz.) | 100 | .1 |
| (Breakstone) | 1 T. (.5 oz.) | 100 | <.1 |
| (Breakstone) whipped | 1 T. (9 grams) | 67 | .1 |
| (Meadow Gold) | 1 tsp. | 35 | 0. |

**BUTTER BEAN (See BEAN, LIMA)**

(USDA): United States Department of Agriculture
(HEW/FAO): Health, Education and Welfare/Food and Agriculture Organization
* Prepared as Package Directs

| Food and Description | Measure or Quantity | Calories | Carbo-hydrates (grams) |
|---|---|---|---|
| **BUTTERFISH, raw (USDA):** | | | |
| Gulf: | | | |
| Whole | 1 lb. (weighed whole) | 220 | 0. |
| Meat only | 4 oz. | 108 | 0. |
| Northern: | | | |
| Whole | 1 lb. (weighed whole) | 391 | 0. |
| Meat only | 4 oz. | 192 | 0. |
| **BUTTER FLAVORING,** imitation (Durkee) | 1 tsp. | 3 | |
| **BUTTERMILK (See MILK)** | | | |
| **BUTTERNUT (USDA):** | | | |
| Whole | 1 lb. (weighed in shell) | 399 | 5.3 |
| Shelled | 4 oz. | 713 | 9.5 |
| **BUTTER PECAN ICE CREAM** (Breyer's) | ¼ pt. | 180 | 15.0 |
| **BUTTERSCOTCH MORSELS** (Nestle) | 1 oz. | 150 | 19.0 |
| **BUTTERSCOTCH PUDDING** (See PUDDING, Butterscotch) | | | |

# C

| Food and Description | Measure or Quantity | Calories | Carbo-hydrates (grams) |
|---|---|---|---|
| **CABBAGE:** | | | |
| White (USDA): | | | |
| Raw: | | | |
| Whole | 1 lb. (weighed untrimmed) | 86 | 19.3 |
| Finely shredded or chopped | 1 cup (3.2 oz.) | 22 | 4.9 |
| Coarsely shredded or sliced | 1 cup (2.5 oz.) | 17 | 3.8 |
| Wedge | 3½″ x 4½″ | 24 | 5.4 |

| Food and Description | Measure or Quantity | Calories | Carbo-hydrates (grams) |
|---|---|---|---|
| Boiled: | | | |
| Shredded, in small amount of water, short time, drained | ½ cup (2.6 oz.) | 15 | 3.1 |
| Wedges, in large amount of water, long time, drained | ½ cup (3.2 oz.) | 17 | 3.7 |
| Dehydrated | 1 oz. | 87 | 20.9 |
| Red: | | | |
| Raw (USDA) whole | 1 lb. (weighed untrimmed) | 111 | 24.7 |
| Canned (Comstock) sweet & sour, solids & liq. | ½ cup | 60 | 13.0 |
| Savory, raw (USDA) whole | 1 lb. (weighed untrimmed) | 86 | 16.5 |
| **CABBAGE, CHINESE or CELERY, raw (USDA):** | | | |
| Whole | 1 lb. (weighed untrimmed) | 62 | 13.2 |
| 1″ pieces, leaves with stalk | ½ cup (1.3 oz.) | 5 | 1.1 |
| **CABBAGE, STUFFED,** frozen (Green Giant) with beef in tomato sauce | ½ of 14-oz. pkg. | 209 | 16.5 |
| **CABERNET SAUVIGNON WINE:** | | | |
| (Inglenook) Estate, 12% alcohol | 3 fl. oz. | 58 | .3 |
| (Louis M. Martini) 12½% alcohol | 3 fl. oz. | 90 | .2 |
| *CAFE COMFORT,* 55 proof | 1 fl. oz. | 79 | 8.8 |
| **CAKE:** | | | |
| Plain: | | | |
| Home recipe, with butter & boiled white icing | ⅑ of 9″ square | 401 | 70.5 |

(USDA): United States Department of Agriculture
(HEW/FAO): Health, Education and Welfare/Food and Agriculture Organization
* Prepared as Package Directs

| *Food and Description* | *Measure or Quantity* | *Calories* | *Carbo-hydrates (grams)* |
|---|---|---|---|
| Home recipe, with butter & chocolate icing | 1/9 of 9" square | 453 | 73.1 |
| Angel food, home recipe | 1/12 of 8" cake | 108 | 24.1 |
| Apple walnut, frozen (Sara Lee) | 1/8 of cake (1.6 oz.) | 165 | 21.6 |
| Banana, frozen (Sara Lee) | 1/8 of cake | 175 | 26.8 |
| Banana, frozen (Sara Lee) *Light'n Luscious* | 1/8 of cake | 105 | 19.1 |
| Banana nut layer, frozen (Sara Lee) | 1/8 of cake | 233 | 26.5 |
| Black forest, frozen (Sara Lee) | 1/8 of cake | 203 | 27.9 |
| Caramel: | | | |
| Home recipe, without icing | 1/9 of 9" square | 331 | 46.2 |
| Home recipe, with caramel icing | 1/9 of 9" square | 322 | 50.2 |
| Carrot, frozen (Sara Lee) | 1/8 of cake | 152 | 18.9 |
| Cheesecake, frozen: | | | |
| (Morton): | | | |
| Cherry, *Great Little Desserts* | 6½-oz. cake | 476 | 53.6 |
| Cream, *Great Little Desserts* | 6½-oz. cake | 489 | 46.2 |
| Pineapple, *Great Little Desserts* | 6½-oz. cake | 484 | 55.4 |
| Strawberry, *Great Little Desserts* | 6½-oz. cake | 491 | 57.2 |
| (Rich's) | 1/16 of cake | 212 | 19.6 |
| (Sara Lee): | | | |
| Blueberry cream cheese | 1/6 of cake | 233 | 34.9 |
| Cherry cream cheese | 1/6 of cake | 229 | 30.3 |
| Cream cheese, small | 1/3 of cake | 289 | 28.3 |
| Cream cheese, large | 1/6 of cake | 242 | 23.8 |
| French cream cheese | 1/8 of cake | 274 | 24.9 |
| Strawberry cream cheese | 1/6 of cake | 228 | 30.0 |
| Strawberry French cream cheese | 1/8 of cake | 258 | 27.5 |
| Chocolate: | | | |
| Home recipe, with chocolate icing, 2-layer | 1/12 of 9" cake | 365 | 55.2 |
| Frozen (Sara Lee): | | | |
| Regular | 1/8 of cake | 185 | 24.3 |

| Food and Description | Measure or Quantity | Calories | Carbo-hydrates (grams) |
|---|---|---|---|
| German | ⅛ of cake | 173 | 19.3 |
| Layer, 'n cream | ⅛ of cake | 214 | 23.8 |
| Layer, double chocolate | ⅛ of cake | 217 | 24.0 |
| *Light'n Luscious* | ⅛ of cake | 120 | 19.6 |
| Chocolate bavarian, frozen (Sara Lee) | ⅛ of cake | 285 | 22.6 |
| Coconut, frozen (Sara Lee) | ⅛ of cake | 144 | 17.5 |
| Coffee: | | | |
| (Tastykake) *Koffee Kakes*, creme filled | 1-oz. cake | 124 | DNA |
| Frozen (Sara Lee): | | | |
| Almond | ⅛ of cake | 168 | 19.3 |
| Almond light round | ⅛ of cake | 126 | 13.5 |
| Almond ring | ⅛ of cake | 148 | 16.0 |
| Blueberry light round | ⅛ of cake | 118 | 14.6 |
| Blueberry ring | ⅛ of cake | 134 | 17.6 |
| Butter streusel | ⅛ of 11½-oz. cake | 172 | 16.6 |
| Cinnamon streusel | ⅛ of cake | 159 | 18.1 |
| Danish, apple | 1.3-oz. cake | 120 | 17.4 |
| Danish, cheese | 1.3-oz. cake | 130 | 13.9 |
| Danish, cinnamon raisin | 1.3-oz. cake | 146 | 17.4 |
| Maple crunch ring | ⅛ of cake | 138 | 17.3 |
| Maple light round | ⅛ of cake | 131 | 12.6 |
| Pecan, large | ⅛ of cake | 165 | 18.0 |
| Pecan, small | ¼ of cake | 191 | 20.8 |
| Raspberry light round | ⅛ of cake | 119 | 14.9 |
| Raspberry ring | ⅛ of cake | 143 | 18.2 |
| Crumb: | | | |
| (Hostess) | 1¼-oz. piece | 131 | 21.7 |
| Frozen (Sara Lee): | | | |
| Blueberry | 1 cake | 161 | 23.9 |
| French | 1 cake | 177 | 27.0 |
| Devil's food: | | | |
| Home recipe, without icing | 3″ x 2″ x 1½″ piece | 201 | 28.6 |
| Home recipe, with chocolate icing, 2-layer | 1/16 of 9″ cake | 277 | 41.8 |

(USDA): United States Department of Agriculture
(HEW/FAO): Health, Education and Welfare/Food and Agriculture
Organization
• Prepared as Package Directs

| Food and Description | Measure or Quantity | Calories | Carbohydrates (grams) |
|---|---|---|---|
| Fruit, home recipe: | | | |
| Dark | 1/30 of 8" loaf | 57 | 9.0 |
| Light, made with butter | 1/30 of 8" loaf | 58 | 8.6 |
| Honey (Holland Honey Cake), low sodium: | | | |
| Fruit and raisin | 1/2" slice (.9 oz.) | 80 | 19.0 |
| Orange and premium unsalted | 1/2" slice (.9 oz.) | 70 | 17.0 |
| Orange, frozen (Sara Lee) | 1/8 of cake | 179 | 25.3 |
| Pound: | | | |
| Home recipe, equal weights flour, sugar, butter and eggs | 3½" x 3½" slice (1.1 oz.) | 142 | 14.1 |
| Home recipe, traditional, made with butter | 3½" x 3½" slice (1.1 oz.) | 123 | 16.4 |
| Frozen (Sara Lee): | | | |
| Regular | 1/10 of cake | 126 | 13.7 |
| Banana nut | 1/10 of cake | 117 | 15.1 |
| Chocolate | 1/10 of cake | 122 | 14.5 |
| Chocolate swirl | 1/10 of cake | 130 | 17.9 |
| Family size | 1/15 of cake | 127 | 14.8 |
| Home style | 1/10 of cake | 109 | 12.7 |
| Raisin | 1/10 of cake | 129 | 20.1 |
| Sponge, home recipe | 1/12 of 10" cake | 196 | 35.7 |
| Strawberry 'n cream, frozen (Sara Lee) layer | 1/8 of cake | 217 | 27.4 |
| Strawberry shortcake, frozen (Sara Lee) | 1/8 of cake | 193 | 25.9 |
| Torte, frozen (Sara Lee): | | | |
| Apple 'n cream | 1/8 of cake | 200 | 26.3 |
| Fudge nut | 1/8 of cake | 200 | 21.0 |
| Walnut, frozen (Sara Lee) layer | 1/8 of cake | 217 | 22.3 |
| White: | | | |
| Home recipe, made with butter, without icing, 2-layer | 1/9 of 9" wide, 3" high cake | 353 | 50.8 |
| Home recipe, made with butter, with coconut icing, 2-layer | 1/12 of 9" wide, 3" high cake | 386 | 63.1 |

| Food and Description | Measure or Quantity | Calories | Carbo-hydrates (grams) |
|---|---|---|---|
| Yellow: | | | |
| Home recipe, made with butter, without icing, 2-layer | 1/19 of cake | 351 | 56.3 |
| Frozen (Sara Lee) *Light 'n Luscious* | 1/8 of cake | 122 | 21.7 |
| **CAKE ICING:** | | | |
| Butter pecan (Betty Crocker) ready to spread, *Creamy Deluxe* | 1/12 of can | 170 | 27.0 |
| Caramel, home recipe (USDA) | 4-oz. | 408 | 86.8 |
| Cherry (Betty Crocker) ready to spread, *Creamy Deluxe* | 1/12 of can | 170 | 28.0 |
| Chocolate: | | | |
| Home recipe (USDA) | 4 oz. | 426 | 76.4 |
| (Betty Crocker): | | | |
| Ready to spread, *Creamy Deluxe* | 1/12 of can | 170 | 25.0 |
| Milk, ready to spread, *Creamy Deluxe* | 1/12 of can | 170 | 26.0 |
| Nut, ready to spread, *Creamy Deluxe* | 1/12 of can | 170 | 24.0 |
| Sour cream, ready to spread, *Creamy Deluxe* | 1/12 of can | 170 | 25.0 |
| (Pillsbury): | | | |
| Fudge, ready to spread | 1/12 container | 160 | 24.0 |
| Milk, ready to spread | 1/12 container | 160 | 24.0 |
| Coconut, home recipe (USDA) | 4 oz. | 413 | 84.9 |
| Dark dutch (Betty Crocker) ready to spread, *Creamy Deluxe* | 1/12 of can | 160 | 24.0 |
| Double dutch (Pillsbury) ready to spread | 1/12 of container | 160 | 24.0 |

(USDA): United States Department of Agriculture
(HEW/FAO): Health, Education and Welfare/Food and Agriculture Organization
* Prepared as Package Directs

| Food and Description | Measure or Quantity | Calories | Carbohydrates (grams) |
|---|---|---|---|
| Lemon (Betty Crocker) *Sunkist,* ready to spread, *Creamy Deluxe* | ½₂ of can | 170 | 28.0 |
| Lemon (Pillsbury) ready to spread | ½₂ of container | 160 | 27.0 |
| Orange (Betty Crocker) ready to spread, *Creamy Deluxe* | ½₂ of can | 170 | 28.0 |
| Strawberry (Pillsbury) ready to spread | ½₂ of container | 160 | 27.0 |
| Vanilla: | | | |
| (Betty Crocker) ready to spread | ½₂ of can | 170 | 28.0 |
| (Pillsbury) read to spread | ½₂ of container | 160 | 27.0 |
| White: | | | |
| Home recipe (USDA) boiled | 4 oz. | 358 | 91.1 |
| Home recipe (USDA) uncooked | 4 oz. | 426 | 92.5 |
| (Betty Crocker) ready-to-spread, *Creamy Deluxe* | ½₂ of can | 160 | 27.0 |
| **\*CAKE ICING MIX:** | | | |
| Banana (Betty Crocker) *Chiquita,* creamy | ½₂ of cake's icing | 170 | 30.0 |
| *Butter Brickle* (Betty Crocker) creamy | ½₂ of cake's icing | 170 | 30.0 |
| Butter pecan (Betty Crocker) creamy | ½₂ of cake's icing | 170 | 30.0 |
| Carmel (Pillsbury) *Rich 'n Easy* | ½₂ of cake's icing | 170 | 29.0 |
| Cherry (Betty Crocker) creamy | ½₂ of cake's icing | 170 | 30.0 |
| Chocolate: | | | |
| Fudge: | | | |
| Home recipe (USDA) | 4 oz. | 429 | 76.0 |

| Food and Description | Measure or Quantity | Calories | Carbohydrates (grams) |
|---|---|---|---|
| Home recipe (USDA) prepared with water (Betty Crocker): | 4 oz. | 384 | 84.6 |
| Creamy | 1/12 of cake's icing | 180 | 32.0 |
| Dark | 1/12 of cake's icing | 170 | 30.0 |
| Sour cream | 1/12 of cake's icing | 170 | 30.0 |
| (Pillsbury) *Rich 'n Easy* | 1/12 of cake's icing | 170 | 30.0 |
| Milk: | | | |
| (Betty Crocker) creamy | 1/12 of cake's icing | 170 | 30.0 |
| (Pillsbury) *Rich 'n Easy* | 1/12 of cake's icing | 170 | 29.0 |
| Coconut almond (Pillsbury) | 1/12 of cake's icing | 170 | 17.0 |
| Coconut pecan: | | | |
| (Betty Crocker) creamy | 1/12 of cake's icing | 140 | 18.0 |
| (Pillsbury) | 1/12 of cake's icing | 150 | 20.0 |
| Double Dutch (Pillsbury) *Rich 'n Easy* | 1/12 of cake's icing | 170 | 30.0 |
| Fudge (See Chocolate) Strawberry (Pillsbury) *Rich 'n Easy* | 1/12 of cake's icing | 170 | 29.0 |
| Vanilla (Pillsbury) *Rich 'n Easy* | 1/12 of cake's icing | 170 | 29.0 |
| White: (Betty Crocker): | | | |
| Creamy | 1/12 of cake's icing | 190 | 33.0 |

(USDA): United States Department of Agriculture
(HEW/FAO): Health, Education and Welfare/Food and Agriculture Organization
* Prepared as Package Directs

| Food and Description | Measure or Quantity | Calories | Carbohydrates (grams) |
|---|---|---|---|
| Fluffy | 1/12 of cake's icing | 60 | 16.0 |
| Sour cream, creamy | 1/12 of cake's icing | 170 | 30.0 |
| (Pillsbury) fluffy | 1/12 of cake's icing | 70 | 17.0 |
| **CAKE MIX:** | | | |
| Angel food: | | | |
| *(USDA) | 1/12 of 10" cake | 137 | 31.5 |
| (Betty Crocker): | | | |
| Chocolate | 1/12 pkg. | 140 | 32.0 |
| Confetti | 1/12 pkg. | 150 | 34.0 |
| Lemon custard | 1/12 pkg. | 140 | 32.0 |
| One-step | 1/12 pkg. | 140 | 32.0 |
| Strawberry | 1/12 pkg. | 150 | 34.0 |
| Traditional | 1/12 pkg. | 130 | 30.0 |
| (Duncan Hines) | 1/12 pkg. | 124 | 28.9 |
| *(Pillsbury): | | | |
| Raspberry | 1/12 of cake | 140 | 33.0 |
| White | 1/12 of cake | 140 | 33.0 |
| Applesauce (Betty Crocker) raisin, *Snackin' Cake* | 1/9 pkg. | 200 | 34.0 |
| Banana nut (Duncan Hines) *Moist & Easy Snack Cake* | 1/6 pkg. | 196 | 31.0 |
| Banana walnut (Betty Crocker) *Snackin' Cake* | 1/9 pkg. | 200 | 33.0 |
| *Butter Brickle* (Betty Crocker) layer, *Super Moist* | 1/12 of cake | 260 | 35.0 |
| *Butter pecan* (Betty Crocker) layer, *Super Moist* | 1/12 of cake | 260 | 32.0 |
| Cheesecake: | | | |
| *(Jell-O) | 1/8 of 8" cake | 250 | 33.0 |
| *(Pillsbury) no bake | 1/8 of cake | 260 | 34.0 |
| *(Royal) | 1/8 of cake | 230 | 31.0 |
| *Cherry chip* (Betty Crocker) layer, *Super Moist* | 1/12 of cake | 210 | 34.0 |
| Chocolate: | | | |
| (Betty Crocker): | | | |
| Almond, *Snackin' Cake* | 1/9 of pkg. | 210 | 33.0 |

| *Food and Description* | *Measure or Quantity* | *Calories* | *Carbo-hydrates (grams)* |
|---|---|---|---|
| Chip, *Snackin' Cake* | 1/9 of cake | 220 | 35.0 |
| Fudge chip, *Snackin' Cake* | 1/9 of cake | 220 | 34.0 |
| *Fudge supreme, layer, *Supermoist* | 1/12 of cake | 270 | 32.0 |
| *German chocolate, layer, *Supermoist* | 1/12 of cake | 270 | 34.0 |
| *Milk, layer, *Supermoist* | 1/12 of cake | 260 | 34.0 |
| *Pudding | 1/6 of cake | 230 | 45.0 |
| *(Pillsbury): | | | |
| Dark, *Pillsbury Plus* | 1/12 of cake | 260 | 33.0 |
| German, *Bundt Basic* | 1/12 of cake | 260 | 35.0 |
| German, *Pillsbury Plus* | 1/12 of cake | 260 | 33.0 |
| German, *Streusel Swirl* | 1/12 of cake | 350 | 50.0 |
| Macaroon, *Bundt* ring | 1/12 of cake | 320 | 47.0 |
| *Cinnamon (Pillsbury) Streusel Swirl | 1/12 of cake | 330 | 51.0 |
| Coffee cake: | | | |
| *(Aunt Jemima) | 1/8 of cake | 170 | 29.0 |
| *(Pillsbury): | | | |
| Apple cinnamon | 1/8 of cake | 230 | 40.0 |
| Blueberry | 1/8 of cake | 230 | 39.0 |
| Butter pecan | 1/8 of cake | 310 | 39.0 |
| Cinnamon streusel | 1/8 of cake | 250 | 41.0 |
| Sour cream | 1/8 of cake | 270 | 35.0 |
| Date nut (Betty Crocker) *Snackin' Cake* | 1/9 of pkg. | 210 | 32.0 |
| Devil's food: | | | |
| *(USDA) with chocolate icing | 1/16 of 9" cake | 234 | 40.2 |
| *(Betty Crocker) layer, *Super Moist* | 1/12 of cake | 270 | 34.0 |
| *(Betty Crocker) chocolate with chocolate frosting, *Stir N' Frost* | 1/6 of cake | 280 | 44.0 |
| (Duncan Hines) | 1/12 of pkg. | 190 | 33.0 |

(USDA): United States Department of Agriculture
(HEW/FAO): Health, Education and Welfare/Food and Agriculture Organization
* Prepared as Package Directs

| Food and Description | Measure or Quantity | Calories | Carbohydrates (grams) |
|---|---|---|---|
| (Duncan Hines) pudding recipe | ½₂ of pkg. | 187 | 34.8 |
| *(Pillsbury): | | | |
| Bundt Basic | ½₂ of cake | 260 | 34.0 |
| Pillsbury Plus | ½₂ of cake | 260 | 33.0 |
| Streusel Swirl | ½₂ of cake | 330 | 50.0 |
| *Fudge (Pillsbury): | | | |
| Bundt ring, nut crown | ½₂ of cake | 290 | 41.0 |
| Bundt ring, triple fudge | ½₂ of cake | 300 | 42.0 |
| Pillsbury Plus, marble | ½₂ of cake | 270 | 36.0 |
| Streusel Swirl, marble | ½₂ of cake | 340 | 51.0 |
| Lemon: | | | |
| *(Betty Crocker): | | | |
| Chiffon, & lemon frosting, Stir N' Frost | ⅛ of cake | 190 | 35.0 |
| Layer, Supermoist & lemon frosting, Stir N' Frost | ⅛ of cake | 230 | 38.0 |
| Pudding | ⅛ of cake | 230 | 45.0 |
| (Duncan Hines) pudding recipe | ½₂ of pkg. | 183 | 36.1 |
| *(Pillsbury): | | | |
| Bundt Basic | ½₂ of cake | 260 | 35.0 |
| Bundt ring, blueberry | ½₂ of cake | 280 | 42.0 |
| Pillsbury Plus | ½₂ of cake | 260 | 33.0 |
| Streusel Swirl | ½₂ of cake | 340 | 51.0 |
| Marble: | | | |
| *(Betty Crocker) layer, Supermoist | ½₂ of cake | 290 | 38.0 |
| *(Pillsbury) supreme, Bundt ring | ½₂ of cake | 330 | 51.0 |
| *Orange (Betty Crocker) layer, Supermoist | ½₂ of cake | 270 | 34.0 |
| Pound: | | | |
| *(Betty Crocker) golden | ½₂ of cake | 190 | 27.0 |
| *(Dromedary) | ¾" slice | 210 | 29.0 |
| *(Pillsbury) Bundt ring | ½₂ of cake | 310 | 45.0 |
| *Sour cream chocolate supreme (Betty Crocker) layer, Supermoist | ½₂ of cake | 270 | 32.0 |
| *Sour cream white (Betty Crocker) layer, Supermoist | ½₂ of cake | 200 | 33.0 |

| Food and Description | Measure or Quantity | Calories | Carbo-hydrates (grams) |
|---|---|---|---|
| Spice (Betty Crocker): | | | |
| *Layer, *Supermoist* | 1/12 of cake | 270 | 33.0 |
| Raisin, *Snackin' Cake* | 1/9 of pkg. | 200 | 34.0 |
| *With vanilla frosting, *Stir N' Frost* | 1/8 of cake | 270 | 47.0 |
| *Strawberry (Betty Crocker) layer, *Supermoist* | 1/12 of cake | 270 | 34.0 |
| *Upside down cake (Betty Crocker) pineapple | 1/9 of cake | 270 | 42.0 |
| White: | | | |
| *(USDA) made with egg whites and water with chocolate icing, 2-layer | 1/16 of 9" cake | 249 | 44.6 |
| *(Betty Crocker): | | | |
| Layer, *Supermoist* | 1/12 of cake | 190 | 34.0 |
| With milk chocolate frosting, *Stir N' Frost* | 1/8 of cake | 290 | 46.0 |
| (Duncan Hines) | 1/12 of pkg. | 187 | 34.8 |
| (Duncan Hines) pudding recipe | 1/12 of pkg. | 183 | 36.5 |
| *(Pillsbury) *Pillsbury Plus* | 1/12 of cake | 177 | 36.2 |
| Yellow: | | | |
| *(USDA) made with eggs and water with chocolate icing, 2-layer | 1/16 of 9" cake | 253 | 43.2 |
| *(Betty Crocker): | | | |
| With chocolate frosting, *Stir N' Frost* | 1/8 of cake | 230 | 37.0 |
| Layer, *Supermoist* | 1/12 of cake | 270 | 35.0 |
| (Duncan Hines) | 1/12 of pkg. | 185 | 35.7 |
| (Duncan Hines) pudding recipe | 1/12 of pkg. | 183 | 37.0 |
| *(Pillsbury): | | | |
| *Bundt Basic* | 1/12 of cake | 260 | 36.0 |
| *Pillsbury Plus* | 1/12 of cake | 260 | 33.0 |
| *Pillsbury Plus*, butter recipe | 1/12 of cake | 240 | 33.0 |

(USDA): United States Department of Agriculture
(HEW/FAO): Health, Education and Welfare/Food and Agriculture
         Organization

* Prepared as Package Directs

| Food and Description | Measure or Quantity | Calories | Carbo-hydrates (grams) |
|---|---|---|---|
| *Dietetic (Dia-Mel) all flavors | 1/10 of cake | 100 | 18.0 |
| **CAMPARI,** 45 proof | 1 fl. oz. (1.1 oz.) | 66 | 7.1 |

**CANADIAN WHISKY** (See **DISTILLED LIQUOR**)

**CANDIED FRUIT** (See individual kinds)

**CANDY.** The following values of candies from the U.S. Department of Agriculture are representative of the types sold commercially. These values may be useful when individual brands or sizes are not known:

| | | | |
|---|---|---|---|
| Almond: | | | |
|    Chocolate-coated | 1 cup (6.3 oz.) | 1024 | 71.3 |
|    Chocolate-coated | 1 oz. | 161 | 11.2 |
|    Sugar-coated or Jordan | 1 oz. | 129 | 19.9 |
| Butterscotch | 1 oz. | 113 | 26.9 |
| Candy corn | 1 oz. | 103 | 25.4 |
| Caramel: | | | |
|    Plain | 1 oz. | 113 | 21.7 |
|    Plain with nuts | 1 oz. | 121 | 20.0 |
|    Chocolate | 1 oz. | 113 | 21.7 |
|    Chocolate with nuts | 1 oz. | 121 | 20.0 |
|    Chocolate-flavored roll | 1 oz. | 112 | 23.4 |
| Chocolate: | | | |
|    Bittersweet | 1 oz. | 135 | 13.3 |
|    Milk: | | | |
|       Plain | 1 oz. | 147 | 16.1 |
|       With almonds | 1 oz. | 151 | 14.5 |
|       With peanuts | 1 oz. | 154 | 12.6 |
|    Semisweet | 1 oz. | 144 | 16.2 |
|    Sweet | 1 oz. | 150 | 16.4 |
| Chocolate discs, sugar-coated | 1 oz. | 132 | 20.6 |
| Coconut center, chocolate-coated | 1 oz. | 124 | 20.4 |

| Food and Description | Measure or Quantity | Calories | Carbo-hydrates (grams) |
|---|---|---|---|
| Fondant, plain | 1 oz. | 103 | 25.4 |
| Fondant, chocolate-covered | 1 oz. | 116 | 23.0 |
| Fudge: | | | |
| Chocolate fudge | 1 oz. | 113 | 21.3 |
| Chocolate fudge, chocolate-coated | 1 oz. | 122 | 20.7 |
| Chocolate fudge with nuts | 1 oz. | 121 | 19.6 |
| Chocolate fudge with nuts, chocolate-coated | 1 oz. | 128 | 19.1 |
| Vanilla fudge | 1 oz. | 113 | 21.2 |
| Vanilla fudge with nuts | 1 oz. | 120 | 19.5 |
| With peanuts & caramel, chocolate-coated | 1 oz. | 130 | 16.6 |
| Gum drops | 1 oz. | 98 | 24.8 |
| Hard | 1 oz. | 109 | 27.6 |
| Honeycombed hard candy, with peanut butter, chocolate-covered | 1 oz. | 131 | 20.0 |
| Jelly beans | 1 oz. | 104 | 26.4 |
| Marshmallows | 1 oz. | 90 | 22.8 |
| Mints, uncoated | 1 oz. | 103 | 25.4 |
| Nougat & caramel, chocolate-covered | 1 oz. | 118 | 20.6 |
| Peanut bar | 1 oz. | 146 | 13.4 |
| Peanut brittle | 1 oz. | 119 | 23.0 |
| Peanuts, chocolate-covered | 1 oz. | 159 | 11.1 |
| Raisins, chocolate-covered | 1 oz. | 120 | 20.0 |
| Vanilla creams, chocolate-covered | 1 oz. | 123 | 19.9 |

**CANDY, COMMERCIAL:**

Regular:

| | | | |
|---|---|---|---|
| Almond, chocolate covered (Hershey's) *Golden Almond* | 1 oz. | 163 | 12.4 |
| *Baby Ruth* (Curtiss) | 1.8-oz. bar | 260 | 31.0 |
| *Breath Saver* (Life Savers) | 1 piece (1.6 grams) | 7 | 1.7 |

(USDA): United States Department of Agriculture
(HEW/FAO): Health, Education and Welfare/Food and Agriculture Organization
* Prepared as Package Directs

| Food and Description | Measure or Quantity | Calories | Carbohydrates (grams) |
|---|---|---|---|
| Bridge mix (Nabisco) | 1 piece (2 grams) | 8 | 1.4 |
| *Bun Bars* (Wayne), vanilla or maple | 1 oz. | 133 | 17.0 |
| *Butterfinger* | 1.6-oz. bar | 220 | 28.0 |
| *Butterscotch Skimmers* (Nabisco) | 1 piece (6 grams) | 25 | 5.7 |
| Candy corn (Curtiss) | 1 piece (2 grams) | 4 | 1.0 |
| Caramel: | | | |
| *Caramel Flipper* (Wayne) | 1 oz. | 128 | 19.0 |
| *Caramel Nip* (Pearson) | 1 piece | 29 | 5.6 |
| (Curtiss) chocolate | 1 piece | 29 | 5.0 |
| (Curtiss) vanilla | 1 piece | 29 | 5.0 |
| *Milk Duds* (Holloway) | 1 oz. | 111 | DNA |
| Carob bar (Joan's Natural) | ¾-oz. bar | 116 | 10.5 |
| *Charleston Chew* | 1½-oz. bar | 179 | 32.6 |
| Cherry, chocolate-covered: | | | |
| (Nabisco) dark | 1 piece (.6 oz.) | 67 | 13.0 |
| *Welch's,* dark | 1 piece | 67 | 13.0 |
| *Welch's,* milk | 1 piece | 66 | 13.1 |
| *Cherry-A-Let* (Hoffman) | 1 piece | 215 | DNA |
| *Chewees* (Curtiss) | 1 oz. | 116 | 24.1 |
| Chocolate bar: | | | |
| *Choco-Lite* (Nestlé) | .35-oz. minature | 52 | 6.3 |
| *Choco-Lite* (Nestlé) | 1-oz. bar | 150 | 18.0 |
| *Choco-Lite* (Nestlé) | 5-oz. bar | 750 | 75.0 |
| *Crunch* (Nestlé) | .35-oz. minature | 52 | 6.3 |
| *Crunch* (Nestlé) | 1¹⁄₁₆-oz. bar | 244 | 29.3 |
| *Crunch* (Nestlé) | 2½-oz. bar | 375 | 45.0 |
| *Crunch* (Nestlé) | 5-oz. bar | 750 | 90.0 |
| Milk: | | | |
| (Hershey's) | .35-oz. miniature | 55 | 5.7 |
| (Hershey's) | 1.2-oz. bar | 187 | 19.4 |
| (Hershey's) | 4-oz. bar | 623 | 64.7 |
| (Hershey's) | 8-oz. bar | 1246 | 129.3 |
| (Nestlé) | .35-oz. miniature | 52 | 6.0 |
| (Nestlé) | 1¹⁄₁₆-oz. bar | 244 | 27.6 |
| (Nestlé) | 2½-oz. bar | 375 | 42.5 |
| (Nestlé) | 5-oz. bar | 750 | 85.0 |
| *Special Dark* (Hershey's) | 1.05-oz. bar | 160 | 18.4 |

| Food and Description | Measure or Quantity | Calories | Carbohydrates (grams) |
|---|---|---|---|
| *Special Dark* (Hershey's) | 4-oz. bar | 611 | 70.2 |
| Chocolate bar with almonds: | | | |
| (Hershey's) milk | .35-oz. miniature | 55 | 5.4 |
| (Hershey's) milk | 1.15-oz. bar | 180 | 17.6 |
| (Hershey's) milk | 4-oz. bar | 625 | 61.4 |
| (Nestlé) | 1-oz. serving | 150 | 17.0 |
| *Chocolate Parfait* (Pearson's) | 1 piece | 31 | 5.2 |
| *Choc-Shop* (Hoffman) | 1 piece | 241 | DNA |
| *Chuckles* | 1 oz. | 92 | 23.0 |
| *Chunky* | 1 oz. | 131 | DNA |
| Cinnamon Hearts (Curtiss) | 10 pieces (3.1 grams) | 12 | 3.0 |
| Circus peanuts (Curtiss) | 1 piece (6 grams) | 19 | 6.0 |
| *Clark Bar* | .7-oz. bar | 94 | 14.2 |
| *Clark Bar* | 1.4-oz. bar | 188 | 28.4 |
| *Clark Bar* | 1.65-oz. bar | 222 | 33.4 |
| Cluster (Nabisco): | | | |
| Crispy | 1 piece (.6 oz.) | 65 | 14.0 |
| *Royal Clusters* | 1 piece (.6 oz.) | 78 | 7.5 |
| *Coco-Mello* (Nabisco) | 1 piece (.7 oz.) | 91 | 13.8 |
| Coconut: | | | |
| (Curtiss): | | | |
| Bar | 1 oz. | 124 | 20.0 |
| Squares | 1 piece (.4 oz.) | 53 | 9.0 |
| *Welch's*, squares | 1 piece (.4 oz.) | 64 | 12.3 |
| *Coffee Nips* (Pearson's) | 1 piece | 29 | 5.6 |
| *Coffioca* (Pearson's) | 1 piece (6.5 grams) | 31 | 5.2 |
| *Crispy Bar* (Clark) | 1¼-oz. bar | 187 | 24.2 |
| *Crispy Bar* (Clark) | 1.4-oz. bar | 209 | 27.1 |
| *Crows* (Mason) | 1 piece | 11 | 2.7 |
| *Dots* (Mason) | 1 piece | 11 | 2.7 |
| *Dutch Treat Bar* (Clark) | 1¹⁄₁₆-oz. bar | 160 | 20.3 |
| *Dutch Treat Bar* (Clark) | 1.3-oz. bar | 196 | 24.9 |

(USDA): United States Department of Agriculture
(HEW/FAO): Health, Education and Welfare/Food and Agriculture Organization
* Prepared as Package Directs

| Food and Description | Measure or Quantity | Calories | Carbo-hydrates (grams) |
|---|---|---|---|
| Eggs (Nabisco) *Chuckles* | 1 piece (2 grams) | 10 | 2.3 |
| *Expresso Discs* (Curtiss) | 1 piece (5.5 grams) | 21 | 5.0 |
| *Forever Yours* (M&M/Mars) | 1.37-oz. bar | 171 | 28.6 |
| *Frappe*, Welch's | 1 piece (1.1 oz.) | 132 | 23.5 |
| *Fruit Gems* (Sunkist) | 1 piece | 31 | 8.2 |
| Fruit roll (Sahadi): | | | |
|   Apple, cherry or plain | 1-oz. piece | 90 | 20.0 |
|   Apricot, grape, raspberry | 1-oz. piece | 90 | 21.0 |
|   Strawberry | 1-oz. piece | 100 | 22.0 |
| Fudge: | | | |
|   (Kraft) chocolate fudgies | 1 piece | 35 | 6.2 |
|   (Nabisco): | | | |
|     Bar, *Home Style* | 1 bar (.7 oz.) | 90 | 13.9 |
|     Nut, bar or square | ½-oz. serving | 71 | 10.2 |
|   *Welch's*, bar | 1.1-oz. piece | 144 | 20.5 |
| *Good & Plenty* | 1 oz. | 100 | 24.8 |
| Hard candy: | | | |
|   (Bonomo) | 1 oz. | 112 | DNA |
|   (H-B) | 1 piece | 12 | 2.9 |
|   (Peerless Maid) | 1 piece | 22 | 5.6 |
|   Butterscotch: | | | |
|     (Curtiss) drops | 1 piece | 21 | 5.0 |
|     (Reed's) | 1 piece | 17 | DNA |
|   Cinnamon (Reed's) | 1 piece | 17 | DNA |
|   Cinnamon balls (Curtiss) | 1 piece (7 grams) | 27 | 7.0 |
|   Fruit drops (Curtiss) | 1 piece (5.5 grams) | 21 | 5.0 |
|   Lemon drops (Curtiss) | 1 piece (4 grams) | 15 | 4.8 |
|   *Root Beer Barrels* | 1 piece (6.5 grams) | 25 | 5.0 |
|   *Sherbit* (F&F) | 1 piece | 9 | 2.2 |
|   Sour apples (Curtiss) | 1 piece (7 grams) | 27 | 7.0 |
|   *Stix Bars* (Jolly Rancher) | 1 oz. | 102 | 25.5 |
|   *Stix Kisses* (Jolly Rancher) | 1 piece | 27 | 7.0 |
|   *Stix Pak* (Jolly Rancher) | 1 piece | 18 | 4.0 |

| Food and Description | Measure or Quantity | Calories | Carbohydrates (grams) |
|---|---|---|---|
| Washington cherries (Curtiss) | 1 piece (7 grams) | 27 | 7.0 |
| *Hollywood* | 1½-oz. bar | 183 | 28.9 |
| Jelly (See also individual flavors and brand names in this section): | | | |
| (Curtiss): | | | |
| Bar | 1 piece (.6 oz.) | 59 | 15.0 |
| Beans | 1 piece (3.5 grams) | 12 | 3.0 |
| Feature jellies | 1 piece | 49 | 12.0 |
| Fruit slices | 1 piece (.4 oz.) | 34 | 9.0 |
| Strings | 1 piece (3.5 grams) | 12 | 3.0 |
| (Nabisco) rings, *Chuckles* | 1 piece (.4 oz.) | 37 | 9.0 |
| Jujubes, assorted (Nabisco) *Chuckles* | 1 piece | 13 | 3.3 |
| *Ju Jus* (Curtiss) assorted | 1 piece (2 grams) | 7 | 2.0 |
| *Ju Jus* (Curtiss) coins or raspberries | 1 piece (4.3 grams) | 15 | 4.0 |
| *Kisses* (Hershey) milk chocolate | 1 piece (5 grams) | 27 | 2.8 |
| *Kit Kat* (Hershey's) | 1⅛-oz. bar | 179 | 21.0 |
| *Krackel Bar* (Hershey's) | .35-oz. miniature | 52 | 5.9 |
| *Krackel Bar* (Hershey's) | 1.2-oz. bar | 178 | 20.3 |
| Licorice: | | | |
| *Chuckles* | 1 piece (.4 oz.) | 36 | 9.0 |
| (Curtiss) black | 1 piece (.4 oz.) | 27 | 6.0 |
| *Licorice Nip* (Pearson's) | 1 piece (6.5 grams) | 29 | 5.6 |
| *Life Savers* (Beech-Nut): | | | |
| Drop | 1 piece (3 grams) | 10 | 2.4 |
| Mint | 1 piece (2 grams) | 7 | 1.7 |
| *Log Rolls* (Curtiss) | 1 piece (7 grams) | 29 | 5.0 |
| Lollipop (Life Savers) | 1 piece (.9 oz.) | 99 | 24.0 |
| Lollipop (Life Savers) | 1 piece (.6 oz.) | 69 | 16.7 |

(USDA): United States Department of Agriculture
(HEW/FAO): Health, Education and Welfare/Food and Agriculture Organization
* Prepared as Package Directs

| Food and Description | Measure or Quantity | Calories | Carbo-hydrates (grams) |
|---|---|---|---|
| *Mallo Cup* (Boyer) | ⁹⁄₁₆-oz. cup | 54 | 11.2 |
| *Mallo Cup* (Boyer) | 1.2-oz. cup | 114 | 23.9 |
| Malted milk crunch (Nabisco) | 1 piece (2 grams) | 9 | .9 |
| *Marathon* (M&M/Mars, Snack-master) | .4-oz. bar | 58 | 8.5 |
| *Marathon* (M&M/Mars, Snack-master) | 1.37-oz. bar | 180 | 26.5 |
| *Mars Almond Bar* (M&M/Mars) | 1.25-oz. bar | 172 | 22.1 |
| Marshmallow: | | | |
| (Campfire) | 1 oz. | 111 | 24.9 |
| *Chuckles,* egg | 1 piece | 38 | 9.3 |
| (Curtiss) | 1 piece | 19 | 6.0 |
| (Curtiss) egg | 1 oz. | 133 | 35.0 |
| *Mary Jane* (Miller) | ¼-oz. piece | 18 | 3.3 |
| *Milk Duds* (Clark) | .75-oz. box | 89 | 17.8 |
| *Milk Duds* (Clark) | 1.25-oz. box | 148 | 29.6 |
| *Milk Duds* (Clark) | 1.4-oz. box | 166 | 33.2 |
| *Milky Way* (M&M/Mars) | .8-oz. bar | 103 | 15.5 |
| *Milky Way* (M&M/Mars) | 1.81-oz. bar | 233 | 35.1 |
| *Milky Way* (M&M/Mars) | 2.25-oz. bar | 290 | 43.7 |
| Mint or peppermint: | | | |
| *Jamaica Mint* (Nabisco) | 1 piece | 24 | 5.8 |
| *Liberty Mint* (Nabisco) | 1 piece | 24 | 5.8 |
| *Mighty Mint* (Life Savers) | 1 piece | 2 | .4 |
| *Mint Parfait* (Pearson's) | 1 piece | 31 | 5.2 |
| Pattie, chocolate-covered: | | | |
| *Junior* mint pattie (Nabisco) | 1 piece (.1 oz.) | 10 | 2.0 |
| Peppermint (Nabisco) | 1 piece | 64 | 12.5 |
| Wafer (Nabisco) | 1 piece | 10 | 1.0 |
| *M&M's* (M&M/Mars): | | | |
| Peanut | 1-oz. serving | 144 | 16.3 |
| Peanut | 1.56-oz. serving | 225 | 25.5 |
| Peanut | 1.87-oz. serving | 270 | 30.5 |
| Plain | 1-oz. serving | 140 | 19.3 |
| Plain | 1.5-oz. serving | 210 | 28.9 |
| Plain | 1.87-oz. serving | 262 | 36.1 |
| *Mr. Goodbar* (Hershey's) | .35-oz. miniature | 54 | 4.9 |
| *Mr. Goodbar* (Hershey's) | 1.5-oz. bar | 233 | 20.8 |

| Food and Description | Measure or Quantity | Calories | Carbo-hydrates (grams) |
|---|---|---|---|
| Mr. Goodbar (Hershey's) | 4-oz. bar | 620 | 55.6 |
| Munch, peanut bar (M&M/Mars, Snack-master) | 1½-oz. bar | 230 | 19.0 |
| Nougat centers, Chuckles | 1 piece (4.5 grams) | 17 | 4.2 |
| Nutty Crunch (Nabisco) | 1 piece | 71 | 10.2 |
| $100,000 Bar (Nestlé) | 1⅛-oz. bar | 158 | 21.4 |
| $100,000 Bar (Nestlé) | 1¼-oz. bar | 175 | 23.8 |
| Orange slices: Chuckles | 1 piece (8 grams) | 29 | 7.2 |
| (Curtiss) | 1 piece (.6 oz.) | 55 | 14.4 |
| Peanut, chocolate-covered: (Curtiss) | 1 piece | 5 | 1.0 |
| (Curtiss) French burnt | 1 piece (2 grams) | 4 | 1.0 |
| (Nabisco) | 1 piece (4 grams) | 24 | 1.6 |
| Peanut brittle (Planters): Jumbo Peanut Block Bar, regular size | 1-oz. bar | 119 | 23.0 |
| Jumbo Peanut Block Bar, fun size | 1 piece (.4 oz.) | 61 | 12.0 |
| Pom Poms (Nabisco) | 1 piece (3 grams) | 14 | 2.3 |
| Raisin, chocolate-covered: (Curtiss) | 1 oz. | 120 | 20.0 |
| (Nabisco) | 1 piece (<1 gram) | 4 | .6 |
| Reggie Bar | 2-oz. bar | 290 | 29.0 |
| Rolo (Hershey's) | 1 piece (6 grams) | 30 | 4.1 |
| Rolo (Hershey's) | 1.74-oz. roll | 245 | 33.5 |
| Saf-T-Pops (Curtiss) | 1 piece | 37 | 9.0 |
| Sesame crunch (Sahadi) | ¾-oz. bar | 120 | 9.0 |
| Sesame crunch (Sahadi) | 10 pieces from 6-oz. jar | 90 | 6.5 |

(USDA): United States Department of Agriculture
(HEW/FAO): Health, Education and Welfare/Food and Agriculture Organization
* Prepared as Package Directs

| Food and Description | Measure or Quantity | Calories | Carbo-hydrates (grams) |
|---|---|---|---|
| Snickers (M&M/Mars) | .8-oz. fun size | 103 | 14.5 |
| Snickers (M&M/Mars) | 1.81-oz. bar | 234 | 32.9 |
| Snickers (M&M/Mars) | 2.25-oz. bar | 291 | 41.0 |
| Spearmint leaves (Curtiss) | 1 piece (.7 oz.) | 32 | 8.0 |
| Spearmint leaves Chuckles | 1 piece (8 grams) | 27 | 6.6 |
| Spice flavored sticks & drops, Chuckles | 1 piece | 13 | 3.4 |
| Spice flavored strings, Chuckles | 1 piece | 18 | 4.6 |
| Starburst (M&M/Mars) | 1-oz. serving | 113 | 26.7 |
| Starburst (M&M/Mars) | 1.68-oz. serving | 190 | 44.9 |
| Stars, chocolate (Nabisco) | 1 piece (3 grams) | 15 | 1.6 |
| Sugar Babies (Nabisco) | 1 piece (1.5 grams) | 6 | 1.3 |
| Sugar Daddy (Nabisco): | | | |
| Giant sucker | 1 piece (1 lb.) | 1809 | 398.6 |
| Junior sucker | 1 piece (.4 oz.) | 50 | 11.1 |
| Junior sucker, chocolate flavored | 1 piece (.4 oz.) | 51 | 10.6 |
| Nugget | 1 piece (7 grams) | 27 | 6.0 |
| Sucker, caramel | 1 piece (1.1 oz.) | 121 | 26.4 |
| Sugar Mama (Nabisco) | 1 piece (.8 oz.) | 101 | 18.6 |
| Summit, cookie bar (M&M/Mars) | .4-oz. serving | 70 | 7.0 |
| Summit, cookie bar (M&M/Mars) | 1.37-oz. bar | 217 | 21.9 |
| Taffy, Turkish (Bonomo): | | | |
| Chocolate: | | | |
| Bar | 10-oz. bar | 108 | 24.4 |
| Drop | .2-oz. drop | 18 | 4.1 |
| Flavored: | | | |
| Bar | 1-oz. bar | 109 | 24.7 |
| Drop | .2-oz. drop | 18 | 4.1 |
| Plain: | | | |
| Bar | 1-oz. bar | 110 | 27.6 |
| Drop | .2-oz. drop | 18 | 4.6 |
| 3 Musketeers Bar (M&M/Mars) | .8-oz. fun bar | 98 | 17.4 |
| 3 Musketeers Bar (M&M/Mars) | 2.06-oz. bar | 252 | 44.7 |

| Food and Description | Measure or Quantity | Calories | Carbo-hydrates (grams) |
|---|---|---|---|
| *Tootsie Roll:* | | | |
| Regular: | | | |
| Chocolate | .23-oz. midgee | 26 | 5.3 |
| Chocolate | .63-oz. bar | 73 | 14.3 |
| Chocolate | .75-oz. bar | 86 | 17.2 |
| Chocolate | 1-oz. bar | 115 | 22.9 |
| Chocolate | 1.25-oz. bar | 144 | 28.6 |
| Flavored | .16-oz. sq. | 19 | 3.8 |
| Flavored | .23-oz. midgee | 27 | 5.4 |
| Pop: | | | |
| Caramel | .49-oz. pop | 55 | 12.5 |
| Chocolate | .49-oz. pop | 54 | 12.7 |
| Flavored | .49-oz. pop | 55 | 12.9 |
| Pop drop: | | | |
| Caramel | .17-oz. piece | 19 | 4.2 |
| Chocolate | .17-oz. piece | 18 | 4.3 |
| Flavored | .17-oz. piece | 19 | 4.4 |
| *Twix*, cookie bar (M&M/Mars) | .6-oz. serving | 79 | 10.0 |
| *Twix*, cookie bar (M&M/Mars) | 1.75-oz. serving | 246 | 31.3 |
| *Twizzler:* | | | |
| Cherry | 1 oz. | 100 | 22.0 |
| Chocolate | 1 oz. | 100 | 21.0 |
| Licorice | 1 oz. | 90 | 20.0 |
| Strawberry | 1 oz. | 100 | 22.0 |
| *Whatchamacallit* (Hershey's) | 1.15-oz. bar | 180 | 19.0 |
| *Whirligigs* (Nabisco) | 1 piece (6 grams) | 26 | 5.1 |
| *World Series Bar* | 1 oz. | 128 | 21.3 |
| *Zagnut Bar* (Clark) | .7-oz. bar | 92 | 14.6 |
| *Zagnut Bar* (Clark) | 1⅜-oz. bar | 180 | 28.7 |
| *Zagnut Bar* (Clark) | 1⅝-oz. bar | 213 | 33.9 |
| Dietetic or low calorie: | | | |
| Assorted, *Sug'r Like* | 1 piece | 12 | 3.0 |
| Chocolate bar with almonds (Estee) | ¾-oz. bar | 110 | 9.6 |
| Chocolate bar with | | | |

(USDA): United States Department of Agriculture
(HEW/FAO): Health, Education and Welfare/Food and Agriculture Organization
* Prepared as Package Directs

| Food and Description | Measure or Quantity | Calories | Carbo-hydrates (grams) |
|---|---|---|---|
| almonds (Estee) | 1 section of 3-oz. bar | 37 | 3.2 |
| Chocolate bar, bitter-sweet (Estee) | 1 section of 3-oz. bar | 38 | 3.3 |
| Chocolate bar, bitter-sweet (Estee) | 3-oz. bar | 460 | 40.0 |
| Chocolate bar, crunch (Estee) | ⅝-oz. bar | 90 | 8.8 |
| Chocolate bar, crunch (Estee) | 1 section of 2½-oz. bar | 30 | 2.9 |
| Chocolate bar, fruit-nut (Estee) | 1 section of 3-oz. bar | 37 | 3.2 |
| Chocolate bar, milk (Estee) | ¾-oz. bar | 110 | 10.2 |
| Chocolate bar, milk (Estee) | 1 section of 3-oz. bar | 37 | 3.4 |
| *Estee-Ets*, peanut | 1.4-gram piece | 7 | .7 |
| *Estee-Ets*, plain | 1.2-gram piece | 6 | .6 |
| Gum drops (Estee) fruit and licorice | 1 piece (2 grams) | 3 | .8 |
| Hard Candy: | | | |
| (Estee) all flavors | 1 piece (3 grams) | 12 | 3.0 |
| *Sug'r Like* | 1 piece | 12 | 3.0 |
| Mint: | | | |
| (Estee) all flavors | 1 piece | 4 | 1.0 |
| *Sug'r Like*, all flavors | 1 piece | 6 | DNA |
| (Sunkist): | | | |
| Mini mint | 1 piece (.23 grams) | <1 | .2 |
| Roll mint | 1 piece (.89 grams) | 4 | .9 |
| Peanut butter cup (Estee) | 1 cup (8 grams) | 45 | 2.9 |
| Raisin, chocolate-covered (Estee) | 1 piece (1 gram) | 6 | .7 |
| TV mix (Estee) | 1 piece (2 grams) | 9 | .7 |
| **CANE SYRUP (USDA)** | 1 T. (.7 oz.) | 55 | 14.0 |

| Food and Description | Measure or Quantity | Calories | Carbohydrates (grams) |
|---|---|---|---|
| **CANNELONI FLORENTINE,** frozen (Weight Watchers) casserole | 13-oz. meal | 448 | 45.8 |
| **CANTALOUPE,** fresh (USDA): | | | |
| Whole, medium | 1 lb. (weighed with skin & cavity contents) | 68 | 17.0 |
| Cubed | ½ cup (2.9 oz.) | 24 | 6.1 |
| **CAPICOLA or CAPACOLA SAUSAGE** (USDA) | 1 oz. | 141 | 0. |
| *CAP'N CRUNCH,* cereal (Quaker): | | | |
| Crunchberries | ¾ cup (1 oz.) | 120 | 22.9 |
| Peanut butter | ¾ cup (1 oz.) | 127 | 20.9 |
| Regular | ¾ cup (1 oz.) | 121 | 22.9 |
| **CAPPELLA WINE** (Italian Swiss Colony) 13% alcohol | 3 fl. oz. (2.9 oz.) | 64 | 1.5 |
| **CARAMBOLA,** raw (USDA): | | | |
| Whole | 1 lb. (weighed whole) | 149 | 34.1 |
| Flesh only | 4 oz. | 40 | 9.1 |
| **CARAWAY SEED** (French's) | 1 tsp. | 8 | .8 |
| **CARDAMOM SEED** (French's) | 1 tsp. | 6 | 1.3 |
| **CARISSA or NATAL PLUM,** raw (USDA): | | | |
| Whole | 1 lb. (weighed whole) | 273 | 62.4 |
| Flesh only | 4 oz. | 79 | 18.1 |

(USDA): United States Department of Agriculture
(HEW/FAO): Health, Education and Welfare/Food and Agriculture Organization
* Prepared as Package Directs

| Food and Description | Measure or Quantity | Calories | Carbohydrates (grams) |
|---|---|---|---|
| *CARNATION INSTANT BREAKFAST: | | | |
| Chocolate | 8 fl. oz. | 280 | 35.0 |
| Chocolate Malt | 8 fl. oz. | 280 | 35.0 |
| Coffee | 8 fl. oz. | 280 | 35.0 |
| Eggnog | 8 fl. oz. | 280 | 34.0 |
| Strawberry | 8 fl. oz. | 280 | 34.0 |
| Vanilla | 8 fl. oz. | 280 | 33.0 |
| | | | |
| CARP, raw (USDA): | | | |
| Whole | 1 lb. (weighed whole) | 156 | 0. |
| Meat only | 4 oz. | 130 | 0. |
| | | | |
| CARROT: | | | |
| Raw (USDA): | | | |
| Whole | 1 lb. (weighed with full tops) | 112 | 26.0 |
| Partially trimmed | 1 lb. (weighed without tops, with skins) | 156 | 36.1 |
| Trimmed | 5½″ x 1″ carrot (1.8 oz.) | 21 | 4.8 |
| Trimmed | 25 thin strips (1.8 oz.) | 21 | 4.8 |
| Chunks | ½ cup (2.4 oz.) | 29 | 6.7 |
| Diced | ½ cup (2.5 oz.) | 30 | 7.0 |
| Grated or shredded | ½ cup (1.9 oz.) | 23 | 5.3 |
| Slices | ½ cup (2.2 oz.) | 27 | 6.2 |
| Strips | ½ cup (2 oz.) | 24 | 5.6 |
| Boiled (USDA): | | | |
| Chunks, drained | ½ cup (2.9 oz.) | 25 | 5.8 |
| Diced, drained | ½ cup (2.5 oz.) | 24 | 5.2 |
| Slices, drained | ½ cup (2.7 oz.) | 24 | 5.4 |
| Canned, regular pack: | | | |
| (USDA) diced, solids & liq. | ½ cup (4.3 oz.) | 34 | 8.0 |
| (Del Monte): | | | |
| Diced, drained | ½ cup | 35 | 6.8 |
| Sliced, drained | ½ cup | 37 | 7.4 |
| (Libby's): | | | |
| Diced, solids & liq. | ½ cup | 19 | 4.1 |
| Sliced, solids & liq. | ½ cup | 24 | 5.3 |

| Food and Description | Measure or Quantity | Calories | Carbo-hydrates (grams) |
|---|---|---|---|
| (Stokely-Van Camp): | | | |
| Diced, solids & liq. | ½ cup (4.3 oz.) | 30 | 6.0 |
| Sliced, solids & liq. | ½ cup (4.3 oz.) | 25 | 5.0 |
| Canned, dietetic pack: | | | |
| (USDA) low sodium, solids & liq. | 4 oz. | 25 | 5.7 |
| (USDA) low sodium, drained | ½ cup (2.8 oz.) | 20 | 4.5 |
| (Blue Boy) sliced, solids & liq. | ½ of 8¼-oz. can | 35 | 6.4 |
| (Featherweight) sliced, solids & liq. | ½ cup | 25 | 6.0 |
| (Tillie Lewis) *Tasti Diet* | ½ cup (4.3 oz.) | 30 | 6.2 |
| Dehydrated (USDA) | 1 oz. | 97 | 23.0 |
| Frozen: | | | |
| (Birds Eye) with brown sugar glaze | ⅓ of 10-oz. pkg. | 81 | 14.6 |
| (Green Giant) nuggets in butter sauce | ⅓ of 10-oz. pkg. | 46 | 6.0 |
| (McKenzie) whole | 3.3-oz. serving | 39 | 8.1 |
| (Seabrook Farms) whole | 3.3-oz. serving | 39 | 8.1 |
| **CASABA MELON, fresh (USDA):** | | | |
| Whole | 1 lb. (weighed whole) | 61 | 14.7 |
| Flesh | 4 oz. | 31 | 7.4 |
| **CASHEW NUT:** | | | |
| (USDA) | 1 oz. | 159 | 8.3 |
| (USDA) | ½ cup (2.5 oz.) | 393 | 20.5 |
| (USDA) | 5 large or 8 med. | 60 | 3.1 |
| (A&P) dry roasted | 1 oz. | 173 | 8.5 |
| (Frito-Lay's) | 1 oz. | 168 | 8.7 |
| (Planters): | | | |
| Dry roasted | 1 oz. | 160 | 9.0 |
| Oil roasted | 1 oz. | 170 | 8.0 |
| Unsalted | 1 oz. | 160 | 9.0 |

(USDA): United States Department of Agriculture
(HEW/FAO): Health, Education and Welfare/Food and Agriculture Organization
* Prepared as Package Directs

| Food and Description | Measure or Quantity | Calories | Carbo-hydrates (grams) |
|---|---|---|---|
| **CATAWBA WINE:** | | | |
| (Great Western) pink, 12% alcohol | 3 fl. oz. | 111 | 11.3 |
| (Taylor) 12% alcohol | 3 fl. oz. | 96 | 9.0 |
| **CATFISH, freshwater, raw** fillet (USDA) | 4 oz. | 117 | 0. |
| **CATSUP:** | | | |
| Regular pack: | | | |
| (USDA) | 1 T. (.6 oz.) | 19 | 4.6 |
| (USDA) | ½ cup (.5 oz.) | 149 | 35.8 |
| (Blue Boy) | 1 T. | 23 | 5.5 |
| (Del Monte) | 1 T. (.7 oz.) | 24 | 5.5 |
| (Smucker's) | 1 T. (.6 oz.) | 21 | 4.5 |
| Dietetic pack: | | | |
| (Dia-Mel) | 1 T. (14 grams) | 7 | 1.5 |
| (Featherweight) | 1 T. (.6 oz.) | 7 | 1.2 |
| (Tillie Lewis) *Tasti Diet* | 1 T. | 20 | 6.0 |
| **CAULIFLOWER:** | | | |
| Raw (USDA): | | | |
| Whole | 1 lb. (weighed untrimmed) | 48 | 9.2 |
| Flowerbuds | ½ cup (1.8 oz.) | 14 | 2.6 |
| Slices | ½ cup (1.5 oz.) | 11 | 2.2 |
| Boiled (USDA) flowerbuds, drained | ½ cup (2.2 oz.) | 14 | 2.5 |
| Frozen: | | | |
| (USDA) unthawed | 10-oz. pkg. | 62 | 12.2 |
| (USDA) boiled, drained | ½ cup (3.4 oz.) | 16 | 3.0 |
| (Birds Eye) 5-minute | ⅓ of 10-oz. pkg. | 25 | 3.7 |
| (Green Giant): | | | |
| In cheese sauce, *Bake 'n Serve* | ⅛ of 10-oz. pkg. | 80 | 5.6 |
| In cheese sauce, boil-in-bag | ⅛ of 10-oz. pkg. | 49 | 5.2 |
| Cuts | ¼ of 18-oz. pkg. | 28 | 4.1 |
| (Kounty Kist) cut | ⅕ of 20-oz. pkg. | 25 | 3.6 |
| (McKenzie) | 3.3-oz. serving | 27 | 4.5 |
| (Mrs. Paul's) & cheese, batter fried | ⅓ of 8-oz. pkg. | 136 | 15.4 |
| (Seabrook Farms) | 3.3-oz. serving | 27 | 4.5 |
| (Stouffer's) au gratin | ⅓ of 10-oz. pkg. | 104 | 7.2 |

| Food and Description | Measure or Quantity | Calories | Carbohydrates (grams) |
|---|---|---|---|
| **CAVIAR, STURGEON** (USDA): | | | |
| Pressed | 1 oz. | 90 | 1.4 |
| Whole eggs | 1 T. (.6 oz.) | 42 | .5 |
| **CELERIAC ROOT,** raw (USDA): | | | |
| Whole | 1 lb. (weighed unpared) | 156 | 39.2 |
| Pared | 4 oz. | 45 | 9.6 |
| **CELERY,** all varieties (USDA): Fresh: | | | |
| Whole | 1 lb. (weighed untrimmed) | 58 | 13.3 |
| 1 large outer stalk | 8" x 1½" at root end (1.4 oz.) | 7 | 1.6 |
| Diced, chopped or cut in chunks | ½ cup (2.1 oz.) | 10 | 2.3 |
| Slices | ½ cup (1.9 oz.) | 9 | 2.1 |
| Boiled, drained solids: | | | |
| Diced or cut in chunks | ½ cup (2.7 oz.) | 10 | 2.4 |
| Slices | ½ cup (3 oz.) | 12 | 2.6 |
| **CELERY CABBAGE (See CABBAGE, CHINESE)** | | | |
| **CELERY SALT** (French's) | 1 tsp. (4.6 grams) | 2 | <.5 |
| **CELERY SEED** (French's) | 1 tsp. (2.4 grams) | 11 | 1.1 |
| **CELERY SOUP,** cream of: (USDA) condensed | 8 oz. (by wt.) | 163 | 16.8 |
| *(USDA) prepared with equal volume water | 1 cup (8.5 oz.) | 86 | 8.9 |
| *(USDA) prepared with equal volume milk | 1 cup (8.4 oz.) | 169 | 15.2 |

(USDA): United States Department of Agriculture
(HEW/FAO): Health, Education and Welfare/Food and Agriculture Organization

* Prepared as Package Directs

| Food and Description | Measure or Quantity | Calories | Carbohydrates (grams) |
|---|---|---|---|
| *(Ann Page) condensed cream of | 1 cup | 63 | 8.3 |
| *(Campbell) condensed | 10-oz. serving | 120 | 10.0 |
| **CEREAL** (See kind of cereal, such as **CORN FLAKES**, or brand name such as **KIX**) | | | |
| **CERTS** (Warner-Lambert) | 1 piece | 6 | 1.5 |
| **CERVELAT** (USDA): | | | |
| Dry | 1 oz. | 128 | .5 |
| Soft | 1 oz. | 87 | .5 |
| **CHABLIS WINE:** | | | |
| (Great Western) 12% alcohol | 3 fl. oz. | 70 | 2.3 |
| (Great Western) Diamond, 12% alcohol | 3 fl. oz. | 69 | 2.0 |
| (Inglenook) Navalle, 12% alcohol | 3 fl. oz. | 59 | .5 |
| (Inglenook) Vintage, 12% alcohol | 3 fl. oz. | 56 | .2 |
| (Italian Swiss Colony) Gold, 12% alcohol | 3 fl. oz. | 66 | 3.0 |
| (Italian Swiss Colony) Pink, 12% alcohol | 3 fl. oz. | 67 | 3.2 |
| (Taylor) 12% alcohol | 3 fl. oz. | 72 | 1.3 |
| **CHAMPAGNE:** | | | |
| (Great Western) 12% alcohol | 3 fl. oz. | 71 | 2.4 |
| (Great Western) brut, 12% alcohol | 3 fl. oz. | 74 | 3.4 |
| (Great Western) extra dry, 12.5% alcohol | 3 fl. oz. | 78 | 4.3 |
| (Great Western) pink, 12% alcohol | 3 fl. oz. | 81 | 4.9 |
| (Lejon) 12% alcohol | 3 fl. oz. | 66 | 2.5 |
| (Taylor) brut, 12.5% alcohol | 3 fl. oz. | 75 | 3.3 |
| (Taylor) dry, 12.5% alcohol | 3 fl. oz. | 78 | 3.9 |
| (Taylor) pink, 12.5% alcohol | 3 fl. oz. | 81 | 4.8 |

| Food and Description | Measure or Quantity | Calories | Carbo-hydrates (grams) |
|---|---|---|---|
| **CHARD**, Swiss (USDA): | | | |
| Raw, whole | 1 lb. (weighed untrimmed) | 104 | 19.2 |
| Raw, trimmed | 4 oz. | 28 | 5.2 |
| Boiled, drained solids | ½ cup (3.4 oz.) | 17 | 3.2 |
| **CHARLOTTE RUSSE**, with ladyfingers, whipped cream filling, home recipe (USDA) | 4 oz. | 324 | 38.0 |
| *CHATEAU LA GARDE CLARET*, French red Bordeaux (Chanson) 11½% alcohol | 3 fl. oz. | 60 | 6.3 |
| **CHATEAUNEUF-DU-PAPE**, French red Rhone: (Barton & Guestier) | | | |
| 13.5% alcohol | 3 fl. oz. | 70 | .5 |
| (Chanson) 13% alcohol | 3 fl. oz. | 90 | 6.3 |
| *CHATEAU OLIVIER BLANC*, French white Graves (Chanson) 11½% alcohol | 3 fl. oz. | 60 | 6.3 |
| *CHATEAU OLIVIER ROUGE*, French red Graves (Chanson) 11½% alcohol | 3 fl. oz. | 60 | 6.3 |
| *CHATEAU PONTET CANET* (Cruse) 12% alcohol | 3 fl. oz. | 72 | |
| *CHATEAU RAUSAN SEGLA*, French red Bordeaux (Chanson) 11½% alcohol | 3 fl. oz. | 60 | 6.3 |
| *CHATEAU ST. GERMAIN*, French red Bordeaux (Chanson) 11½% alcohol | 3 fl. oz. | 60 | 6.3 |

(USDA): United States Department of Agriculture
(HEW/FAO): Health, Education and Welfare/Food and Agriculture
　　　　　　　Organization
* Prepared as Package Directs

| Food and Description | Measure or Quantity | Calories | Carbo-hydrates (grams) |
|---|---|---|---|
| **CHATEAU VOIGNY**, French Sauternes (Chanson) 13% alcohol | 3 fl. oz. | 96 | 7.5 |
| **CHAYOTE**, raw (USDA): | | | |
| Whole | 1 lb. (weighed unpared) | 108 | 27.4 |
| Pared | 4 oz. | 32 | 8.1 |
| *CHEDDAR CHEESE SOUP (Campbell) condensed | 11-oz. serving | 180 | 14.0 |
| *CHEERI-AID mix (Ann Page) all flavors | 1 serving (.8 oz.) | 85 | 21.1 |
| **CHEERIOS** (General Mills): | | | |
| Honey-nut | 1¾ cups (1 oz.) | 110 | 23.0 |
| Regular | 1¼ cups (1 oz.) | 110 | 20.0 |
| **CHEESE:** | | | |
| American or cheddar: | | | |
| (USDA) natural | 1″ cube (.6 oz.) | 68 | .4 |
| (USDA) process | 1″ cube (.6 oz.) | 65 | .3 |
| (USDA) natural, diced | 1 cup (4.6 oz.) | 521 | 2.8 |
| (USDA) natural, grated or shredded | 1 cup (3.9 oz.) | 442 | 2.3 |
| (USDA) natural, grated or shredded | 1 T. (.7 grams) | 27 | .1 |
| (Borden): | | | |
| Process | ¾-oz. slice | 83 | 1.2 |
| Process, *Miracle Melt* | 1 T. (.5 oz.) | 38 | .6 |
| Process, *Vera Sharp* | 1 oz. | 104 | .6 |
| (Fisher) process | 1 oz. | 110 | 1.0 |
| (Frigo) | 1 oz. | 110 | 1.0 |
| (Kraft) natural | 1 oz. | 113 | .6 |
| (Kraft) *Cracker Barrel* | 1 oz. | 116 | .5 |
| *Laughing Cow*, baby | 1 oz. | 110 | Tr. |
| Bleu or blue: | | | |
| (USDA) natural | 1″ cube (.6 oz.) | 64 | .3 |
| (Borden) *Blufort* | 1 oz. | 105 | .5 |
| (Frigo) | 1 oz. | 100 | 1.0 |
| (Kraft) cold pack or natural | 1 oz. | 99 | .5 |
| *Laughing Cow* | ⅛-oz. cube | 12 | .1 |

| Food and Description | Measure or Quantity | Calories | Carbohydrates (grams) |
|---|---|---|---|
| *Laughing Cow* | ¾-oz. wedge | 55 | .5 |
| *Laughing Cow* | 1 oz. | 74 | .7 |
| Bonbel, *Laughing Cow* | ¾-oz. serving | 71 | Tr. |
| Bonbel, *Laughing Cow* | 1 oz. | 94 | Tr. |
| Bonbino, *Laughing Cow* | 1 oz. | 104 | Tr. |
| Brick: | | | |
| (USDA) natural | 1 oz. | 105 | .5 |
| (Kraft) natural | 1 oz. | 103 | .3 |
| (Kraft) process, slices | 1 oz. | 101 | .4 |
| Camembert, domestic: | | | |
| (USDA) natural | 1 oz. | 85 | .5 |
| (Borden) | 1 oz. | 86 | .5 |
| (Kraft) natural | 1 oz. | 85 | .5 |
| Cheddar (See American) | | | |
| Colby: | | | |
| (Fisher) | 1 oz. | 110 | 1.0 |
| (Frigo) | 1 oz. | 110 | 1.0 |
| (Kraft) natural | 1 oz. | 111 | .6 |
| Cottage: | | | |
| Creamed, unflavored: | | | |
| (USDA) large or small curd | 1 T. (.5 oz.) | 16 | .4 |
| (Borden) | 8-oz. container | 240 | 6.6 |
| (Bordon) *Lite Line,* low fat | 1 cup | 189 | 7.0 |
| (Breakstone) California | 8-oz. container | 216 | 4.8 |
| (Dean) | 8-oz. container | 218 | 5.4 |
| (Foremost Blue Moon) | 1 oz. | 27 | .9 |
| (Foremost Blue Moon) | 8 oz. | 216 | 7.2 |
| (Frigo) | 1 oz. | 30 | .8 |
| (Frigo) | 8 oz. | 240 | 6.4 |
| (Kraft) | 1 oz. | 27 | .9 |
| (Meadow Gold) | 1 cup | 240 | 8.0 |
| (Sealtest) | ½ cup | 120 | 4.0 |
| (Sealtest) extra creamy, 6% fat | ½ cup | 120 | 3.0 |
| (Sealtest) *Light n' Lively* | 1 cup (7.9 oz.) | 155 | 5.6 |

(USDA): United States Department of Agriculture
(HEW/FAO): Health, Education and Welfare/Food and Agriculture Organization
* Prepared as Package Directs

| Food and Description | Measure or Quantity | Calories | Carbo-hydrates (grams) |
|---|---|---|---|
| (Viva) low fat, 2% fat | 1 cup | 200 | 8.0 |
| Creamed, flavored: | | | |
| (Breakstone) chive | 8-oz. container | 216 | 4.8 |
| (Sealtest): | | | |
| Chive-pepper | 1 cup (8 oz.) | 206 | 5.4 |
| Garden Salad | ½ cup | 120 | 5.0 |
| Garden Salad, Light 'n Lively | ½ cup | 90 | 5.0 |
| Peach-pineapple | 1 cup (7.9 oz.) | 228 | 17.9 |
| Peach-pineapple, Light n' Lively | ½ cup | 100 | 11.0 |
| Pineapple | 1 cup (7.9 oz.) | 222 | 16.1 |
| Uncreamed: | | | |
| (Breakstone) potstyle | 1 T. (.6 oz.) | 12 | .3 |
| (Dean) | 8-oz. container | 191 | 3.6 |
| (Frigo) part skim milk | 1 oz. | 24 | .8 |
| (Kraft) | 1 oz. | 26 | .6 |
| (Sealtest) | 1 cup (7.9 oz.) | 179 | 1.6 |
| Cream cheese: | | | |
| Plain, unwhipped: | | | |
| (Borden) | 1 oz. | 101 | 1.5 |
| (Frigo) | 1 oz. | 100 | 1.0 |
| (Kraft) Hostess | 1 oz. | 98 | .6 |
| (Kraft) Philadelphia Brand | 1 oz. | 104 | .9 |
| (Kraft) imitation, Philadelphia Brand | 1 oz. | 52 | 1.9 |
| Plain, whipped: | | | |
| (Breakstone) Temp-Tee | 1 oz. | 98 | .6 |
| (Kraft) Philadelphia Brand | 1 oz. | 99 | 1.1 |
| Flavored, unwhipped: | | | |
| (Borden) chive | 1 oz. | 96 | .6 |
| (Borden) pimiento | 1 oz. | 76 | .6 |
| Flavored, whipped (Kraft) Philadelphia Brand: | | | |
| With bacon & horse-radish | 1 oz. | 93 | 1.3 |
| With chive | 1 oz. | 93 | 1.3 |
| With onion | 1 oz. | 86 | 1.9 |

| Food and Description | Measure or Quantity | Calories | Carbo-hydrates (grams) |
|---|---|---|---|
| With pimiento | 1 oz. | 86 | 1.8 |
| With smoked salmon | 1 oz. | 92 | 1.1 |
| Edam: | | | |
| (House of Gold) | 1 oz. | 100 | 1.0 |
| (Kraft) natural | 1 oz. | 104 | .3 |
| *Laughing Cow* | 1 oz. | 100 | Tr. |
| Farmer: | | | |
| (Dean) | 1 oz. | 46 | .7 |
| *Dutch Garden Brand* | 1 oz. | 100 | 1.0 |
| *Wispride* | 1 oz. | 100 | 1.0 |
| Fontina (Kraft) natural | 1 oz. | 113 | .6 |
| Frankenmuth, natural (Kraft) | 1 oz. | 113 | .7 |
| Gjetost (Kraft) natural | 1 oz. | 134 | 13.0 |
| Gorgonzola (Foremost Blue Moon) | 1 oz. | 110 | Tr. |
| Gouda: | | | |
| (Borden) Dutch Maid | 1 oz. | 86 | .5 |
| (Frigo) | 1 oz. | 100 | 1.0 |
| (Kraft) natural | 1 oz. | 107 | .5 |
| *Laughing Cow*, natural | 1 oz. | 110 | Tr. |
| Gruyère: | | | |
| (Borden) process | 1 oz. | 93 | 1.4 |
| (Kraft) natural | 1 oz. | 110 | .6 |
| *Swiss Knight* | 1 oz. | 101 | <1.0 |
| Jack-dry, natural (Kraft) | 1 oz. | 101 | .4 |
| Jack-fresh, natural (Kraft) | 1 oz. | 95 | .4 |
| *Kisses*, milk (Borden) | 1 piece (6 grams) | 18 | .5 |
| Lagerkase, natural (Kraft) | 1 oz. | 107 | .3 |
| Leyden, natural (Kraft) | 1 oz. | 80 | .7 |
| Liederkranz (Borden) | 1 oz. | 86 | .4 |
| Limburger, natural (USDA) | 1 oz. | 98 | .6 |
| *Lite-Line* (Borden) | ¾-oz. slice | 38 | .8 |
| Monterey Jack: | | | |
| (Borden) | 1 oz. | 103 | .6 |
| (Frigo) | 1 oz. | 100 | 1.0 |
| (Kraft) natural | 1 oz. | 102 | .4 |

(USDA): United States Department of Agriculture
(HEW/FAO): Health, Education and Welfare/Food and Agriculture Organization
* Prepared as Package Directs

| Food and Description | Measure or Quantity | Calories | Carbo-hydrates (grams) |
|---|---|---|---|
| Mozzarella: | | | |
| (Borden) | 1 oz. | 96 | .8 |
| (Fisher) part skim milk, low moisture | 1 oz. | 90 | 1.0 |
| (Frigo) part skim milk | 1 oz. | 80 | 1.0 |
| (Kraft) shredded | 1 oz. | 79 | .3 |
| Muenster: | | | |
| (Borden) natural | 1 oz. | 85 | .7 |
| (Kraft) natural | 1 oz. | 100 | .3 |
| (Kraft) process, slices | 1 oz. | 102 | .6 |
| Neufchâtel: | | | |
| (Borden) process | 1 oz. | 73 | 6.5 |
| (Kraft) loaf | 1 oz. | 69 | .7 |
| Nuworld (Kraft) natural | 1 oz. | 103 | .7 |
| Old English, process | | | |
| (Kraft) loaf or slices | 1 oz. | 105 | .5 |
| Parmesan: | | | |
| Natural: | | | |
| (USDA) | 1 oz. | 111 | .8 |
| (Frigo) | 1 oz. | 110 | 1.0 |
| (Kraft) | 1 oz. | 107 | .8 |
| Grated: | | | |
| (USDA) loosely packed | 1 cup (3.7 oz.) | 494 | 3.6 |
| (USDA) loosely packed | 1 T. (7 grams) | 31 | .2 |
| (Borden) | 1 oz. | 143 | 8.8 |
| (Frigo) | 1 T. (6 grams) | 23 | Tr. |
| (Kraft) | 1 oz. | 127 | 1.0 |
| Shredded (Kraft) | 1 oz. | 114 | .9 |
| Parmesan & Romano, grated: | | | |
| (Borden) | 1 oz. | 135 | 2.2 |
| (Kraft) | 1 oz. | 130 | 1.0 |
| Pimiento American, process: | | | |
| (USDA) | 1 oz. | 105 | .5 |
| (Borden) | 1 oz. | 104 | .5 |
| (Kraft) loaf or slices | 1 oz. | 103 | .4 |
| Pizza: | | | |
| (Borden) | 1 oz. | 85 | .8 |
| (Kraft) | 1 oz. | 73 | .3 |
| Port du Salut (Kraft) natural | 1 oz. | 100 | .3 |
| Primost (Kraft) natural | 1 oz. | 134 | 13.0 |

| Food and Description | Measure or Quantity | Calories | Carbo- hydrates (grams) |
|---|---|---|---|
| Provolone: | | | |
| (Borden) | 1 oz. | 93 | 1.0 |
| (Frigo) | 1 oz. | 90 | 1.0 |
| (Kraft) natural | 1 oz. | 99 | .5 |
| *Laughing Cow* | ⅙-oz. cube | 12 | .1 |
| *Laughing Cow* | ¾-oz. wedge | 55 | .5 |
| *Laughing Cow* | 1 oz. | 74 | .7 |
| Ricotta: | | | |
| (Frigo) part skim milk, moist | 1 oz. | 43 | .9 |
| (Kraft) natural | 1 oz. | 47 | 1.3 |
| Romano: | | | |
| Natural: | | | |
| (Borden) Italian pecorino | 1 oz. | 114 | .8 |
| (Frigo) | 1 oz. | 100 | 1.0 |
| Grated: | | | |
| (Frigo) | 1 T. (6 grams) | 21 | Tr. |
| (Kraft) | 1 oz. | 134 | 1.0 |
| Shredded (Kraft) | 1 oz. | 121 | .9 |
| Romano & parmesan, plain (Kraft) | 1 oz. | 133 | 1.0 |
| Roquefort, natural: | | | |
| (USDA) | 1 oz. | 104 | .6 |
| (Kraft) | 1 oz. | 105 | .5 |
| Sage (Kraft) natural | 1 oz. | 113 | .6 |
| Sap Sago (Kraft) natural | 1 oz. | 76 | 1.7 |
| Sardo Romano, natural (Kraft) | 1 oz. | 109 | .8 |
| Scamorze: | | | |
| (Frigo) | 1 oz. | 79 | .3 |
| (Kraft) natural | 1 oz. | 100 | .3 |
| Stirred curd (Frigo) | 1 oz. | 110 | 1.0 |
| Swiss: | | | |
| Domestic: | | | |
| (Borden) process | ¾-oz. slice | 72 | .8 |
| (Fisher) | 1 oz. | 100 | 0. |
| (Frigo) natural | 1 oz. | 100 | 0. |

(USDA): United States Department of Agriculture
(HEW/FAO): Health, Education and Welfare/Food and Agriculture
       Organization
* Prepared as Package Directs

| Food and Description | Measure or Quantity | Calories | Carbohydrates (grams) |
|---|---|---|---|
| (Kraft): | | | |
| Natural | 1 oz. | 105 | .5 |
| Process, loaf | 1 oz. | 93 | .5 |
| Process, slices | 1 oz. | 95 | .6 |
| (Sealtest) natural | 1 oz. | 105 | .5 |
| Imported (Borden): | | | |
| Natural, Finland | 1 oz. | 104 | .5 |
| Natural, Switzerland | 1 oz. | 104 | .5 |
| Washed curd (Frigo) | 1 oz. | 110 | 1.0 |
| **CHEESE CAKE and CHEESE CAKE MIX** (See **CAKE** and **CAKE MIX**, Cheesecake) | | | |
| **CHEESE DIP** (See **DIP**) | | | |
| **CHEESE FONDUE:** | | | |
| Home recipe (USDA) | 4 oz. | 301 | 11.3 |
| (Borden) | 6-oz. serving | 354 | 15.3 |
| *Swiss Knight* | 4-oz. serving | 240 | 4.0 |
| **CHEESE FOOD, process:** | | | |
| American or cheddar: | | | |
| (Borden) | 1" x 1" x 1" piece (.8 oz.) | 71 | 2.5 |
| (Borden) grated | 1 oz. | 129 | 8.4 |
| (Fisher) | 1 oz. | 90 | 2.0 |
| (Kraft) slices | 1 oz. | 94 | 2.4 |
| (Pauly) | .8-oz. slice | 74 | 1.6 |
| (Weight Watchers) colored or white | 1-oz. slice | 50 | 1.0 |
| *Wispride*, cheddar: | | | |
| Plain | 1 oz. | 100 | 7.0 |
| & blue cheese | 1 oz. | 100 | 2.0 |
| & port wine | 1 oz. | 90 | 2.0 |
| & Swiss | 1 oz. | 100 | 7.0 |
| *Cheez'n Bacon* (Kraft) | ¾-oz. slice | 76 | .8 |
| *Cheez'n Crackers*, process (Kraft) | 1.1-oz. piece | 127 | 9.3 |
| *Cheez-ola* (Fisher) process | 1 oz. | 90 | .5 |
| Colby (Pauly) low sodium | 1 oz. | 115 | .6 |

| Food and Description | Measure or Quantity | Calories | Carbo- hydrates (grams) |
|---|---|---|---|
| Links (Kraft) *Handi- Snack:* | | | |
| Bacon | 1 oz. | 93 | 2.2 |
| Jalapeno | 1 oz. | 92 | 2.2 |
| *Nippy* | 1 oz. | 92 | 2.2 |
| *Smokelle* | 1 oz. | 93 | 2.2 |
| *Swiss* | 1 oz. | 90 | 1.4 |
| Loaf, *Count-Down* (Fisher) | 1 oz. | 40 | 3.0 |
| *Mun-chee* (Pauly) chunk | 1 oz. | 100 | 2.0 |
| Pimiento (Borden) | 1 oz. | 91 | 2.0 |
| Pimiento (Pauly) | .8-oz. slice | 73 | .8 |
| *Pizzalone* loaf (Kraft) | 1 oz. | 90 | .5 |
| Salami (Kraft) slices | 1 oz. | 93 | 2.6 |
| Sharp (Pauly) | 1-oz. slice | 100 | .8 |
| Super blend loaf (Kraft) | 1 oz. | 92 | 1.6 |
| Swiss (Borden) cold pack | .7-oz. slice | 62 | 1.1 |
| Swiss, slices (Kraft) | 1 oz. | 92 | 2.3 |
| Swiss (Pauly) | .8-oz. slice | 74 | 1.6 |
| Swiss, *Wispride* | 1 oz. | 100 | 6.0 |
| **CHEESE PUFF**, frozen (Durkee) | 1 piece (.5 oz.) | 59 | 3.0 |
| **CHEESE SPREAD:** | | | |
| American, process: | | | |
| (USDA) | 1 T. (.5 oz.) | 50 | 1.1 |
| (Borden) | .7-oz. | 57 | 1.5 |
| (Fisher) | 1 oz. | 80 | 2.0 |
| (Kraft) | 1 oz. | 78 | 1.9 |
| (Nabisco) *Snack Mate* | 1 tsp. (6 grams) | 16 | .4 |
| Bacon (Borden) cheese & bacon | 1 oz. | 72 | 1.8 |
| Bacon (Kraft) process | 1 oz. | 64 | .5 |
| Cheddar (Nabisco) *Snack Mate* | 1 tsp. (6 grams) | 16 | .4 |
| Cheddar (Nabisco) *Snack Mate*, sharp | 1 tsp. | 16 | .4 |
| Cheddar, *Wispride*, sharp | 1 oz. | 80 | 2.0 |

(USDA): United States Department of Agriculture
(HEW/FAO): Health, Education and Welfare/Food and Agriculture Organization
* Prepared as Package Directs

| Food and Description | Measure or Quantity | Calories | Carbo-hydrates (grams) |
|---|---|---|---|
| Cheese & bacon (Nabisco) *Snack Mate* | 1 tsp. (6 grams) | 16 | .4 |
| *Cheez Whiz* (Kraft) process | 1 oz. | 78 | 1.8 |
| Chive & green onion (Nabisco) *Snack Mate* | 1 tsp. (6 grams) | 16 | .4 |
| *Count Down* (Fisher) | 1 oz. | 30 | 3.0 |
| Garlic (Borden) process | 1 oz. | 72 | 1.8 |
| Imitation (Fisher) *Chef's Delight* | 1 oz. | 40 | 3.0 |
| Imitation (Kraft) *Calorie-Wise* | 1 oz. | 48 | 3.6 |
| Jalapeno (Kraft) *Cheez Whiz* | 1 oz. | 76 | 1.9 |
| Limburger (Kraft) | 1 oz. | 69 | .4 |
| Neufchatel: | | | |
| (Borden) olive & pimiento | 1 T. (.5 oz.) | 36 | 1.8 |
| (Borden) pineapple | 1 T. (.5 oz.) | 36 | 1.8 |
| (Kraft) Jalapeno peppers | 1 oz. | 68 | 2.2 |
| (Kraft) olive & pimiento | 1 oz. | 68 | 1.9 |
| (Kraft) pimiento | 1 oz. | 68 | 2.3 |
| (Kraft) pineapple | 1 oz. | 70 | 3.0 |
| (Kraft) relish | 1 oz. | 72 | 3.2 |
| Pimiento: | | | |
| (Borden) *Country Store* | 1 T. (.5 oz.) | 36 | 1.7 |
| (Kraft) *Cheez Whiz* | 1 oz. | 76 | 1.7 |
| (Kraft) *Squeez-a-Snak* | 1 oz. | 86 | .6 |
| (Nabisco) *Snack Mate* | 1 tsp. (.5 oz.) | 16 | .4 |
| (Pauly) | ¾-oz. serving | 66 | .9 |
| Sharp (Kraft) *Old English* | 1 oz. | 85 | .5 |
| Sharp (Pauly) | .8-oz. serving | 77 | .9 |
| Swiss (Pauly) process | .8-oz. serving | 76 | 1.2 |
| *Velveeta* (Kraft) process | 1 oz. | 85 | 2.5 |
| **CHEESE STRAW:** | | | |
| (USDA) | 5" x ⅜" x ⅜" piece (6 grams) | 27 | 2.1 |
| (Durkee) frozen | 1 piece | 29 | 1.0 |
| **CHELOIS WINE** (Great Western) | | | |
| 12% alcohol | 3 fl. oz. | 70 | 2.2 |

| Food and Description | Measure or Quantity | Calories | Carbo-hydrates (grams) |
|---|---|---|---|
| **CHERRY:** | | | |
| Sour: | | | |
| Fresh (USDA): | | | |
| Whole | 1 lb. (weighed with stems) | 213 | 52.5 |
| Whole | 1 lb. (weighed without stems) | 242 | 59.7 |
| Pitted | ½ cup (2.7 oz.) | 45 | 11.1 |
| Canned, syrup pack, pitted (USDA): | | | |
| Light syrup | 4 oz. (with liq.) | 84 | 21.2 |
| Heavy syrup | ½ cup (with liq.) | 116 | 29.5 |
| Extra heavy syrup | 4 oz. (with liq.) | 127 | 32.4 |
| Canned, water pack, pitted, solids & liq. (USDA) | ½ cup (4.3 oz.) | 52 | 13.1 |
| Frozen, pitted (USDA): | | | |
| Sweetened | ½ cup (4.6 oz.) | 146 | 36.1 |
| Unsweetened | 4 oz. | 62 | 15.2 |
| Sweet: | | | |
| Fresh (USDA): | | | |
| Whole | 1 lb. (weighed with stems) | 286 | 71.0 |
| Whole, with stems | ½ cup (2.3 oz.) | 41 | 10.2 |
| Pitted | ½ cup (2.9 oz.) | 57 | 14.3 |
| Canned, syrup pack: (USDA) | | | |
| Light syrup, pitted | 4 oz. (with liq.) | 74 | 18.7 |
| Heavy syrup, pitted | ½ cup (with liq., 4.2 oz.) | 96 | 24.2 |
| Extra heavy syrup, pitted | 4 oz. (with liq.) | 113 | 29.0 |
| (Del Monte): | | | |
| Dark, solids & liq. | ½ cup (4.3 oz.) | 106 | 25.2 |
| Royal Anne, solids & liq. | ½ cup (4.3 oz.) | 111 | 26.8 |
| (Stokely-Van Camp) pitted, solids & liq. | ½ cup (4.2 oz.) | 50 | 11.0 |

(USDA): United States Department of Agriculture
(HEW/FAO): Health, Education and Welfare/Food and Agriculture
        Organization
* Prepared as Package Directs

| Food and Description | Measure or Quantity | Calories | Carbo-hydrates (grams) |
|---|---|---|---|
| Canned, dietetic or water pack: | | | |
| (Diet Delight) solids & liq. | ½ cup | 73 | 16.9 |
| (Featherweight) dark, solids & liq. | ½ cup | 57 | 13.0 |
| (Featherweight) light, solids & liq. | ½ cup | 48 | 11.0 |
| (Tillie Lewis) *Tasti Diet*, light | ½ cup | 58 | 14.5 |
| **CHERRY BRANDY (See BRANDY, FLAVORED)** | | | |
| **CHERRY, CANDIED** (USDA) | 1 oz. | 96 | 24.6 |
| **CHERRY DRINK:** Canned: | | | |
| (Ann Page) | 1 cup (8.7 oz.) | 124 | 30.9 |
| (Hi-C) | 6 fl. oz. (6.3 oz.) | 93 | 23.0 |
| (Lincoln) cherry berry | 6 fl. oz. | 95 | 23.9 |
| *Mix (Hi-C) | 6 fl. oz. | 76 | 19.0 |
| **CHERRY EXTRACT (Ehlers)** imitation | 1 tsp. | 16 | |
| **CHERRY HEERING,** Danish liqueur, 49 proof | 1 fl. oz. | 80 | 10.0 |
| **CHERRY JELLY:** Sweetened (Smucker's) | 1 T. (.7 oz.) | 53 | 13.5 |
| Dietetic or low calorie: (Featherweight) | 1 T. | 18 | 4.0 |
| (Featherweight) artificially sweetened | 1 T. | 10 | 2.0 |
| (Slenderella) | 1 T. | 24 | 6.0 |
| **CHERRY KIJAFA,** Danish wine, 17.5% alcohol | 3 fl. oz. | 148 | 15.3 |
| **CHERRY LIQUEUR:** | | | |
| (DeKuyper) 50 proof | 1 fl. oz. | 75 | 8.5 |
| (Hiram Walker) 60 proof | 1 fl. oz. | 82 | 8.2 |
| (Leroux) 60 proof | 1 fl. oz. | 80 | 7.6 |

| Food and Description | Measure or Quantity | Calories | Carbohydrates (grams) |
|---|---|---|---|
| **CHERRY, MARASCHINO** (USDA) | 1 oz. (with liq.) | 33 | 8.3 |
| **CHERRY PIE** (See PIE, Cherry) | | | |
| **CHERRY PIE FILLING** (See PIE FILLING, Cherry) | | | |
| **CHERRY PRESERVE or JAM:** | | | |
| Sweetened (Smucker's) | 1 T. (.7 oz.) | 53 | 13.5 |
| Dietetic or low calorie: | | | |
| (Dia-Mel) | 1 T. | 6 | 0. |
| (Louis Sherry) | 1 T. (.5 oz.) | 6 | 1.5 |
| (Smucker's) | 1 T. | 24 | 6.0 |
| **CHERRY TURNOVER,** refrigerated (Pillsbury) | 1 turnover | 180 | 25.0 |
| **CHERVIL,** raw (USDA): | 1 oz. | 16 | 3.3 |
| **CHESTNUT** (USDA): | | | |
| Fresh, in shell | 1 lb. (weighed in shell) | 713 | 154.7 |
| Fresh, shelled | 4 oz. | 220 | 47.7 |
| Dried, in shell | 1 lb. (weighed in shell) | 1402 | 292.4 |
| Dried, shelled | 4 oz. | 428 | 89.1 |
| **CHESTNUT FLOUR** (See FLOUR, Chestnut) | | | |
| **CHEWING GUM:** | | | |
| Sweetened: | | | |
| (USDA) | 1 piece (3 grams) | 10 | 2.9 |
| *Bazooka*, bubble, 1¢ size | 1 piece | 18 | 4.5 |
| *Bazooka*, bubble, 5¢ size | 1 piece | 85 | 21.2 |
| *Beechies* | 1 tablet (2 grams) | 6 | 1.6 |
| *Beech-Nut* | 1 stick | 10 | 2.3 |

(USDA): United States Department of Agriculture
(HEW/FAO): Health, Education and Welfare/Food and Agriculture Organization
* Prepared as Package Directs

| Food and Description | Measure or Quantity | Calories | Carbohydrates (grams) |
|---|---|---|---|
| *Beemans* | 1 stick | 9 | 2.3 |
| *Big Red* | 1 stick | 10 | 2.3 |
| *Black Jack* | 1 stick | 9 | 2.3 |
| *Chiclets* | 1 piece | 6 | 1.1 |
| *Cinnamint* | 1 stick | 10 | 2.3 |
| *Clove* | 1 stick | 9 | 2.3 |
| *Dentyne* | 1 piece | 4 | 1.2 |
| *Doublemint* (Wrigley's) | 1 stick (3 grams) | 10 | 2.3 |
| *Freedent* (Wrigley's) | 1 stick | 10 | 2.3 |
| *Fruit Punch* | 1 stick | 10 | 2.3 |
| *Juicy Fruit* (Wrigley's) | 1 stick | 10 | 2.3 |
| *Orbit*, all flavors | 1 stick | 8 | Tr. |
| Peppermint (Clark) | 1 piece | 6 | 2.3 |
| Sour (Warner-Lambert) | 1 stick | 10 | DNA |
| Sour lemon (Clark) | 1 stick | 10 | 2.3 |
| *Spearmint* (Wrigley's) | 1 stick (3 grams) | 10 | 2.3 |
| *Teaberry* | 1 stick | 10 | 2.3 |
| Unsweetened or dietetic: | | | |
| *Bazooka*, bubble | 1 piece | 16 | Tr. |
| *Care*Free* (Beech-Nut) | 1 stick (3 grams) | 7 | Tr. |
| (Clark) all flavors | 1 stick | 7 | 1.7 |
| (Estee) all flavors | 1 section | 3 | 1.0 |
| *Sug'r Like*, all flavors | 1 piece | 4 | .6 |
| **CHIANTI WINE** (Italian Swiss Colony) 13% alcohol | 3 fl. oz. | 64 | 1.5 |
| **CHICKEN** (See also CHICKEN, CANNED): (USDA): | | | |
| Broiler, cooked, meat only | 4 oz. | 154 | 0. |
| Capon, raw, with bone | 1 lb. (weighed ready-to-cook) | 937 | 0. |
| Fryer: | | | |
| Raw: | | | |
| Ready-to-cook | 1 lb. (weighed ready-to-cook) | 382 | 0. |
| Breast | 1 lb. (weighed with bone) | 394 | 0. |
| Leg or drumstick | 1 lb. (weighed with bone) | 313 | 0. |
| Thigh | 1 lb. (weighed with bone) | 435 | 0. |

| Food and Description | Measure or Quantity | Calories | Carbohydrates (grams) |
|---|---|---|---|
| Fried. A 2½-lb. chicken (Weighed before cooking with bone) will give you: | | | |
| Back | 1 back (2.2 oz.) | 139 | 2.7 |
| Breast | ½ breast (3⅓ oz.) | 154 | 1.1 |
| Leg or drumstick | 1 leg (2 oz.) | 87 | .4 |
| Neck | 1 neck (2.1 oz.) | 121 | 1.9 |
| Rib | 1 rib (.7 oz.) | 42 | .8 |
| Thigh | 1 thigh (2¼ oz.) | 118 | 1.2 |
| Wing | 1 wing (1¾ oz.) | 78 | .8 |
| Fried skin | 1 oz. | 119 | 2.6 |
| Hen and cock: | | | |
| Raw | 1 lb. (weighed ready-to-cook) | 987 | 0. |
| Stewed: | | | |
| Meat only | 4 oz. | 236 | 0. |
| Chopped | ½ cup (2.5 oz.) | 150 | 0. |
| Diced | ½ cup (2.4 oz.) | 139 | 0. |
| Ground | ½ cup (2 oz.) | 116 | 0. |
| Roaster: | | | |
| Raw: | 1 lb. (weighed ready-to-cook) | 791 | 0. |
| Roasted: | | | |
| Dark meat without skin | 4 oz. | 209 | 0. |
| Light meat without skin | 4 oz. | 206 | 0. |
| **CHICKEN A LA KING:** | | | |
| Home recipe (USDA) | 1 cup (8.6 oz.) | 468 | 12.3 |
| Canned (Swanson) | ½ of 10½-oz. can | 180 | 9.0 |
| Frozen: | | | |
| (Banquet) cooking bag | 5-oz. bag | 138 | 10.4 |
| (Green Giant) *Toast Topper* | 5-oz. serving | 162 | 7.7 |
| (Stouffer's) with rice | 9½-oz. pkg. | 331 | 37.8 |

(USDA): United States Department of Agriculture
(HEW/FAO): Health, Education and Welfare/Food and Agriculture Organization
* Prepared as Package Directs

| Food and Description | Measure or Quantity | Calories | Carbohydrates (grams) |
|---|---|---|---|
| **CHICKEN & BISCUITS,** frozen (Green Giant) | ½ of 14-oz. pkg. | 196 | 18.7 |
| **CHICKEN BOUILLON/ BROTH,** cube or powder (See also **CHICKEN SOUP**): | | | |
| (Herb-Ox) | 1 cube (4 grams) | 6 | .6 |
| (Herb-Ox) | 1 packet (5 grams) | 12 | 2.0 |
| (Maggi) | 1 cube | 7 | 1.0 |
| *MBT* | 1 packet (.2 oz.) | 12 | 2.0 |
| **CHICKEN, CANNED, BONED:** | | | |
| (USDA) | ½ cup (3 oz.) | 168 | 0. |
| (Swanson): | | | |
| Chunk | ½ of 5-oz. can | 110 | 0. |
| Chunk, mixin' style | ½ of 5-oz. can | 120 | 0. |
| Chunk, thigh | ½ of 5-oz. can | 120 | 0. |
| Chunk, white | ½ of 5-oz. can | 110 | 0. |
| **CHICKEN, CREAMED,** frozen (Stouffer's) | 6½-oz. pkg. | 300 | 5.9 |
| **CHICKEN CROQUETTE DINNER,** frozen (Morton) | 10¼-oz. dinner | 413 | 46.5 |
| **CHICKEN DINNER or ENTREE:** | | | |
| Canned (Swanson) & dumplings | 7½-oz. serving | 230 | 18.0 |
| Frozen: | | | |
| (Banquet): | | | |
| & dumplings, buffet | 2-lb. bag | 1209 | 128.2 |
| & dumplings, dinner | 12-oz. dinner | 282 | 36.4 |
| Fried | 11-oz. dinner | 530 | 48.4 |
| *Man Pleaser* | 17-oz. dinner | 1026 | 89.2 |
| & noodles | 12-oz. dinner | 374 | 50.7 |
| (Morton): | | | |
| Boneless | 10-oz. dinner | 222 | 22.8 |
| Boneless, King Size | 17-oz. dinner | 546 | 53.1 |

| Food and Description | Measure or Quantity | Calories | Carbo-hydrates (grams) |
|---|---|---|---|
| & dumplings | 11-oz. dinner | 272 | 31.2 |
| Fried | 11-oz. dinner | 450 | 50.0 |
| Fried, *Country Table* | 15-oz. dinner | 692 | 94.8 |
| Fried, *Country Table* | 12-oz. entree | 583 | 27.3 |
| Fried, King Size | 17-oz. dinner | 859 | 91.8 |
| & noodles | 10.3-oz. dinner | 252 | 41.0 |
| (Stouffer's): | | | |
| Cacciatore with spaghetti | 11½-oz. entree | 313 | 28.8 |
| Divan | 8½-oz. pkg. | 336 | 14.0 |
| (Swanson): | | | |
| Boneless, *Hungry Man* | 19-oz. dinner | 730 | 74.0 |
| Fried | 11½-oz. dinner | 570 | 28.0 |
| Fried, barbecue-flavored | 11¼-oz. dinner | 530 | 47.0 |
| Fried, crisp | 10¾-oz. dinner | 650 | 51.0 |
| Fried, *Hungry Man* | 15¾-oz. dinner | 910 | 78.0 |
| Fried, *Hungry Man*, barbecue flavored | 16½-oz. dinner | 760 | 72.0 |
| Fried, 3-course | 15-oz. dinner | 630 | 64.0 |
| & noodle | 10¼-oz. dinner | 390 | 53.0 |
| In white wine sauce | 8¼-oz. entree | 370 | 10.0 |
| (Weight Watchers): | | | |
| Creole style | 13-oz. meal | 256 | 11.8 |
| Divan | 9-oz. meal | 251 | 7.9 |
| Liver, chicken, & onions | 10½-oz. meal | 210 | 11.0 |
| Oriental style | 15-oz. meal | 346 | 32.0 |
| Parmigiana, 2-compartment | 9-oz. meal | 184 | 8.9 |
| With stuffing | 16-oz. meal | 411 | 36.8 |
| White meat | 9-oz. meal | 291 | 13.0 |

**CHICKEN & DUMPLINGS**
(See CHICKEN DINNER
or ENTREE)

(USDA): United States Department of Agriculture
(HEW/FAO): Health, Education and Welfare/Food and Agriculture
Organization
* Prepared as Package Directs

| Food and Description | Measure or Quantity | Calories | Carbo-hydrates (grams) |
|---|---|---|---|
| **CHICKEN FRICASSEE,** home recipe (USDA) | 1 cup (8.5 oz.) | 386 | 7.7 |
| **CHICKEN, FRIED,** frozen: | | | |
| (Banquet) | 2-lb. pkg. | 2591 | 117.3 |
| (Morton) | ⅛ of 32-oz. pkg. | 298 | 32.7 |
| (Morton) breast portion | ¼ of 22-oz. pkg. | 367 | 31.2 |
| (Swanson): | | | |
| Assorted pieces | 3.2-oz. serving | 260 | 10.0 |
| Assorted pieces | 16-oz. pkg. | 1250 | 40.0 |
| Assorted pieces | 32-oz. pkg. | 2600 | 100.0 |
| Breast portion | 3.2-oz. serving | 250 | 8.0 |
| Breast portion | 22-oz. pkg. | 1719 | 55.0 |
| Nibbler (wings) | 3.2-oz. serving | 290 | 12.0 |
| Nibbler (wings) | 28-oz. pkg. | 2538 | 105.0 |
| Take-out style | 4-oz. serving | 260 | 8.0 |
| Thighs & drumsticks | 3.2-oz. serving | 260 | 7.0 |
| Thighs & drumsticks | 28-oz. pkg. | 2275 | 55.7 |
| **CHICKEN GIZZARD** (USDA): | | | |
| Raw | 2 oz. | 64 | .4 |
| Simmered | 2 oz. | 84 | .4 |
| **CHICKEN LIVER** (See LIVER) | | | |
| **CHICKEN LIVER PUFF,** frozen (Durkee) | 1 piece | 48 | 3.0 |
| **CHICKEN & NOODLES:** | | | |
| Home recipe (USDA) | 1 cup (8.5 oz.) | 367 | 25.7 |
| Frozen: | | | |
| (Banquet) buffet | 2-lb. pkg. | 764 | 79.1 |
| (Green Giant) | 9-oz. pkg. | 245 | 21.5 |
| (Stouffer's): | | | |
| Escalloped | ½ of 11½-oz. pkg. | 252 | 15.8 |
| Paprikash, with egg noodles | 10½-oz. pkg. | 381 | 31.9 |
| **CHICKEN, PACKAGED** (Eckrich) sliced | 1-oz. slice | 47 | 1.3 |

| Food and Description | Measure or Quantity | Calories | Carbo-hydrates (grams) |
|---|---|---|---|
| **CHICKEN PIE:** | | | |
| Home recipe, baked (USDA) | 8-oz. pie (4¼" dia.) | 533 | 41.5 |
| Frozen: | | | |
| (Banquet) | 8-oz. pie | 427 | 39.0 |
| (Morton) | 8-oz. pie | 345 | 29.5 |
| (Stouffer's) | 10-oz. pie | 493 | 39.8 |
| (Swanson) | 8-oz. pie | 450 | 44.0 |
| (Swanson) *Hungry Man* | 16-oz. pie | 780 | 66.0 |
| (Van de Kamp's) | 7½-oz. pie | 520 | 47.0 |
| **CHICKEN PUFF,** frozen (Durkee) | 1 piece | 49 | 3.0 |
| **CHICKEN SALAD** (Carnation) *Spreadable* | 1½-oz. serving | 94 | 2.6 |
| **CHICKEN SOUP:** | | | |
| Canned, regular pack: | | | |
| (USDA): | | | |
| Consomme, condensed | 8 oz. (by wt.) | 41 | 3.4 |
| *Consomme, prepared with equal volume water | 1 cup (8.5 oz.) | 22 | 1.9 |
| Cream of, condensed | 8 oz. (by wt.) | 179 | 15.2 |
| *Cream of, prepared with equal volume milk | 1 cup (8.6 oz.) | 179 | 14.5 |
| *Cream of, prepared with equal volume water | 1 cup (8.5 oz.) | 94 | 7.9 |
| Gumbo, condensed | 8 oz. (by wt.) | 104 | 13.8 |
| *Gumbo, prepared with equal volume water | 1 cup (8.5 oz.) | 55 | 7.4 |
| & noodle, condensed | 8 oz. (by wt.) | 120 | 15.0 |
| *& noodle, prepared with equal volume water | 1 cup (8.5 oz.) | 65 | 8.2 |

(USDA): United States Department of Agriculture
(HEW/FAO): Health, Education and Welfare/Food and Agriculture Organization
* Prepared as Package Directs

| Food and Description | Measure or Quantity | Calories | Carbo-hydrates (grams) |
|---|---|---|---|
| & rice, condensed | 8 oz. (by wt.) | 89 | 10.7 |
| *& rice, prepared with equal volume water | 1 cup (8.5 oz.) | 48 | 5.8 |
| & vegetable, condensed | 8 oz. (by wt.) | 141 | 17.5 |
| *& vegetable, prepared with equal volume water | 1 cup (8.6 oz.) | 76 | 9.6 |
| (Ann Page): | | | |
| *Cream of | 1 cup | 104 | 9.3 |
| *& noodle | 1 cup | 66 | 8.7 |
| *& *Noodle-O's* style | 1 cup | 47 | 1.4 |
| *& rice | 1 cup | 47 | 1.4 |
| *& stars | 1 cup | 56 | 7.4 |
| *& vegetable | 1 cup | 75 | 8.6 |
| (Campbell): | | | |
| *Alphabet, condensed | 10-oz. serving | 110 | 14.0 |
| *Broth, condensed | 10-oz. serving | 50 | 4.0 |
| *Broth & noodle, condensed | 10-oz. serving | 80 | 10.0 |
| *Broth & rice, condensed | 10-oz. serving | 60 | 8.0 |
| *Broth & vegetables, condensed | 10-oz. serving | 30 | 4.0 |
| *Chunky* | 10¾-oz. can | 230 | 22.0 |
| *Chunky* | 19-oz. can | 400 | 40.0 |
| *Cream of, condensed | 10-oz. serving | 140 | 10.0 |
| *& dumplings, condensed | 10-oz. serving | 100 | 11.0 |
| *Gumbo, condensed | 10-oz. serving | 70 | 10.0 |
| *& noodle, condensed | 10-oz. serving | 90 | 11.0 |
| *& noodle, *Soup For One*, semicondensed | 7¾-oz. can | 130 | 14.0 |
| *NoodleO's* | 10-oz. serving | 90 | 12.0 |
| & rice, *Chunky* | 19-oz. can | 320 | 32.0 |
| With stars, condensed | 10-oz. serving | 80 | 9.0 |
| *& vegetables, condensed | 10-oz. serving | 90 | 10.0 |
| & vegetables, *Chunky* | 10¾-oz. can | 150 | 25.0 |
| (College Inn) broth | 1 cup | 30 | 0. |
| (Progresso): | | | |
| With escarole | 8-oz. serving | 25 | 1.0 |
| *Chickarina* | 8-oz. serving | 100 | 8.0 |
| (Swanson) broth | ½ of 13¾-oz. can | 20 | 1.0 |

| Food and Description | Measure or Quantity | Calories | Carbo-hydrates (grams) |
|---|---|---|---|
| Canned, dietetic or low calorie: | | | |
| (Campbell) *Chunky,* low sodium | 7¾-oz. can | 160 | 14.0 |
| *(Dia-Mel) broth | 8-oz. serving | 18 | 1.0 |
| *(Dia-Mel) & noodle | 8-oz. serving | 50 | 7.0 |
| (Featherweight) & noodle, low sodium | 8-oz. can | 120 | 16.0 |
| Mix: | | | |
| (Ann Page) & noodle | 2-oz. pkg. | 203 | 28.6 |
| (Lipton): | | | |
| *Broth, *Cup-a-Broth* | 6 fl. oz. | 25 | 3.0 |
| *Cream of, *Cup-a-Soup* | 1 pkg. | 80 | 10.0 |
| *Giggle Noodle* | 1 cup | 80 | 12.0 |
| *Giggle Noodle, Cup-a-Soup* | 6 fl. oz. | 40 | 8.0 |
| *& noodle, with broth | 1 cup | 60 | 8.0 |
| *& noodle, with meat | 1 cup | 70 | 9.0 |
| *& noodle, with meat, *Cup-a-Soup* | 6 fl. oz. | 45 | 6.0 |
| *& rice | 1 cup | 60 | 8.0 |
| *& rice, *Cup-a-Soup* | 6 fl. oz. | 50 | 9.0 |
| *Ring-o-Noodle* | 1 cup | 50 | 9.0 |
| *Ring-o-Noodle, Cup-a-Soup* | 6 fl. oz. | 50 | 9.0 |
| *Ripple Noodle* — | 1 cup | 80 | 12.0 |
| *& vegetable, *Cup-a-Soup* | 6 fl. oz. | 40 | 7.0 |
| *(Nestle): | | | |
| Cream of, *Souptime* | 6 fl. oz. | 100 | 8.0 |
| & noodle, *Souptime* | 6 fl. oz. | 30 | 4.0 |
| **CHICKEN SPREAD:** | | | |
| (Swanson) | 1-oz. serving | 70 | 1.0 |
| (Underwood) | 1-oz. serving | 63 | 1.1 |
| **CHICKEN STEW:** | | | |
| Canned, regular pack: | | | |
| (Bounty) | 7½-oz. can | 175 | 17.5 |

(USDA): United States Department of Agriculture
(HEW/FAO): Health, Education and Welfare/Food and Agriculture
        Organization
* Prepared as Package Directs

| Food and Description | Measure or Quantity | Calories | Carbohydrates (grams) |
|---|---|---|---|
| (Libby's) with dumplings | ⅓ of 24-oz. can | 194 | 20.2 |
| (Swanson) | 7½-oz. serving | 160 | 16.0 |
| Canned, dietetic or low calorie: | | | |
| (Dia-Mel) | 8-oz. can | 150 | 19.0 |
| (Featherweight) | 7¼-oz. can | 160 | 21.0 |
| **CHICKEN STOCK BASE** (French's) | 1 tsp. (3 grams) | 8 | 1.0 |
| **CHICK PEAS or GARBANZOS,** dry (USDA) | 1 cup (7.1 oz.) | 720 | 122.0 |
| **CHICORY GREENS,** raw (USDA): | | | |
| Untrimmed | ½ lb. (weighed untrimmed) | 37 | 7.0 |
| Trimmed | 4 oz. | 23 | 4.3 |
| **CHICORY, WITLOOF,** Belgian or French endive, raw, bleached head (USDA): | | | |
| Untrimmed | ½ lb. (weighed untrimmed) | 30 | 6.4 |
| Trimmed, cut | ½ cup (1.6 oz.) | 7 | 1.4 |
| **CHILI or CHILI CON CARNE:** | | | |
| Canned, beans only: | | | |
| (Blue Boy) | 1 cup | 290 | 46.0 |
| (Van Camp) Mexican style | 1 cup | 250 | 43.0 |
| Canned, with beans: | | | |
| (USDA) | 1 cup (8.8 oz.) | 339 | 31.1 |
| (A&P) | ½ of 15-oz. can | 404 | 28.3 |
| (Bounty) | 7¾-oz. can | 310 | 29.3 |
| (Hormel) *Short Orders,* regular | 7½-oz. can | 300 | 24.0 |
| (Hormel) *Short Orders,* hot | 7½-oz. can | 300 | 23.0 |
| (Libby's) | ½ of 15-oz. can | 293 | 32.2 |

| Food and Description | Measure or Quantity | Calories | Carbohydrates (grams) |
|---|---|---|---|
| (Morton House) | 7½-oz. can | 340 | 27.0 |
| (Nalley's) mild or hot | 8-oz. serving | 314 | 27.3 |
| (Swanson) | ½ of 15½-oz. can | 310 | 28.0 |
| Canned, dietetic or low sodium with beans: | | | |
| (Dia-Mel) | 8-oz. can | 360 | 31.0 |
| (Featherweight) | 8-oz. can | 300 | 26.0 |
| Canned, regular pack, without beans: | | | |
| (USDA) | 1 cup (9 oz.) | 510 | 14.8 |
| (Hormel) *Short Orders* | 7½-oz. serving | 370 | 11.0 |
| (Libby's) | ½ of 15-oz. can | 276 | 32.2 |
| (Morton House) | ½ of 15-oz. can | 340 | 14.0 |
| (Nalley's) | 8-oz. serving | 209 | 15.9 |
| (Nalley's) *Big Chunk* | 7½-oz. can | 383 | 19.2 |
| Frozen (Stouffer's) with beans | 8¾-oz. pkg. | 272 | 25.9 |
| **CHILI BEEF SOUP, canned:** | | | |
| *(Campbell) | 11-oz. serving | 180 | 23.0 |
| (Campbell) *Chunky* | 11-oz. can | 300 | 37.0 |
| (Campbell) *Chunky* | 19½-oz. can | 520 | 64.0 |
| **CHILI SAUCE:** | | | |
| (USDA) | 1 T. (.5 oz.) | 16 | 3.7 |
| (USDA) low sodium | 1 T. (.5 oz.) | 16 | 3.7 |
| (Ortega) green | 1-oz. serving | 7 | 1.2 |
| Dietetic (Featherweight) | 1 T. (.5 oz.) | 8 | 1.5 |
| **CHILI SEASONING MIX:** | | | |
| (Ann Page) | 1¾-oz. pkg. | 147 | 29.8 |
| (Durkee) | 1.7-oz. pkg. | 148 | 33.0 |
| *(Durkee) | 1 cup | 465 | 31.3 |
| (French's) *Chili-O* | 1¾-oz. pkg. | 150 | 30.0 |

**CHINESE DATE (See JUJUBE)**

---

(USDA): United States Department of Agriculture
(HEW/FAO): Health, Education and Welfare/Food and Agriculture Organization
* Prepared as Package Directs

| Food and Description | Measure or Quantity | Calories | Carbo-hydrates (grams) |
|---|---|---|---|
| **CHINESE DINNER,** frozen (See individual listings such as **CHOP SUEY, CHOW MEIN,** etc.) | | | |
| **CHIPS** (See **POTATO CHIPS** and **CRACKERS,** Corn Chips) | | | |
| **CHIVES,** raw (USDA) | ½ lb. | 64 | 13.2 |
| *CHOCO-DILES* (Hostess) | 1 piece (2.2 oz.) | 259 | 37.5 |
| **CHOCOLATE, BAKING:** | | | |
| Bitter or unsweetened: | | | |
| (Baker's) | 1 oz. (1 sq.) | 176 | 8.6 |
| (Baker's) *Redi Blend* | 1-oz. square | 140 | 8.0 |
| (Hershey's) | 1-oz. block | 188 | 6.8 |
| (Nestlé) *Choco-Bake* | 1-oz. packet | 170 | 12.0 |
| Sweetened: | | | |
| (Baker's): | | | |
| *German's* | 1 oz. | 153 | 16.7 |
| Semisweet | 1 oz. | 153 | 16.7 |
| Semisweet, chips | 2½ tsp. (1 oz.) | 147 | 19.7 |
| (Hershey's): | | | |
| Dark, chips, regular & mini | 1 oz. | 151 | 17.8 |
| Milk, chips | 1 oz. | 148 | 18.2 |
| Semisweet, chips | 1 oz. | 150 | 17.3 |
| (Nestlé): | | | |
| Milk, morsels | 1 oz. | 150 | 17.0 |
| Semisweet, morsels | 1 oz. | 150 | 18.0 |
| **CHOCOLATE CAKE** (See **CAKE,** chocolate) | | | |
| **CHOCOLATE CAKE MIX** (See **CAKE MIX,** Chocolate) | | | |
| **CHOCOLATE CANDY** (See **CANDY**) | | | |

| Food and Description | Measure or Quantity | Calories | Carbo-hydrates (grams) |
|---|---|---|---|
| **CHOCOLATE DRINK MIX:** | | | |
| (USDA) hot | 1 cup (4.9 oz.) | 545 | 102.7 |
| (USDA) hot | 1 oz. | 111 | 21.0 |
| *(Sealtest) dry | 1 cup | 180 | 24.0 |
| **CHOCOLATE EXTRACT** | | | |
| (Ehlers) imitation | 1 tsp. | 10 | |
| **CHOCOLATE, HOT,** home recipe (USDA) | 1 cup (8.8 oz.) | 238 | 26.0 |
| **CHOCOLATE ICE CREAM** (See also individual brands): | | | |
| (Dean) 11.7% fat | 1 cup (5.6 oz.) | 352 | 38.4 |
| (Meadow Gold) | ¼ pt. | 140 | 18.0 |
| (Sealtest) | ¼ pt. | 140 | 17.0 |
| (Swift's) sweet cream | ½ cup (2.3 oz.) | 129 | 15.8 |
| **CHOCOLATE PIE** (See **PIE,** Chocolate) | | | |
| **CHOCOLATE PUDDING or PIE FILLING** (See **PUDDING or PIE FILLING,** Chocolate) | | | |
| **CHOCOLATE SYRUP:** | | | |
| Sweetened: | | | |
| (USDA): | | | |
| Fudge | 1 T. (.7 oz.) | 63 | 10.3 |
| Thin type | 1 T. (.7 oz.) | 47 | 11.9 |
| (Hershey's) | 1 T. (.5 oz.) | 37 | 8.3 |
| *Milk Mate* | 1½ T. (1 oz.) | 75 | 18.0 |
| Dietetic or low calorie: | | | |
| (Dia-Mel) | 1 T. | 15 | 3.3 |
| (No-Cal) | 1 tsp. | 2 | 0. |

(USDA): United States Department of Agriculture
(HEW/FAO): Health, Education and Welfare/Food and Agriculture
Organization
* Prepared as Package Directs

| Food and Description | Measure or Quantity | Calories | Carbohydrates (grams) |
|---|---|---|---|
| **CHOP SUEY:** | | | |
| Home recipe (USDA) with meat | 1 cup (8.8 oz.) | 300 | 12.8 |
| Canned (USDA) with meat | 1 cup (8.8 oz.) | 155 | 10.5 |
| Frozen: | | | |
| (Banquet): | | | |
| Beef, buffet | 2-lb. pkg. | 418 | 39.1 |
| Beef, cooking bag | 7-oz. bag | 73 | 9.5 |
| Beef dinner | 12-oz. dinner | 282 | 38.8 |
| (Stouffer's) beef, with rice | 12-oz. pkg. | 355 | 47.7 |
| Mix: | | | |
| (Durkee) | 1⅝-oz. pkg. | 128 | 19.0 |
| *(Durkee) | 1¾ cups | 557 | 21.0 |
| **CHOW CHOW (USDA):** | | | |
| Sour | 1 oz. | 8 | 1.2 |
| Sweet | 1 oz. | 33 | 7.7 |
| **CHOW MEIN:** | | | |
| Home recipe (USDA) chicken, without noodles | 8-oz. serving | 231 | 9.1 |
| Canned: | | | |
| (USDA) without noodles | 8-oz. serving | 86 | 16.2 |
| (Chun King): | | | |
| Beef, *Divider-Pak* | 8-oz. serving | 60 | 5.3 |
| Chicken | 8-oz. serving | 60 | 6.7 |
| Chicken, *Divider-Pak* | ¼ of 42-oz. can | 80 | 9.0 |
| Pork, *Divider-Pak* | ¼ of 42-oz. can | 110 | 7.0 |
| Shrimp, *Divider-Pak* | ¼ of 42-oz. can | 70 | 8.0 |
| (La Choy): | | | |
| Beef | 1 cup | 72 | 5.7 |
| *Beef, bi-pack | 1 cup | 83 | 10.3 |
| Chicken | 1 cup | 68 | 5.0 |
| *Chicken, bi-pack | 1 cup | 101 | 9.3 |
| Meatless | 1 cup (1-lb. can) | 47 | 5.9 |
| *Mushroom, bi-pack | 1 cup | 85 | 10.7 |
| Pepper oriental | 1 cup | 89 | 10.2 |
| *Pepper oriental, bi-pack | 1 cup | 89 | 11.1 |
| *Pork, bi-pack | 1 cup | 120 | 10.6 |
| Shrimp | 1 cup | 61 | 5.7 |
| *Shrimp, bi-pack | 1 cup | 110 | 9.7 |

| Food and Description | Measure or Quantity | Calories | Carbo- hydrates (grams) |
|---|---|---|---|
| **Frozen:** | | | |
| (Banquet): | | | |
| Chicken, buffet | 2-lb. pkg. | 345 | 36.4 |
| Chicken, cooking bag | 7-oz. bag | 89 | 9.7 |
| Chicken dinner | 12-oz. dinner | 282 | 38.8 |
| (Chun King): | | | |
| Chicken dinner | 11-oz. dinner | 320 | 43.0 |
| Chicken, pouch | ½ of 12-oz. pouch | 90 | 12.0 |
| Chicken with sweet and sour pork | 13-oz. dinner | 390 | 52.0 |
| Shrimp dinner | 11-oz. dinner | 300 | 43.0 |
| Shrimp dinner with beef pepper oriental | 13-oz. dinner | 350 | 51.0 |
| Shrimp pouch | ½ of 12-oz. pouch | 80 | 10.0 |
| (Green Giant) chicken, without noodles | 9-oz. entree | 126 | 14.8 |
| (La Choy): | | | |
| Beef, 5-compartment | 11-oz. dinner | 337 | 52.8 |
| Chicken | 11-oz. dinner | 356 | 53.8 |
| Pepper oriental, 5-compartment | 11-oz. dinner | 333 | 54.6 |
| Shrimp, 5-compartment | 11-oz. dinner | 324 | 55.4 |
| (Stouffer's) chicken, without noodles | 8-oz. pkg. | 145 | 10.0 |

**CHOW MEIN NOODLES (See NOODLES, CHOW MEIN)**

| | | | |
|---|---|---|---|
| **CHUB, raw (USDA):** | | | |
| Whole | 1 lb. (weighed whole) | 217 | 0. |
| Meat only | 4 oz. | 164 | 0. |

**CIDER (See APPLE CIDER)**

| | | | |
|---|---|---|---|
| **CINNAMON, GROUND:** | | | |
| (USDA) | 1 tsp. (2.3 grams) | 6 | 1.8 |
| (French's) | 1 tsp. (1.7 grams) | 6 | 1.4 |

(USDA): United States Department of Agriculture
(HEW/FAO): Health, Education and Welfare/Food and Agriculture Organization
* Prepared as Package Directs

| Food and Description | Measure or Quantity | Calories | Carbo- hydrates (grams) |
|---|---|---|---|
| **CINNAMON LIFE**, cereal (Quaker) | ⅔ cup (1 oz.) | 105 | 19.7 |
| **CINNAMON SUGAR** (French's) | 1 tsp. | 16 | 4.0 |
| **CITRON, CANDIED** (USDA) | 1 oz. | 89 | 22.7 |
| **CITRUS COOLER**, canned: | | | |
| (Ann Page) | 1 cup (8.7 oz.) | 118 | 29.4 |
| (Hi-C) | 6 fl. oz. (6.3 oz.) | 93 | 23.0 |
| **CITRUS SALAD**, canned (See GRAPEFRUIT & ORANGE SECTIONS) | | | |
| **CLAM:** | | | |
| Raw, hard or round (USDA): | | | |
| Meat & liq. | 1 lb. (weighed in shell) | 71 | 6.1 |
| Meat only | 1 cup (8 oz.) | 182 | 13.4 |
| Raw, soft (USDA) meat & liq. | 1 lb. (weighed in shell) | 142 | 5.3 |
| Raw, soft (USDA) meat only | 1 cup (8 oz.) | 186 | 3.0 |
| Canned, all kinds (Doxsee): | | | |
| Chopped, solids & liq. | 4 oz. | 66 | DNA |
| Chopped & minced, solids & liq. | 4 oz. | 59 | 3.2 |
| Chopped, meat only | 4 oz. | 111 | 2.1 |
| Steamed, meat & broth | 1 pt. (8 fl. oz.) | 152 | DNA |
| Steamed, meat only | 1 pt. (8 fl. oz.) | 66 | DNA |
| Whole | 4 oz. | 62 | DNA |
| Frozen (Mrs. Paul's): | | | |
| Deviled | 3-oz. piece | 179 | 14.4 |
| Fried | ½ of 5-oz. pkg. | 264 | 24.1 |
| **CLAMATO COCKTAIL** (Mott's) | 6 fl. oz. | 80 | 19.0 |
| **CLAM CAKE**, frozen (Mrs. Paul's) thins | 2½-oz. cake | 158 | 16.6 |

| Food and Description | Measure or Quantity | Calories | Carbo-hydrates (grams) |
|---|---|---|---|
| **CLAM CHOWDER:** | | | |
| Manhattan, canned: | | | |
| *(Campbell) condensed | 10-oz. serving | 90 | 15.0 |
| (Campbell) *Chunky* | 19-oz. can | 320 | 46.0 |
| (Crosse & Blackwell) | 6½-oz. serving | 50 | 9.0 |
| *(Doxsee) | 1 cup (8.6 oz.) | 112 | 17.7 |
| (Progresso) | 1 cup (8 oz. by wt.) | 100 | 16.0 |
| (Snow) | 8-oz. serving | 87 | 10.4 |
| New England, canned: | | | |
| *(Campbell) condensed | 10-oz. serving | 100 | 12.0 |
| *(Campbell) *Soup For One*, semicondensed, made with equal volume milk | 11-oz. serving | 190 | 22.0 |
| *(Campbell) *Soup For One*, semicondensed, made with equal volume water | 11-oz. serving | 120 | 17.0 |
| (Crosse & Blackwell) | 6½-oz. serving | 90 | 14.0 |
| *(Doxsee) | 1 cup (8.6 oz.) | 214 | 27.0 |
| (Snow) | ½ of 15-oz. can | 129 | 18.3 |
| **CLAM JUICE, canned:** | | | |
| (USDA) | 1 cup (8.3 oz.) | 45 | 5.0 |
| (Doxsee) | 8 oz. | 54 | DNA |
| (Snow) | ½ cup (4 fl. oz.) | 15 | 1.2 |
| **CLAM STICKS, frozen (Mrs. Paul's) breaded & fried** | .8-oz. stick | 49 | 6.5 |
| **CLARET WINE:** | | | |
| (Gold Seal) 12% alcohol | 3 fl. oz. | 82 | .4 |
| (Inglenook) Navalle, 12% alcohol | 3 fl. oz. | 60 | .3 |
| (Louis M. Martini) 12.5% alcohol | 3 fl. oz. | 90 | .2 |
| (Taylor) 12.5% alcohol | 3 fl. oz. | 72 | 2.4 |

(USDA): United States Department of Agriculture
(HEW/FAO): Health, Education and Welfare/Food and Agriculture Organization

* Prepared as Package Directs

| Food and Description | Measure or Quantity | Calories | Carbo-hydrates (grams) |
|---|---|---|---|
| **CLARISTINE LIQUEUR** | | | |
| (Leroux) 86 proof | 1 fl. oz. | 114 | 10.8 |
| **CLORETS:** | | | |
| Chewing gum | 1 piece | 6 | 1.3 |
| Mint | 1 piece | 6 | 1.6 |
| **CLOVE, GROUND:** | | | |
| (USDA) | 1 tsp. (2.1 grams) | 7 | 1.3 |
| (French's) | 1 tsp. (1.7 grams) | 7 | 1.2 |
| **CLUB SODA (See SOFT DRINK)** | | | |
| **COCKTAIL HOST COCKTAIL, liquid mix** | | | |
| (Holland House) | 1½ fl. oz. | 70 | 18.0 |
| **COCOA:** | | | |
| Dry: | | | |
| (USDA): | | | |
| Low fat | 1 T. (5 grams) | 10 | 3.1 |
| Medium-low fat | 1 T. (5 grams) | 12 | 2.9 |
| Medium-high fat | 1 T. (5 grams) | 14 | 2.8 |
| High fat | 1 T. | 16 | 2.6 |
| (Hershey's) unsweetened American process | ⅓ cup (1 oz.) | 116 | 13.0 |
| (Sultana) unsweetened | 1 T. (7 grams) | 30 | 3.5 |
| Home recipe (USDA) | 1 cup (8.8 oz.) | 242 | 27.2 |
| Mix, regular: | | | |
| *(Alba '66) instant, low fat, regular and chocolate and marshmallow flavor | 6 fl. oz. | 60 | 11.0 |
| (Carnation): | | | |
| Instant, chocolate & artificial marshmallow | 1-oz. pkg. | 112 | 22.0 |
| Instant, milk chocolate | 1-oz. pkg. | 112 | 22.0 |
| Instant, rich chocolate | 1-oz. pkg. | 112 | 22.0 |
| (Hershey's): | | | |
| Hot | 1-oz. packet | 115 | 21.0 |
| Instant | 3 T. (¾ oz.) | 76 | 17.0 |
| (Nestlé): | | | |
| Hot | 1-oz. packet | 110 | 22.0 |

| Food and Description | Measure or Quantity | Calories | Carbo- hydrates (grams) |
|---|---|---|---|
| Hot, with mini marshmallows | 1 oz. | 110 | 23.0 |
| (Ovaltine) hot | 1.1-oz. pkg. | 130 | 24.0 |
| *Swiss Miss:* | | | |
| Instant | 1 oz. | 115 | 21.9 |
| Instant, double rich | 1 oz. | 120 | 20.0 |
| Instant, with mini marshmallows | 1.1 oz. | 110 | 22.0 |
| Mix, dietetic or low calorie: | | | |
| (Carnation) *70 Calorie,* with mini marshmallows or rich chocolate | .73-oz. packet | 70 | 15.0 |
| (Ovaltine) reduced calorie | .45-oz. pkg. | 50 | 8.0 |
| *Swiss Miss,* Lite | 3 T. | 70 | 17.0 |
| **COCOA KRISPIES,** cereal | | | |
| (Kellogg's) | ¾ cup (1 oz.) | 110 | 26.0 |
| **COCOA PUFFS,** cereal | | | |
| (General Mills) | 1 cup (1 oz.) | 110 | 25.0 |
| **COCONUT:** | | | |
| Fresh (USDA): | | | |
| Whole | 1 lb. (weighed in shell) | 816 | 22.2 |
| Meat only | 4 oz. | 392 | 10.7 |
| Meat only | 2″ x 2″ x ½″ piece (1.6 oz.) | 156 | 4.2 |
| Grated or shredded, loosely packed | ½ cup (1.4 oz.) | 225 | 6.1 |
| Dried, canned or packaged: | | | |
| (Baker's): | | | |
| *Angel Flake* | ¼ cup (.7 oz.) | 95 | 7.9 |
| Cookie | ¼ cup (1 oz.) | 137 | 12.2 |
| Premium shred | ¼ cup (.8 oz.) | 100 | 9.0 |
| Premium shred, Southern style | ¼ cup (.74 oz.) | 99 | 8.2 |
| (Durkee) shredded | ¼ cup | 69 | 2.0 |

(USDA): United States Department of Agriculture
(HEW/FAO): Health, Education and Welfare/Food and Agriculture Organization
* Prepared as Package Directs

| Food and Description | Measure or Quantity | Calories | Carbo-hydrates (grams) |
|---|---|---|---|
| **COCO WHEATS**, cereal | 3 T. (1.3 oz.) | 131 | 27.7 |
| **COD:** | | | |
| Raw (USDA): | | | |
| Whole | 1 lb. (weighed whole) | 110 | 0. |
| Meat only | 4 oz. | 88 | 0. |
| Broiled (USDA) | 4 oz. | 193 | 0. |
| Canned (USDA) | 4 oz. | 96 | 0. |
| Dehydrated, lightly salted (USDA) | 4 oz. | 425 | 0. |
| Dried, salted (USDA) | 5½" x 1½" x ½" (2.8 oz.) | 104 | 0. |
| **COFFEE:** | | | |
| Ground: | | | |
| *(Chase & Sanborn) drip or electric perk | 5 fl. oz. | 2 | 0. |
| *Max-Pax | 6 fl. oz. | 2 | 0. |
| *(Maxwell House) regular | 6 fl. oz. | 2 | 0. |
| *(Maxwell House) Electra-Perk | 6 fl. oz. | 2 | 0. |
| *Mellow Roast | 6 fl. oz. | 8 | 2.0 |
| *(Yuban) regular or drip | 6 fl. oz. | 2 | 0. |
| *(Yuban) Electra Matic | 6 fl. oz. | 2 | 0. |
| Decaffeinated: | | | |
| *Brim, regular, drip or electric perk | 6 fl. oz. | 2 | 0. |
| *Brim, freeze-dried | 6 fl. oz. | 4 | 1.0 |
| Decaf | 1 tsp. (2 grams) | 4 | 1.0 |
| Nescafé, freeze-dried | 1 slightly rounded tsp. | 4 | 1.0 |
| *Sanka, regular, electric perk | 6 fl. oz. | 2 | 0. |
| *Sanka, freeze-dried or instant | 6 fl. oz. | 4 | 1.0 |
| Taster's Choice, freeze-dried | 1 slightly rounded tsp. (2 grams) | 4 | 1.0 |
| Freeze-dried: | | | |
| *Maxim | 6 fl. oz. | 4 | 1.0 |
| Taster's Choice | 1 slightly rounded tsp. (2 grams) | 4 | 1.0 |

| Food and Description | Measure or Quantity | Calories | Carbo-hydrates (grams) |
|---|---|---|---|
| Instant: | | | |
| (USDA) | 1 rounded tsp. (2 grams) | 1 | .3 |
| *(USDA) | 1 cup (8.4 oz.) | 3 | .9 |
| *(Chase & Sanborn) | 5 fl. oz. | 2 | 0. |
| *(General Foods) | | | |
| International Coffee: | | | |
| Café Français | 6 fl. oz. | 60 | 7.0 |
| Café Vienna | 6 fl. oz. | 60 | 11.0 |
| Irish Mocha Mist | 6 fl. oz. | 50 | 7.0 |
| Orange Cappuccino | 6 fl. oz. | 60 | 7.0 |
| Suisse Mocha | 6 fl. oz. | 60 | 7.0 |
| *(Maxwell House) | 6 fl. oz. | 4 | 1.0 |
| *Mellow Roast | 6 fl. oz. | 8 | 2.0 |
| Nescafé | 1 slightly rounded tsp. (2 grams) | 4 | 1.0 |
| *Sunrise, with chicory | 6 fl. oz. | 6 | 1.0 |
| *(Yuban) | 6 fl. oz. | 4 | 1.0 |
| COFFEE CAKE (See CAKE, Coffee) | | | |
| COFFEE ICE CREAM (Breyer's) | ¼ pt. | 140 | 15.0 |
| COFFEE SOUTHERN, liqueur | 1 fl. oz. | 79 | 8.8 |
| COFFEE SYRUP, dietetic (No-Cal) | 1 tsp. | 2 | .4 |
| COGNAC (See DISTILLED LIQUOR) | | | |
| COLA SOFT DRINK (See SOFT DRINK, Cola) | | | |
| COLA SYRUP, dietetic (No-Cal) | 1 tsp. (5 grams) | 0 | Tr. |

(USDA): United States Department of Agriculture
(HEW/FAO): Health, Education and Welfare/Food and Agriculture Organization
* Prepared as Package Directs

| Food and Description | Measure or Quantity | Calories | Carbohydrates (grams) |
|---|---|---|---|
| **COLD DUCK WINE:** | | | |
| (Great Western) pink, 12% alcohol | 3 fl. oz. | 92 | 7.7 |
| (Taylor) 12.5% alcohol | 3 fl. oz. | 90 | 6.6 |
| **COLESLAW**, solids & liq. (USDA): | | | |
| Prepared with commercial French dressing | 4-oz. serving | 108 | 8.6 |
| Prepared with homemade French dressing | 4-oz. serving | 146 | 5.8 |
| Prepared with mayonnaise | 4-oz. serving | 163 | 5.4 |
| Prepared with mayonnaise-type salad dressing | 1 cup (4.2 oz.) | 119 | 8.5 |
| **COLLARDS:** | | | |
| Raw (USDA): | | | |
| Leaves, including stems | 1 lb. | 181 | 32.7 |
| Leaves only | ½ lb. | 70 | 11.6 |
| Boiled (USDA) drained: | | | |
| Leaves, cooked in large amount of water | ½ cup (3.4 oz.) | 29 | 4.6 |
| Leaves & stems, cooked in small amount of water | ½ cup (3.4 oz.) | 31 | 4.8 |
| Frozen: | | | |
| (USDA) not thawed | 10-oz. pkg. | 91 | 16.4 |
| (USDA) boiled, chopped, drained | ½ cup (3 oz.) | 26 | 4.8 |
| (Birds Eye) chopped | ⅓ of 10-oz. pkg. | 25 | 4.0 |
| (McKenzie) chopped | 3.3-oz. serving | 31 | 4.3 |
| (Seabrook Farms) chopped | ⅓ of 10-oz. pkg. | 31 | 4.3 |
| **COLLINS MIX** (Bar-Tender's) | 1 serving (⅝ oz.) | 70 | 17.4 |
| **COLLINS MIXER** (See **SOFT DRINK**, Tom Collins) | | | |
| **CONCENTRATE**, cereal (Kellogg's) | ⅓ cup (1 oz.) | 110 | 15.0 |
| **CONCORD WINE:** | | | |
| (Gold Seal) 13-14% alcohol | 3 fl. oz. | 125 | 9.8 |
| (Mogen David) 12% alcohol | 3 fl. oz. | 120 | 16.0 |

| Food and Description | Measure or Quantity | Calories | Carbo- hydrates (grams) |
|---|---|---|---|
| (Pleasant Valley) red, 12½% alcohol | 3 fl. oz. | 90 | DNA |
| **CONSOMME MADRILENE,** canned (Crosse & Blackwell) clear or red | 6½-oz. serving | 25 | 4.0 |
| **COOKIE** (listed by type or brand name. See also **COOKIE, DIETETIC, COOKIE DOUGH, COOKIE HOME RECIPE** and **COOKIE MIX**): | | | |
| *Almond Windmill* (Nabisco) | 1 piece | 47 | 7.0 |
| Animal cracker: | | | |
| (USDA) | 1 piece | 11 | 2.1 |
| *Barnum's Animals* (Nabisco) | 1 piece | 12 | 1.9 |
| Apple crisp (Nabisco) | 1 piece | 50 | 7.0 |
| Assortment: | | | |
| (Nabisco): | | | |
| *Baronet,* creme sandwich | 1 piece | 53 | 8.0 |
| *Biscos,* sugar wafer | 1 piece | 50 | 6.7 |
| Butter flavored | 1 piece | 28 | 4.2 |
| *Cameo,* creme sandwich | 1 piece | 75 | 11.0 |
| Kettle cookie | 1 piece | 35 | 5.2 |
| *Lorna Doone* | 1 piece | 40 | 5.0 |
| *Oreo,* chocolate sandwich | 1 piece | 50 | 7.3 |
| (Nabisco) *Mayfair Assortment,* English-style: | | | |
| Crown creme sandwich | 1 piece | 53 | 8.0 |
| Fancy shortbread biscuit | 1 piece | 22 | 3.8 |
| Filigree creme sandwich | 1 piece | 60 | 8.5 |
| *Mayfair* creme sandwich | 1 piece | 65 | 9.0 |
| Tea Rose creme sandwich | 1 piece | 53 | 7.7 |
| Tea Time, biscuit | 1 piece | 25 | 3.7 |

(USDA): United States Department of Agriculture
(HEW/FAO): Health, Education and Welfare/Food and Agriculture Organization
* Prepared as Package Directs

| Food and Description | Measure or Quantity | Calories | Carbo-hydrates (grams) |
|---|---|---|---|
| *Biscos* (Nabisco) waffle creme | 1 piece | 43 | 6.0 |
| Brown edge wafer (Nabisco) | 1 piece | 28 | 4.2 |
| Brownie: | | | |
| (Frito-Lay's) nut fudge | 1.8-oz. piece | 200 | 34.0 |
| (Hostess) large | 2-oz. piece | 251 | 38.6 |
| (Hostess) small | 1¼-oz. piece | 157 | 24.1 |
| (Planters) peanut fudge | 1 oz. | 137 | 14.0 |
| Frozen (Sara Lee) | ⅛ of 13-oz. pkg. | 199 | 25.8 |
| Butter (Nabisco) | 1 piece | 23 | 3.5 |
| Butterscotch chip (Nabisco) *Bakers Bonus* | 1 piece | 80 | 11.0 |
| Caramel peanut log (Nabisco) *Heyday* | 1 piece | 120 | 13.0 |
| *Cheda Nut* (Nabisco) | 1 piece | 38 | 4.5 |
| Cheese peanut butter (Nabisco) | 1 piece | 35 | 4.3 |
| Chocolate & chocolate covered (Nabisco): | | | |
| *Famous* chocolate wafer | 1 piece | 28 | 4.8 |
| *Pinwheels,* cake | 1.1-oz. piece | 140 | 21.0 |
| Snaps | 1 piece | 16 | 2.8 |
| Chocolate chip (Nabisco): | | | |
| *Chips Ahoy!* | 1 piece | 53 | 7.0 |
| Chocolate | 1 piece | 53 | 7.3 |
| *Cookie Little* | 1 piece | 7 | 1.0 |
| Chocolate chip snap (Nabisco) | 1 piece | 20 | 3.3 |
| *Cinnamon Treats* (Nabisco) | 1 piece | 27 | 5.0 |
| Coconut bar (Nabisco) *Bakers Bonus* | 1 piece | 43 | 5.3 |
| Coconut chocolate chip (Nabisco) | 1 piece | 75 | 9.0 |
| Creme wafer stick (Nabisco) | 1 piece | 50 | 6.0 |
| Devil's food cake (Nabisco) | 1 piece | 50 | 10.5 |
| Double chips fudge (Nabisco) *Bakers Bonus* | 1 piece | 80 | 11.0 |
| Fig bar: | | | |
| *Fig Newtons* (Nabisco) | 1 piece | 60 | 11.0 |
| (Nabisco) fig wheats | 1 piece | 60 | 11.5 |
| Fudge (Planters) creme | 1 oz. | 140 | 20.0 |
| Gingersnap (Nabisco) old fashioned | 1 piece | 30 | 5.5 |

| Food and Description | Measure or Quantity | Calories | Carbo-hydrates (grams) |
|---|---|---|---|
| Lemon (Planters) creme | 1 oz. | 140 | 20.0 |
| Macaroon: | | | |
| (Hostess) fudge | 1 piece | 213 | 32.7 |
| (Nabisco) coconut | 1 piece | 95 | 11.5 |
| Marshmallow: | | | |
| *Mallomars* (Nabisco) | 1 piece | 60 | 8.5 |
| (Nabisco) puffs, cocoa covered | 1 piece | 85 | 14.0 |
| (Nabisco) sandwich | 1 piece | 30 | 5.7 |
| (Planters) banana pie | 1 oz. | 127 | 22.0 |
| (Planters) chocolate pie | 1 oz. | 127 | 22.0 |
| *Twirls,* cake (Nabisco) | 1 piece | 130 | 20.0 |
| Molasses (Nabisco) *Pantry* | 1 piece | 60 | 9.5 |
| Oatmeal (Nabisco): | | | |
| Regular | 1 piece | 75 | 11.5 |
| *Bakers Bonus* | 1 piece | 80 | 12.0 |
| *Cookie Little* | 1 piece | 6 | 1.0 |
| Oatmeal raisin bar (Tastykake) | 1¾-oz. pkg. | 267 | DNA |
| *Party Grahams* (Nabisco) | 1 piece | 47 | 6.0 |
| Peanut creme pattie (Nabisco) | 1 piece | 35 | 4.0 |
| Peanut butter, *Nutter Butter* sandwich (Nabisco) | 1 piece | 70 | 9.5 |
| Peanut brittle (Nabisco) | 1 piece | 50 | 6.3 |
| *Piccolo* (Nabisco) | 1 piece | 22 | 3.3 |
| Raisin fruit biscuit (Nabisco) | 1 piece | 60 | 12.0 |
| Sandwich (Nabisco): | | | |
| Brown edge | 1 piece | 80 | 10.0 |
| *Cameo* creme | 1 piece | 70 | 10.5 |
| Cheese flavored | 1 piece | 27 | 3.3 |
| *Cookie Break,* mixed | 1 piece | 53 | 7.3 |
| *Cookie Break,* vanilla | 1 piece | 50 | 7.3 |
| *Gaity,* fudge | 1 piece | 53 | 7.0 |
| *Mystic,* mint | 1 piece | 90 | 11.0 |
| *Oreo,* chocolate | 1 piece | 50 | 7.3 |
| *Oreo,* Double Stuf | 1 piece | 70 | 9.0 |

(USDA): United States Department of Agriculture
(HEW/FAO): Health, Education and Welfare/Food and Agriculture Organization
* Prepared as Package Directs

| Food and Description | Measure or Quantity | Calories | Carbo-hydrates (grams) |
|---|---|---|---|
| Swiss | 1 piece | 50 | 7.7 |
| Shortbread (Nabisco): | | | |
| Cookie Little | 1 piece | 6 | 1.1 |
| Lorna Doone | 1 piece | 40 | 5.0 |
| Melt-A-Way | 1 piece | 70 | 8.0 |
| Pecan | 1 piece | 80 | 8.5 |
| Striped | 1 piece | 50 | 6.3 |
| Social Tea (Nabisco) | 1 piece | 22 | 3.5 |
| Special Wafers (Nabisco) | 1 piece | 33 | 5.8 |
| Sugar rings (Nabisco) | 1 piece | 70 | 10.5 |
| Sugar wafer: | | | |
| Biscos (Nabisco) | 1 piece | 19 | 2.6 |
| (Dutch Treat) | 1 piece | 49 | 6.3 |
| (Dutch Twin) | 1 piece | 48 | 6.2 |
| Vanilla creme (Planters) | 1 oz. | 116 | DNA |
| Vanilla wafer, Nilla (Nabisco) | 1 piece | 19 | 3.0 |
| Waffle creme (Dutch Twin) | 1 piece | 45 | 5.7 |
| **COOKIE, DIETETIC:** | | | |
| Chocolate chip (Estee) | 1 piece | 30 | 4.0 |
| Chocolate chip, Sug'r Like | 1 piece | 40 | 4.0 |
| Chocolate creme wafer, Sug'r Like | 1 piece | 49 | 4.0 |
| Chocolate crescent, Sug'r Like | 1 piece | 40 | 4.0 |
| Chocolate-flavored bar, Sug'r Like | 1 piece | 45 | 4.0 |
| Lemon, Sug'r Like | 1 piece | 41 | 4.0 |
| Lemon thin (Estee) | 1 piece | 25 | 4.0 |
| Oatmeal raisin (Estee) | 1 piece | 30 | 4.0 |
| Peanut butter creme wafer, Sug'r Like | 1 piece | 49 | 3.0 |
| Rice crisp bar, Sug'r Like | 1 piece | 45 | 4.0 |
| Sandwich (Estee) | 1 piece | 50 | 8.0 |
| Sandwich, lemon (Estee) | 1 piece | 60 | 8.0 |
| Vanilla, Sug'r Like | 1 piece | 41 | 4.0 |
| Vanilla creme wafer, Sug'r Like | 1 piece | 49 | 4.0 |
| Vanilla thins (Estee) | 1 piece | 25 | 4.0 |
| Wafer (Estee) assorted | 1 piece | 35 | 4.1 |
| Wafer (Estee) chocolate | 1 piece | 25 | 3.0 |

| Food and Description | Measure or Quantity | Calories | Carbo-hydrates (grams) |
|---|---|---|---|
| Wafer (Estee) chocolate/strawberry | 1 piece | 90 | 10.5 |
| **COOKIE CRISP**, cereal (Ralston-Purina): | | | |
| Chocolate chip | 1 cup (1 oz.) | 110 | 25.0 |
| Oatmeal | 1 cup (1 oz.) | 120 | 24.0 |
| Vanilla | 1 cup (1 oz.) | 110 | 25.0 |
| **COOKIE DOUGH,** refrigerated: | | | |
| Unbaked (USDA) plain | 1 oz. | 127 | 16.7 |
| Baked (USDA) plain (Pillsbury): | 1 oz. | 141 | 18.4 |
| Butterscotch nut | 1 cookie | 53 | 6.7 |
| Chocolate chip | 1 cookie | 50 | 7.3 |
| Oatmeal chocolate chip | 1 piece | 57 | 7.7 |
| Oatmeal raisin | 1 cookie | 60 | 8.7 |
| Peanut butter | 1 cookie | 53 | 6.3 |
| Sugar | 1 cookie | 63 | 8.3 |
| **COOKIE, HOME RECIPE** (USDA): | | | |
| Brownie with nuts | 1¾" x 1¾" x ⅞" | 97 | 10.2 |
| Chocolate chip | 1 oz. | 146 | 17.0 |
| Sugar, soft, thick | 1 oz. | 126 | 19.3 |
| **COOKIE MIX:** Regular: Brownie: *(Betty Crocker): | | | |
| Chocolate chip butterscotch | ⅟₁₆ pkg. | 130 | 20.0 |
| Fudge, family size | ⅟₂₄ pkg. | 130 | 21.0 |
| Fudge, regular size | ⅟₁₆ pkg. | 150 | 22.0 |
| Fudge, supreme | ⅟₂₄ pkg. | 120 | 20.0 |
| German chocolate | ⅟₁₆ pkg. | 150 | 26.0 |
| Walnut, family size | ⅟₂₄ pkg. | 130 | 19.0 |

(USDA): United States Department of Agriculture
(HEW/FAO): Health, Education and Welfare/Food and Agriculture Organization
* Prepared as Package Directs

| Food and Description | Measure or Quantity | Calories | Carbo-hydrates (grams) |
|---|---|---|---|
| Walnut, regular size | 1/16 pkg. | 160 | 22.0 |
| (Duncan Hines) | 1/24 pkg. | 128 | 19.4 |
| *(Pillsbury): | | | |
| Fudge | 1½" sq. | 60 | 9.5 |
| Fudge, family style | 1½" sq. | 65 | 10.0 |
| Walnut | 1½" sq. | 65 | 10.0 |
| Walnut, family style | 1½" sq. | 65 | 10.0 |
| *Chocolate (Betty Crocker) Big Batch, double chocolate | 1 cookie | 70 | 9.5 |
| *Chocolate chip (Betty Crocker) Big Batch | 1 cookie | 75 | 9.0 |
| Date bar (Betty Crocker) | 1/32 pkg. | 60 | 9.0 |
| *Fudge chip (Quaker) | 1 cookie | 75 | 9.5 |
| *Macaroon, coconut (Betty Crocker) | 1/24 pkg. | 80 | 10.0 |
| *Oatmeal (Betty Crocker) Big Batch | 1 cookie | 70 | 9.5 |
| *Oatmeal (Quaker) | 1 cookie | 65 | 9.5 |
| *Peanut butter (Betty Crocker) Big Batch | 1 cookie | 70 | 8.0 |
| *Peanut butter (Quaker) | 1 cookie | 75 | 8.0 |
| *Peanut butter, flavored chip (Betty Crocker) Big Batch | 1 cookie | 70 | 9.0 |
| *Sugar (Betty Crocker) Big Batch | 1 cookie | 65 | 9.0 |
| *Vienna Dream Bar (Betty Crocker) | 1/24 pkg. | 90 | 10.0 |
| *Dietetic (Dia-Mel) chocolate chip & oatmeal | 2" cookie | 50 | 7.0 |

**COOKING FATS** (See **FAT**)

| | | | |
|---|---|---|---|
| **COOKING SPRAY,** Mazola No Stick | 2-second spray | 7 | 0. |

**CORDIAL** (See individual kinds of liqueur by flavor or brand name)

| Food and Description | Measure or Quantity | Calories | Carbohydrates (grams) |
|---|---|---|---|
| **CORDON D' ALSACE,** Alsatian wine, 12% alcohol (Wilm) | 3 fl. oz. | 66 | 3.6 |
| **CORDON DE BORDEAUX,** French Bordeaux, red or white (Chanson) 11½% alcohol | 3 fl. oz. | 60 | 6.3 |
| **CORDON DE BOURGOGNE,** French white Burgundy (Chanson) 11½% alcohol | 3 fl. oz. | 81 | 6.3 |
| **CORDON DU RHONE,** French red Rhone wine (Chanson) 12% alcohol | 3 fl. oz. | 84 | 6.3 |
| **CORIANDER SEED** (French's) | 1 tsp. (1.4 grams) | 6 | .8 |
| **CORN:** Fresh, white or yellow (USDA): | | | |
| Raw, untrimmed, on cob | 1 lb. (weighed in husk) | 157 | 36.1 |
| Raw, trimmed, on cob | 1 lb. (husk removed) | 240 | 55.1 |
| Boiled, kernels; cut from cob, drained | 1 cup (5.8 oz.) | 137 | 31.0 |
| Boiled, whole | 4.9-oz. ear (5" x 1¾") | 70 | 16.2 |
| Canned, regular pack: (USDA): | | | |
| Golden or yellow, whole kernel, solids & liq., vacuum pack | ½ cup (3.7 oz.) | 87 | 21.6 |
| Golden or yellow, whole kernel, wet pack | ½ cup (4.5 oz.) | 84 | 20.1 |

(USDA): United States Department of Agriculture
(HEW/FAO): Health, Education and Welfare/Food and Agriculture Organization
* Prepared as Package Directs

| Food and Description | Measure or Quantity | Calories | Carbo-hydrates (grams) |
|---|---|---|---|
| Golden or yellow, whole kernel, drained solids, wet pack | ½ cup (3 oz.) | 72 | 16.4 |
| White kernel, solids & liq. | ½ cup (4.5 oz.) | 84 | 20.1 |
| White kernel, drained solids | ½ cup (2.8 oz.) | 70 | 16.4 |
| White, whole kernel, drained liq., wet pack | 4 oz. | 29 | 7.8 |
| Cream style | ½ cup (4.4 oz.) | 105 | 25.6 |
| (Del Monte): | | | |
| Cream style, golden, wet pack | ½ cup (4.4 oz.) | 89 | 19.2 |
| Cream style, white, wet pack | ½ cup (4.3 oz.) | 97 | 21.3 |
| Golden, whole kernel, solids & liq. | ½ cup (4 oz.) | 78 | 16.6 |
| Golden, whole kernel, drained solids | ½ cup | 100 | 21.3 |
| Golden or yellow, whole kernel, vacuum pack | ½ cup | 101 | 21.6 |
| White, whole kernel, solids & liq. | ½ cup | 78 | 16.6 |
| White, whole kernel, drained solids | ½ cup | 102 | 21.4 |
| (Green Giant): | | | |
| Cream style, golden kernel | ½ of 8½-oz. can | 103 | 22.3 |
| Golden or yellow kernel, solids & liq. | ¼ of 17-oz. can | 77 | 15.8 |
| Golden or yellow kernel, vacuum pack, Niblets | ½ of 7-oz. can | 82 | 17.1 |
| Golden, whole kernel, solids & liq., Mexicorn, with peppers | ½ of 7-oz. can | 85 | 17.8 |
| (Kounty Kist): | | | |
| Cream style, golden kernel | ½ of 8½-oz. can | 106 | 23.2 |
| Golden, whole kernel, liquid pack, solids & liq. | ½ of 7-oz. can | 106 | 19.4 |

| Food and Description | Measure or Quantity | Calories | Carbo-hydrates (grams) |
|---|---|---|---|
| Golden, whole kernel, vacuum pack | ½ cup | 80 | 17.5 |
| (Le Sueur) golden, whole kernel, solids & liq. | ¼ of 17-oz. can | 84 | 17.3 |
| (Libby's): | | | |
| Cream style | ½ cup | 100 | 21.2 |
| Whole kernel, solids & liq. | ½ cup | 92 | 18.8 |
| (Lindy): | | | |
| Cream style, golden kernel | ½ of 8-oz. can | 106 | 23.2 |
| Golden, whole kernel, liquid pack, solids & liq. | ½ of 7-oz. can | 106 | 19.4 |
| Golden, whole kernel, vacuum pack | ½ cup | 80 | 17.5 |
| (Stokely-Van Camp): | | | |
| Cream style, golden | ½ cup | 105 | 23.5 |
| Cream style, white | ½ cup | 110 | 24.5 |
| Golden or yellow, whole kernel, solids & liq. | ½ cup (4.5 oz.) | 90 | 19.5 |
| Golden, vacuum pack | ½ cup | 120 | 26.5 |
| White, solids & liq. | ½ cup | 95 | 20.5 |
| Canned, dietetic or low calorie: | | | |
| (USDA): | | | |
| Cream style | 4 oz. | 93 | 21.0 |
| White or yellow, whole kernel, solids & liq. | 4 oz. | 65 | 15.4 |
| White or yellow, whole kernel, drained solids | 4 oz. | 86 | 20.4 |
| (Blue Boy): | | | |
| Cream style, solids & liq. | ½ cup | 100 | 22.0 |
| Whole kernel, solids & liq. | ½ cup | 85 | 18.0 |

(USDA): United States Department of Agriculture
(HEW/FAO): Health, Education and Welfare/Food and Agriculture
         Organization
* Prepared as Package Directs

| Food and Description | Measure or Quantity | Calories | Carbo-hydrates (grams) |
|---|---|---|---|
| (Diet Delight) whole kernel, solids & liq. | ½ cup (4.4 oz.) | 71 | 14.6 |
| (Featherweight): | | | |
| Cream style | ½ cup | 80 | 18.0 |
| Whole kernel, solids & liq. | ½ cup | 70 | 16.0 |
| (Tillie Lewis) whole kernel, *Tasti Diet* | ½ cup | 76 | 15.0 |
| Frozen: | | | |
| (USDA) boiled, drained | 4 oz. | 107 | 24.5 |
| (Birds Eye): | | | |
| On the cob | 1 ear (4.9 oz.) | 130 | 28.0 |
| On the cob, *Little Ears* | 1 ear | 70 | 16.0 |
| Kernel, white | ⅓ of 10-oz. pkg. | 112 | 23.2 |
| (Green Giant): | | | |
| On the cob | 5½" ear | 155 | 32.7 |
| On the cob, *Nibblers* | 3" ear | 85 | 18.0 |
| Cream style | ⅓ of 10-oz. pkg. | 72 | 15.2 |
| *Mexicorn*, in butter sauce | ⅓ of 10-oz. pkg. | 86 | 14.2 |
| *Niblets*, in butter sauce | ⅓ of 10-oz. pkg. | 86 | 14.2 |
| Whole kernel, white | ⅕ of 20-oz. pkg. | 105 | 21.7 |
| Whole kernel, white, in butter sauce | ⅓ of 10-oz. pkg. | 89 | 15.2 |
| (Kounty Kist) whole kernel, golden or white | ⅙ of 20-oz. pkg. | 105 | 21.6 |
| (McKenzie or Seabrook Farms): | | | |
| On the cob | 5" ear | 140 | 30.0 |
| Whole kernel | ⅓ of 10-oz. pkg. | 97 | 19.9 |
| (Ore-Ida): | | | |
| On the cob | 1 ear | 140 | 27.0 |
| Whole kernel | ⅒ of 32-oz. pkg. | 106 | 21.3 |
| **CORNBREAD, HOME RECIPE (USDA):** | | | |
| Corn pone, prepared with white, whole-ground cornmeal | 4 oz. | 231 | 41.1 |
| Johnnycake, prepared with yellow, degermed cornmeal | 4 oz. | 303 | 51.6 |

| Food and Description | Measure or Quantity | Calories | Carbo-hydrates (grams) |
|---|---|---|---|
| Southern-style, prepared with degermed cornmeal | 2½″ x 2½″ x 1⅝″ piece | 186 | 28.8 |
| Southern-style, prepared with whole-ground cornmeal | 4 oz. | 235 | 33.0 |
| Spoon bread, prepared with white, whole-ground cornmeal | 4 oz. | 221 | 19.2 |
| **CORNBREAD MIX:** | | | |
| Dry (USDA) | 1 oz. | 122 | 20.1 |
| *(USDA) prepared with egg and milk | 2⅜″ muffin (1.4 oz.) | 130 | 20.0 |
| *(Aunt Jemima) | ⅙ pkg. | 220 | 34.0 |
| *(Dromedary) | 2″ x 2″ piece | 130 | 19.0 |
| *(Pillsbury) *Ballard* | ¹⁄₁₆ of recipe | 160 | 26.0 |
| **CORN CHEX**, cereal (Ralston Purina) | 1 cup (1 oz.) | 110 | 25.0 |
| **CORN CHIPS** (See CRACKERS) | | | |
| **CORNED BEEF:** | | | |
| Uncooked (USDA) boneless, medium fat | 1 lb. | 1329 | 0. |
| Cooked (USDA) medium fat, boneless | 4 oz. | 422 | 0. |
| Canned: | | | |
| (Hormel) | 3-oz. serving | 195 | 0. |
| (Libby's) | ½ of 7-oz. can | 244 | 1.9 |
| Packaged: | | | |
| (Eckrich) sliced | 1 oz. slice | 41 | .9 |
| (Oscar Mayer) jellied loaf | 1 oz. slice | 44 | 0. |
| (Vienna): | | | |
| Brisket | 1 oz. | 88 | 0. |
| Flats | 1 oz. | 49 | .1 |

(USDA): United States Department of Agriculture
(HEW/FAO): Health, Education and Welfare/Food and Agriculture Organization
* Prepared as Package Directs

| Food and Description | Measure or Quantity | Calories | Carbo-hydrates (grams) |
|---|---|---|---|
| **CORNED BEEF HASH:** | | | |
| Canned: | | | |
| (A&P) | ½ of 15-oz. can | 379 | 19.9 |
| (Bounty) | 7½-oz. can | 372 | 22.2 |
| *Mary Kitchen* | 7½-oz. serving | 399 | 21.1 |
| (Libby's) | 1 cup | 454 | 31.1 |
| (Nalley's) | 4-oz. serving | 208 | 10.2 |
| Frozen (Banquet) | 10-oz. dinner | 372 | 42.6 |
| **CORNED BEEF SPREAD** | | | |
| (Underwood) | 1 oz. | 55 | Tr. |
| **CORN FLAKE CRUMBS** | | | |
| (Kellogg's) | ¼ cup | 110 | 25.0 |
| **CORN FLAKES, cereal:** | | | |
| (USDA) | 1 cup (1 oz.) | 112 | 24.7 |
| (USDA) crushed | 1 cup (2.5 oz.) | 270 | 59.7 |
| (USDA) frosted | 1 cup (1.4 oz.) | 154 | 36.5 |
| (General Mills) *Country* | 1 cup (1 oz.) | 110 | 25.0 |
| (Kellogg's) | 1 cup (1 oz.) | 110 | 25.0 |
| *King Kullen* | 1 cup (1 oz.) | 107 | 24.3 |
| *King Kullen,* sugar toasted | ¾ cup (1 oz.) | 108 | 25.3 |
| (Post) *Post Toasties* | 1¼ cups (1 oz.) | 107 | 24.4 |
| *Provigo* | 1 cup (1 oz.) | 107 | 24.3 |
| (Ralston Purina) | 1 cup (1 oz.) | 110 | 24.0 |
| *Rokeach* | 1 cup (1 oz.) | 107 | 24.3 |
| (Van Brode) regular | 1 cup (1 oz.) | 107 | 24.3 |
| (Van Brode) sugar toasted | ¾-cup (1 oz.) | 108 | 25.3 |
| Low Sodium: | | | |
| (Featherweight) | 1 cup (.8 oz.) | 88 | 20.0 |
| *Nature Foods* | 1 cup (.8 oz.) | 88 | 20.0 |
| (Van Brode) | 1¼ cups (1 oz.) | 110 | 25.0 |
| **CORN FRITTER** (See **FRITTER,** Corn) | | | |
| **CORN GRITS** (See **HOMINY**) | | | |
| **CORNMEAL, WHITE or YELLOW:** | | | |
| Dry: | | | |
| Bolted: | | | |
| (USDA) | 1 cup (4.3 oz.) | 442 | 90.9 |
| (Aunt Jemima/Quaker) | 1 cup (4 oz.) | 408 | 84.8 |

| Food and Description | Measure or Quantity | Calories | Carbo-hydrates (grams) |
|---|---|---|---|
| Degermed: | | | |
| (USDA) | 1 cup (4.9 oz.) | 502 | 108.2 |
| (Aunt Jemima/Quaker) | 1 cup (4 oz.) | 404 | 88.8 |
| Self-rising, degermed: | | | |
| (USDA) | 1 cup (5 oz.) | 491 | 105.9 |
| (Aunt Jemima) | 1 cup (6 oz.) | 582 | 126.0 |
| Self-rising, whole ground | | | |
| (USDA) | 1 cup (5 oz.) | 489 | 101.4 |
| Self-rising (Aunt Jemima) | 1 cup (6 oz.) | 594 | 122.4 |
| Whole ground, unbolted | | | |
| (USDA) | 1 cup (4.3 oz.) | 433 | 90.0 |
| Cooked: | | | |
| (USDA) | 1 cup (8.5 oz.) | 120 | 25.7 |
| (Albers) degermed | 1 cup | 119 | 25.5 |
| Mix (Aunt Jemima/Quaker) bolted | 1 cup (4 oz.) | 392 | 80.4 |
| **CORN PUDDING,** home recipe (USDA) | 1 cup (8.6 oz.) | 255 | 31.9 |
| **CORN SALAD,** raw (USDA): | | | |
| Untrimmed | 1 lb. (weighed untrimmed) | 91 | 15.7 |
| Trimmed | 4 oz. | 24 | 4.1 |
| **CORNSTARCH:** | | | |
| (USDA) | 1 cup (4.5 oz.) | 463 | 112.1 |
| (Argo) | 1 T. (9.5 grams) | 34 | 8.3 |
| (Kingsford's) | 1 T. (9.5 grams) | 34 | 8.3 |
| (Duryea's) | 1 T. (8 grams) | 34 | 8.3 |
| **CORN STICK** (See CORNBREAD) | | | |
| **CORN SYRUP** (USDA) light & dark blend | 1 T. (.7 oz.) | 61 | 15.8 |
| **CORN TOTAL,** cereal (General Mills) | 1 cup (1 oz.) | 110 | 24.0 |

(USDA): United States Department of Agriculture
(HEW/FAO): Health, Education and Welfare/Food and Agriculture Organization
* Prepared as Package Directs

| Food and Description | Measure or Quantity | Calories | Carbohydrates (grams) |
|---|---|---|---|
| **CORNY-SNAPS**, cereal (Kellogg's) | 1 cup (1 oz.) | 120 | 24.0 |
| **COTTAGE PUDDING**, home recipe (USDA): | | | |
| Without sauce | 2 oz. | 195 | 30.8 |
| With chocolate sauce | 2 oz. | 180 | 32.1 |
| With strawberry sauce | 2 oz. | 166 | 27.4 |
| **COUGH DROP:** | | | |
| (Beech-Nut) | 1 drop (2 grams) | 10 | 2.5 |
| (H-B) | 1 drop | 8 | 1.9 |
| (Luden's): | | | |
| Honey lemon | 1 drop | 8 | DNA |
| Honey licorice | 1 drop | 8 | DNA |
| Menthol | 1 drop | 9 | 2.1 |
| Wild cherry | 1 drop | 9 | DNA |
| (Pine Bros.) | 1 drop (3 grams) | 8 | 2.0 |
| (Smith Brothers) | 1 drop | 7 | 2.1 |
| **COUNT CHOCULA**, cereal (General Mills) | 1 cup (1 oz.) | 110 | 24.0 |
| **COUNTRY CRISP**, cereal (Post) | ¾ cup (1 oz.) | 114 | 24.4 |
| **COUNTRY MORNING**, cereal (Kellogg's): | | | |
| Regular | ⅓ cup (1 oz.) | 130 | 18.0 |
| With raisins & dates | ⅓ cup (1 oz.) | 130 | 19.0 |
| **COUNTRY-STYLE SAUSAGE**, smoked links (USDA) | 1 oz. | 98 | 0. |
| **COWPEA** (USDA): | | | |
| Immature seeds: | | | |
| Raw, whole | 1 lb. (weighed in pods) | 317 | 54.4 |
| Raw, shelled | ½ cup (2.5 oz.) | 92 | 15.8 |
| Boiled, drained solids | ½ cup (2.9 oz.) | 89 | 15.0 |
| Canned, solids & liq. | 4 oz. | 79 | 14.1 |

| Food and Description | Measure or Quantity | Calories | Carbo- hydrates (grams) |
|---|---|---|---|
| Frozen (See BLACK-EYED PEAS, frozen) | | | |
| Young pods with seeds: | | | |
| Raw, whole | 1 lb. (weighed untrimmed) | 182 | 39.2 |
| Boiled, drained solids | 4 oz. | 39 | 7.9 |
| Mature seeds, dry: | | | |
| Raw | 1 lb. | 1556 | 279.9 |
| Raw | ½ cup (3 oz.) | 292 | 52.4 |
| Boiled | ½ cup (4.4 oz.) | 95 | 17.2 |
| **CRAB, all species:** | | | |
| Fresh (USDA): | | | |
| Steamed, whole | 1 lb. (weighed in shell) | 202 | 1.1 |
| Steamed, meat only | 4 oz. | 105 | .6 |
| Canned: | | | |
| (USDA) drained solids | 4 oz. | 115 | 1.2 |
| (Icy Point) Alaska King, drained solids | 7½-oz. can | 215 | 2.3 |
| (Pillar Rock) Alaska King, drained solids | 7½-oz. can | 215 | 2.3 |
| Frozen: | | | |
| (Ship Ahoy) King crab | 8-oz. pkg. | 211 | .5 |
| (Wakefield's) Alaska King, thawed & drained | 4 oz. | 86 | .7 |
| **CRAB APPLE, fresh (USDA):** | | | |
| Whole | 1 lb. (weighed whole) | 284 | 74.3 |
| Flesh only | 4 oz. | 77 | 20.2 |
| **CRABAPPLE JELLY,** sweetened (Smucker's) | 1 T. | 53 | 13.5 |
| **CRABAPPLE PRESERVE or JAM,** sweetened (Smucker's) | 1 T. | 53 | 13.5 |

(USDA): United States Department of Agriculture
(HEW/FAO): Health, Education and Welfare/Food and Agriculture Organization
* Prepared as Package Directs

| Food and Description | Measure or Quantity | Calories | Carbo- hydrates (grams) |
|---|---|---|---|
| **CRAB CAKE**, frozen (Mrs. Paul's) thins | ½ of 10-oz. pkg. | 324 | 35.3 |
| **CRAB, DEVILED:** | | | |
| Home recipe (USDA) | 1 cup (8.5 oz.) | 451 | 31.9 |
| Frozen (Mrs. Paul's): | | | |
| Breaded & french-fried | 3-oz. cake | 166 | 18.3 |
| Breaded & fried, miniatures | ½ of 7-oz. pkg. | 221 | 25.8 |
| **CRAB IMPERIAL**, home recipe (USDA) | 1 cup (7.8 oz.) | 323 | 8.6 |
| **CRAB SOUP** (Crosse & Blackwell) | ½ of 13-oz. can | 50 | 8.0 |
| **CRACKER, PUFFS and CHIPS:** | | | |
| *American Harvest* (Nabisco) | 1 piece (3 grams) | 16 | 2.0 |
| Arrowroot biscuit (Nabisco) *National* | 1 piece (5 grams) | 20 | 3.5 |
| Bacon 'n Dip (Nabisco) | 1 piece | 21 | .9 |
| Bacon flavored thins (Nabisco) | 1 piece (2 grams) | 11 | 1.3 |
| *Bacon Nips* | 1 oz. | 147 | 15.6 |
| *Bakon Snacks* | 1 oz. | 150 | 14.3 |
| *Betcha Bacon* | 1 oz. | 170 | 18.0 |
| *Bugles* (General Mills) | 15 pieces (1 oz.) | 150 | 17.0 |
| Butter (USDA) | 1 oz. | 130 | 19.1 |
| Butter thins (Nabisco) | 1 piece (3 grams) | 14 | 2.2 |
| Cheese-flavored (See also individual brand names in this grouping): | | | |
| (USDA) | 1 oz. | 136 | 17.1 |
| *Bops* (Nalley's) | 1 oz. | 147 | 13.6 |
| *Cheddar Bitz* (Frito-Lay's) | 1 oz. | 129 | 18.9 |
| Cheddar triangles (Nabisco) | 1 piece | 9 | .9 |
| Cheese'n Crunch (Nabisco) | 1 oz. | 160 | 14.0 |
| Cheese filled (Frito-Lay's) | 1½ oz. | 203 | 25.3 |
| *Chee•Tos*, crunchy | 1 oz. | 160 | 15.0 |
| *Chee•Tos*, puffed | 1 oz. | 160 | 15.0 |
| *Cheez Balls* (Planters) | 1 oz. | 160 | 15.0 |

| Food and Description | Measure or Quantity | Calories | Carbohydrates (grams) |
|---|---|---|---|
| *Cheez Curls* (Planters) | 1 oz. | 160 | 15.0 |
| *Cheez Doodles* (Old London) baked | 1 oz. | 155 | 15.7 |
| Country cheddar 'n sesame (Nabisco) | 1 piece | 9 | 1.0 |
| *Dip In A Chip* (Nabisco) cheese'n chive | 1 piece | 15 | 1.6 |
| *Nips* (Nabisco) | 1 piece | 6 | .7 |
| Parmesan swirl (Nabisco) | 1 piece (2.2 grams) | 11 | 1.2 |
| Sandwich (Planters) | 1 piece | 29 | 3.0 |
| Swiss cheese (Nabisco) | 1 piece (1.9 grams) | 10 | 1.1 |
| *Tid-Bit* (Nabisco) | 1 piece (<1 gram) | 5 | .5 |
| Twists (Bachman) | 1 oz. | 150 | 17.0 |
| Twists (Nalley's) | 1 oz. | 126 | 9.1 |
| Cheese & peanut butter sandwich (USDA) | 1 oz. | 139 | 15.9 |
| *Chicken in a Biskit* (Nabisco) | 1 piece (2 grams) | 11 | 1.1 |
| *Chipos* (General Mills) | 1 oz. | 150 | 17.0 |
| *Chippers* (Nabisco) potato 'n cheese | 1 piece | 15 | 1.7 |
| *Chipsters* (Nabisco) | 1 piece | 2 | .3 |
| Corn chips: | | | |
| (Bachman) | 1 oz. | 160 | 17.0 |
| *Fritos* | 1 oz. | 160 | 16.0 |
| *Fritos*, barbecue-flavored | 1 oz. | 150 | 15.5 |
| (Planters) | 1 oz. | 170 | 15.0 |
| *Corn Nuggets* (Frito-Lay's) | 1 oz. | 128 | 21.2 |
| Corn Nuts (Nalley's) | 1 oz. | 120 | 20.4 |
| Corn & Sesame Chips (Nabisco) | 1 piece | 10 | .9 |
| Creme wafer sticks (Nabisco) | 1 piece | 47 | 6.3 |
| *Crown Pilot* (Nabisco) | 1 piece (.6 oz.) | 75 | 13.0 |
| *Diggers* (Nabisco) | 1 piece | 4 | .5 |
| *Dixies* (Nabisco) | 1 piece | 8 | .9 |
| *Doo Dads* (Nabisco) | 1 piece | 2 | .3 |

(USDA): United States Department of Agriculture
(HEW/FAO): Health, Education and Welfare/Food and Agriculture Organization
* Prepared as Package Directs

| Food and Description | Measure or Quantity | Calories | Carbo-hydrates (grams) |
|---|---|---|---|
| *Escort* (Nabisco) | 1 piece | 21 | 2.7 |
| *Flings* (Nabisco) cheese-flavored curls | 1 piece (2 grams) | 10 | .8 |
| *Goldfish* (Pepperidge Farm): | | | |
| Thins: | | | |
| Cheese | 1 piece (3.5 grams) | 17 | 2.3 |
| Lightly salted | 1 piece (3.5 grams) | 17 | 2.3 |
| Rye | 1 piece (3.5 grams) | 17 | 2.3 |
| Wheat | 1 piece (3.5 grams) | 17 | 2.3 |
| Tiny: | | | |
| Cheddar cheese | ¼-oz. serving | 35 | 4.0 |
| Lightly salted | ¼-oz. serving | 35 | 4.0 |
| Parmesan | ¼-oz. serving | 35 | 4.0 |
| Pizza | ¼-oz. serving | 35 | 4.0 |
| Pretzel | ¼-oz. serving | 30 | 5.0 |
| Graham: | | | |
| (USDA) | 2½" sq. (7 grams) | 27 | 5.2 |
| (Nabisco) *Cinnamon Treats* | 1 piece (.2 oz.) | 28 | 5.0 |
| Chocolate or cocoa-covered: | | | |
| (USDA) | 1 oz. | 135 | 19.2 |
| (Nabisco) | 1 piece | 57 | 7.0 |
| (Nabisco) *Fancy Dip* | 1 piece (.5 oz.) | 65 | 8.5 |
| Sugar-honey coated: | | | |
| (USDA) | 1 oz. | 117 | 21.7 |
| (Nabisco) *Honey Maid* | 1 piece (7 grams) | 30 | 5.5 |
| *Ideal Flatbrod:* | | | |
| Caraway | 1 piece | 19 | 4.0 |
| Ultra thin | 1 piece (3 grams) | 12 | 3.0 |
| Whole grain | 1 piece | 19 | 4.0 |
| *Korkers* (Nabisco) | 1 piece (1.5 grams) | 8 | .8 |
| *Lil' Loaf* (Nabisco) | 1 stick (2.8 grams) | 14 | 1.8 |
| Matzo (See MATZO) | | | |
| Melba toast (See MELBA TOAST) | | | |
| *Munchos* | 1 oz. | 154 | 15.2 |
| Onion flavored: | | | |
| *Funyuns* (Frito-Lay's) | 1 oz. | 137 | 18.9 |
| (Nabisco) French | 1 piece | 12 | 1.5 |
| *Onyums* (General Mills) | 30 pieces (½ oz.) | 79 | 7.7 |

| Food and Description | Measure or Quantity | Calories | Carbohydrates (grams) |
|---|---|---|---|
| Oyster: | | | |
| (USDA) | 10 pieces (.4 oz.) | 33 | 5.3 |
| (USDA) | 1 cup (1 oz.) | 124 | 20.0 |
| (Nabisco): | | | |
| *Dandy* | 1 piece | 3 | .5 |
| *Oysterettes* | 1 piece | 3 | .6 |
| Peanut butter sandwich: | | | |
| (Planters) | 1 piece (7 grams) | 29 | 3.0 |
| (Planters) toasted | 1 piece (7 grams) | 29 | 3.0 |
| Peanut butter toast (Frito-Lay's) | ½ oz. | 73 | 6.7 |
| *Pizza Spins* (General Mills) | 32 pieces (1 oz.) | 150 | 15.0 |
| *Ritz* (Nabisco) | 1 piece (3 grams) | 17 | 2.0 |
| *Royal Lunch* (Nabisco) | 1 piece (1.7 grams) | 55 | 8.0 |
| Rusk (Nabisco) *Holland* | 1 piece | 40 | 7.5 |
| Rye: | | | |
| (Nabisco): | | | |
| Regular | 1 wafer (5.7 grams) | 20 | 4.0 |
| Seasoned | 1 wafer (5.7 grams) | 23 | 4.5 |
| *Wasa Crisp:* | | | |
| Golden | 1 piece | 37 | 8.0 |
| Lite | 1 piece | 30 | 6.0 |
| Seasoned | 1 piece | 34 | 7.0 |
| Saltine (Nabisco) *Premium,* salted or unsalted tops | 1 piece (2.8 oz.) | 12 | 2.0 |
| *Sea Rounds* (Nabisco) | 1 piece | 45 | 7.5 |
| Sesame: | | | |
| (Nabisco): | | | |
| Buttery flavored | 1 piece (3.1 grams) | 17 | 1.9 |
| *Sesame Wheats!* | 1 piece | 17 | 1.8 |
| *Teeko,* glazed crisp | 1 piece (4.7 grams) | 22 | 3.0 |

(USDA): United States Department of Agriculture
(HEW/FAO): Health, Education and Welfare/Food and Agriculture Organization
* Prepared as Package Directs

| Food and Description | Measure or Quantity | Calories | Carbo-hydrates (grams) |
|---|---|---|---|
| *Wasa Crisp* | 1 piece (14 grams) | 60 | 9.0 |
| *Skittle Chips* (Nabisco) | 1 piece (2.8 grams) | 14 | 1.8 |
| *Snacks Ahoy* (Nabisco) | 1 piece | 9 | 1.1 |
| Snack Sticks (Pepperidge Farm): | | | |
| Lightly salted | 1 oz. | 120 | 18.0 |
| Pumpernickel | 1 oz. | 110 | 17.0 |
| Sesame | 1 oz. | 120 | 16.0 |
| Wheat | 1 oz. | 110 | 17.0 |
| *Sociables* (Nabisco) | 1 piece (2 grams) | 9 | 1.3 |
| Soda: | | | |
| (USDA) | 1 oz. | 124 | 20.0 |
| (USDA) | 2½" sq. (6 grams) | 24 | 3.9 |
| *Gitano* (Nabisco) | 1 piece | 15 | 2.5 |
| Taco chip (Nalley's) | 1 oz. | 147 | 17.6 |
| *Tater Puffs* (Nabisco) | 1 piece (1.3 grams) | 7 | .8 |
| Tortilla chip: | | | |
| (Bachman): | | | |
| Nacho cheese flavor | 1 oz. | 150 | 17.0 |
| Taco cheese flavor | 1 oz. | 150 | 17.0 |
| *Buenos* (Nabisco): | | | |
| Nacho cheese flavor | 1 piece (2 grams) | 10 | 1.2 |
| Sour cream & onion flavor | 1 piece | 11 | 1.3 |
| *Doritos:* | | | |
| Nacho cheese flavor | 1 oz. | 140 | 18.0 |
| Taco cheese flavor | 1 oz. | 140 | 18.0 |
| (Nabisco): | | | |
| Regular | 1 piece | 11 | 1.3 |
| Nacho cheese flavor | 1 piece (2.8 grams) | 11 | 1.3 |
| (Nalley's) | 1 oz. | 147 | 17.6 |
| (Planters) | 1 oz. | 130 | 14.0 |
| *Tostitos*, round | 1 oz. | 140 | 17.0 |
| *Triscuit* (Nabisco) | 1 piece (4 grams) | 20 | 3.0 |
| *Twigs* (Nabisco) | 1 stick | 14 | 1.6 |
| *Uneeda Biscuit* (Nabisco) unsalted tops | 1 piece (5 grams) | 22 | 3.7 |
| Vegetable thins (Nabisco) | 1 piece | 11 | 1.3 |

| Food and Description | Measure or Quantity | Calories | Carbo-hydrates (grams) |
|---|---|---|---|
| *Wafer-ets* (Hol-Grain): | | | |
| Rice, salted | 1 piece (3 grams) | 12 | 2.5 |
| Rice, unsalted | 1 piece (3 grams) | 12 | 2.5 |
| Wheat, salted | 1 piece (2 grams) | 7 | 1.4 |
| Wheat, unsalted | 1 piece (2 grams) | 7 | 1.4 |
| *Waverly Wafer* (Nabisco) | 1 piece (4 grams) | 18 | 2.6 |
| Wheat chips (Nabisco) | 1 piece | 4 | .5 |
| *Wheatsworth* (Nabisco) | 1 piece | 14 | 1.8 |
| *Wheat Thins* (Nabisco) | 1 piece (2 grams) | 9 | 1.2 |
| Whole wheat (USDA) | 1 oz. | 114 | 19.3 |
| **CRACKER CRUMBS, GRAHAM:** | | | |
| (USDA) | 1 cup (3 oz.) | 330 | 63.0 |
| (Nabisco) | ⅛ of 9″ pie shell (.6 oz.) | 70 | 12.0 |
| **CRACKER MEAL:** | | | |
| (USDA) | 1 T. (.4 oz.) | 44 | 7.1 |
| (Nabisco) | ½ cup (2 oz.) | 220 | 47.5 |
| **CRACKER PIE CRUST MIX** (See PIE CRUST MIX) | | | |
| *CRANAPPLE* juice drink (Ocean Spray): | | | |
| Regular | 6 fl. oz. | 131 | 32.5 |
| Low calorie | 6 fl. oz. | 32 | 7.8 |
| **CRANBERRY:** | | | |
| Fresh: | | | |
| (USDA): | | | |
| Untrimmed | 1 lb. (weighed with stems) | 200 | 47.0 |
| Trimmed, stems removed | 1 cup (4 oz.) | 52 | 12.2 |
| (Ocean Spray) | ½ cup (2 oz.) | 26 | 6.1 |
| Dehydrated (USDA) | 1 oz. | 104 | 23.9 |

(USDA): United States Department of Agriculture
(HEW/FAO): Health, Education and Welfare/Food and Agriculture Organization
* Prepared as Package Directs

| Food and Description | Measure or Quantity | Calories | Carbohydrates (grams) |
|---|---|---|---|
| **CRANBERRY-APPLE JUICE DRINK,** canned (Ann Page) | ½ cup | 91 | 22.6 |
| **CRANBERRY JUICE COCKTAIL:** | | | |
| (Ann Page) | ½ cup | 79 | 19.8 |
| (Ocean Spray): | | | |
| Regular | 6 fl. oz. | 106 | 26.4 |
| Low calorie | 6 fl. oz. | 36 | 8.3 |
| **CRANBERRY-ORANGE RELISH:** | | | |
| Uncooked (USDA) | 4 oz. | 202 | 51.5 |
| (Ocean Spray) crushed | 1 T. (.6 oz.) | 33 | 8.2 |
| **CRANBERRY SAUCE:** | | | |
| Home recipe (USDA), sweetened, unstrained | 4 oz. | 202 | 51.6 |
| Canned: | | | |
| (USDA) sweetened, strained | ½ cup (4.8 oz.) | 199 | 51.0 |
| (Ocean Spray): | | | |
| Jellied | 2 oz. | 89 | 21.8 |
| Whole berry | 2 oz. | 89 | 22.0 |
| **CRANBREAKER MIX** (Bar-Tender's) | ⅝-oz. serving | 70 | 17.4 |
| *CRANGRAPE,* drink (Ocean Spray) | 6 fl. oz. | 107 | 26.0 |
| *CRANICOT,* drink (Ocean Spray) | 6 fl. oz. | 109 | 26.4 |
| *CRANPRUNE JUICE DRINK* (Ocean Spray) | 6 fl. oz. | 117 | 28.8 |
| **CRAPPIE,** white, raw, meat only (USDA) | 4 oz. | 90 | 0. |
| **CRAYFISH,** freshwater (USDA): | | | |
| Raw, in shell | 1 lb. (weighed in shell) | 39 | .7 |

| Food and Description | Measure or Quantity | Calories | Carbo-hydrates (grams) |
|---|---|---|---|
| Raw, meat only | 4 oz. | 82 | 1.4 |
| **CRAZY COW**, cereal (General Mills): | | | |
| Chocolate | 1 cup (1 oz.) | 110 | 24.0 |
| Strawberry | 1 cup (1 oz.) | 110 | 25.0 |
| **CREAM** (See also **CREAM SUBSTITUTE**): | | | |
| Half & Half: | | | |
| (Meadow Gold) | 1 T. | 30 | .6 |
| (Sealtest) 10.5% fat | 1 T. | 18 | 1.0 |
| Light, table or coffee: | | | |
| (USDA) | 1 T. (.5 oz.) | 32 | .6 |
| (Sealtest) 16% fat | 1 T. (.5 oz.) | 26 | .6 |
| (Sealtest) 18% fat | 1 T. (.5 oz.) | 28 | .6 |
| Light whipping: | | | |
| (USDA) | 1 cup (8.4 oz.) | 717 | 8.6 |
| (USDA) | 1 T. (.5 oz.) | 45 | .5 |
| (Sealtest) 30% fat | 1 T. (.5 oz.) | 45 | 1.0 |
| Whipped topping, pressurized: | | | |
| (USDA) | 1 cup (2.1 oz.) | 155 | .6 |
| (USDA) | 1 T. (3 grams) | 10 | .1 |
| Heavy whipping: | | | |
| Unwhipped (USDA) | 1 cup (8.4 oz.) | 838 | 7.4 |
| (Dean) | 1 T. (.5 oz.) | 51 | .5 |
| (Sealtest) 36% fat | 1 T. (.5 oz.) | 52 | .5 |
| (Sealtest) 40% fat | 1 T. | 60 | .5 |
| Sour: | | | |
| (USDA) | 1 cup (8.1 oz.) | 485 | 9.9 |
| (Axelrod's) | 8-oz. container | 433 | 8.8 |
| (Dean) | 1 T. (.5 oz.) | 28 | .6 |
| (Sealtest) | 1 T. (.5 oz.) | 28 | .5 |
| Sour, imitation: | | | |
| (Dean) *Sour Slim* | 1 T. (1.1 oz.) | 30 | 3.3 |
| (Pet) | 1 T. (.5 oz.) | 25 | 1.0 |

(USDA): United States Department of Agriculture
(HEW/FAO): Health, Education and Welfare/Food and Agriculture
            Organization
* Prepared as Package Directs

| Food and Description | Measure or Quantity | Calories | Carbo-hydrates (grams) |
|---|---|---|---|
| **CREAMIES** (Tastykake): | | | |
| Chocolate | 1 piece | 257 | DNA |
| Spice | 1 piece | 272 | DNA |
| **CREAM PUFF**, home recipe | | | |
| (USDA) with custard filling | 3½″ x 2″ piece (4.6 oz.) | 303 | 26.7 |
| **CREAMSICLE** (Popsicle | | | |
| Industries) | 2½ fl. oz. | 78 | 12.8 |
| **CREAM SUBSTITUTE:** | | | |
| (USDA): | | | |
| Liquid, frozen | 1 T. (.5 oz.) | 20 | 2.0 |
| Powdered | 1 tsp. (2 grams) | 10 | 1.0 |
| (Alba) *Dairy Light* | 2.8-oz. envelope | 10 | 1.0 |
| (Carnation) *Coffee-mate* | 1 tsp. (1.9 grams) | 11 | 1.1 |
| *Coffee Rich*, frozen, liquid | ½ oz. | 22 | 2.1 |
| *N-Rich* | 1½ tsp. (3 grams) | 15 | 1.6 |
| (Pet) nondairy | 1 tsp. (2 grams) | 10 | 1.0 |
| *Poly Rich*, frozen, liquid | ½ oz. | 22 | 2.1 |
| **CREAM OF WHEAT**, cereal: | | | |
| Instant, dry | 2½ T. (1 oz.) | 100 | 21.0 |
| *Mix 'n Eat:* | | | |
| Regular | 1 packet (1 oz.) | 100 | 21.0 |
| Baked apple & cinnamon | 1¼-oz. packet | 130 | 29.0 |
| Banana & spice | 1½-oz. packet | 130 | 29.0 |
| Maple & brown sugar | 1½-oz packet | 130 | 29.0 |
| Quick, dry | 2½ T. (1 oz.) | 100 | 21.0 |
| Regular | 2½ T. (1 oz.) | 100 | 22.0 |
| **CREME DE BANANA** | | | |
| **LIQUEUR** (Mr. Boston) | 1 fl. oz. | 93 | 12.0 |
| **CREME DE CACAO** | | | |
| **LIQUEUR**, brown or white: | | | |
| (Garnier) | 1 fl. oz. | 97 | 13.1 |
| (Hiram Walker) | 1 fl. oz. | 104 | 15.0 |
| (Leroux) brown | 1 fl. oz. | 101 | 14.3 |
| (Leroux) white | 1 fl. oz. | 98 | 13.3 |
| (Mr. Boston) brown | 1 fl. oz. | 102 | 14.3 |
| (Mr. Boston) white | 1 fl. oz. | 93 | 12.0 |

| Food and Description | Measure or Quantity | Calories | Carbo-hydrates (grams) |
|---|---|---|---|
| **CREME DE CAFE LIQUEUR** | | | |
| (Leroux) 60 proof | 1 fl. oz. | 104 | 13.6 |
| **CREME DE CASSIS LIQUEUR:** | | | |
| (Garnier) 36 proof | 1 fl. oz. | 83 | 13.5 |
| (Leroux) | 1 fl. oz. | 88 | 14.9 |
| (Mr. Boston) | 1 fl. oz. | 85 | 14.1 |
| **CREME DE MENTHE LIQUEUR, green or white:** | | | |
| (Garnier) | 1 fl. oz. | 110 | 15.3 |
| (Hiram Walker) | 1 fl. oz. | 94 | 11.2 |
| (Leroux) green | 1 fl. oz. | 110 | 15.2 |
| (Leroux) white | 1 fl. oz. | 101 | 12.8 |
| (Mr. Boston) green | 1 fl. oz. | 109 | 16.0 |
| (Mr. Boston) white | 1 fl. oz. | 97 | 13.0 |
| **CREME DE NOYAUX LIQUEUR** (Mr. Boston) | 1 fl. oz. | 99 | 13.5 |
| **CREPE, frozen:** | | | |
| (Mrs. Paul's): | | | |
| Clam | 5½-oz. pkg. | 286 | 21.6 |
| Crab | 5½-oz. pkg. | 247 | 24.5 |
| Scallop | 5½-oz. pkg. | 220 | 25.2 |
| Shrimp | 5½-oz. pkg. | 252 | 23.8 |
| (Stouffer's): | | | |
| Beef burgundy | 6¼-oz. pkg. | 335 | 24.0 |
| Chicken with mushroom sauce | 8¼-oz. pkg. | 390 | 19.0 |
| Ham & asparagus | 6¼-oz. pkg. | 325 | 21.0 |
| Mushroom | 6¼-oz. pkg. | 255 | 27.0 |
| **CRISP RICE, CEREAL:** | | | |
| Regular: | | | |
| *Breakfast Best* | 1 cup (1 oz.) | 107 | 24.9 |

(USDA): United States Department of Agriculture
(HEW/FAO): Health, Education and Welfare/Food and Agriculture Organization
\* Prepared as Package Directs

| Food and Description | Measure or Quantity | Calories | Carbo-hydrates (grams) |
|---|---|---|---|
| *Breakfast Best*, sugar toasted | ⅝ cup (1 oz.) | 108 | 25.3 |
| (Ralston Purina) | 1 cup (1 oz.) | 110 | 25.0 |
| *Rokeach* | 1 cup (1 oz.) | 107 | 24.9 |
| (Van Brode): | | | |
| Regular | 1 cup (1 oz.) | 107 | 24.9 |
| Cocoa-covered | ¾ cup (1 oz.) | 108 | 25.3 |
| Sugar toasted | ⅝ cup (1 oz.) | 108 | 25.3 |
| Low sodium: | | | |
| (Featherweight) | 1 cup (1 oz.) | 110 | 25.6 |
| *Nature Foods* | 1 cup (1 oz.) | 110 | 25.6 |
| (Van Brode) | 1 cup (1 oz.) | 110 | 25.6 |
| **CRISPY WHEATS 'N RAISINS,** cereal (General Mills) | ¾ cup (1 oz.) | 100 | 23.0 |
| **CROAKER** (USDA): | | | |
| Atlantic: | | | |
| Raw, whole | 1 lb. (weighed whole) | 148 | 0. |
| Raw, meat only | 4 oz. | 109 | 0. |
| Baked | 4 oz. | 151 | 0. |
| White, raw, meat only | 4 oz. | 95 | 0. |
| Yellowfin, raw, meat only | 4 oz. | 101 | 0. |
| **CROQUETTES,** frozen (Mrs. Paul's) seafood | 3-oz. piece | 180 | 23.9 |
| **CROUTON:** | | | |
| (Arnold): | | | |
| American style | ½ oz. | 66 | 8.7 |
| Bavarian rye | ½ oz. | 65 | 9.5 |
| Danish style | ½ oz. | 67 | 8.8 |
| English style | ½ oz. | 66 | 9.5 |
| French style | ½ oz. | 66 | 9.2 |
| Italian or Mexican style | ½ oz. | 66 | 9.1 |
| (Kellogg's) *Croutettes* | .7 oz. | 70 | 15.0 |
| **CRULLER (See DOUGHNUT)** | | | |
| **CUCUMBER,** fresh (USDA): | | | |
| Eaten with skin | ½ lb. (weighed whole) | 32 | 7.4 |

| Food and Description | Measure or Quantity | Calories | Carbo-hydrates (grams) |
|---|---|---|---|
| Eaten without skin | ½ lb. (weighed with skin) | 23 | 5.3 |
| Unpared, 10-oz. cucumber | 7½" x 2" pared cucumber (7.3 oz.) | 29 | 6.6 |
| Pared | 6 slices (2" x ⅛") | 7 | 1.6 |
| Pared and diced | ½ cup (2.5 oz.) | 10 | 2.3 |
| **CUMIN SEED** (French's) | 1 tsp. (1.6 oz.) | 7 | .7 |
| **CUPCAKE:** | | | |
| Home recipe (USDA): | | | |
| Without icing | 1.4-oz. cupcake | 146 | 22.4 |
| With chocolate icing | 1.8-oz. cupcake | 184 | 29.7 |
| With boiled white icing | 1.8-oz. cupcake | 176 | 30.9 |
| With uncooked white icing | 1.8-oz. cupcake | 184 | 31.6 |
| Commercial type: | | | |
| Chocolate: | | | |
| (Hostess) | 1¾-oz. cupcake | 166 | 29.9 |
| (Tastykake) | 1 oz. cupcake | 100 | DNA |
| (Tastykake) creme-filled | 1.12-oz. cupcake | 122 | DNA |
| Chocolate buttercream (Tastykake) | 1.13-oz. cupcake | 120 | DNA |
| Frozen: | | | |
| Chocolate (Sara Lee): | | | |
| Regular | 1 cupcake | 196 | 27.5 |
| Double chocolate | 1 cupcake | 197 | 26.8 |
| Yellow (Sara Lee) | 1 cupcake | 180 | 27.9 |
| ***CUPCAKE MIX** (Flako) | ¹⁄₁₂ of pkg. | 150 | 25.0 |
| **CURACAO LIQUEUR:** | | | |
| (Bols) blue, 64 proof | 1 fl. oz. | 105 | 10.3 |
| (Bols) orange, 64 proof | 1 fl. oz. | 100 | 8.8 |
| (Garnier) 60 proof | 1 fl. oz. | 100 | 12.7 |
| (Hiram Walker) 60 proof | 1 fl. oz. | 84 | 9.5 |
| (Leroux) 60 proof | 1 fl. oz. | 84 | 9.5 |

(USDA): United States Department of Agriculture
(HEW/FAO): Health, Education and Welfare/Food and Agriculture Organization
* Prepared as Package Directs

| Food and Description | Measure or Quantity | Calories | Carbohydrates (grams) |
|---|---|---|---|
| **CURRANT:** | | | |
| Fresh (USDA): | | | |
| Black European: | | | |
| Whole | 1 lb. (weighed with stems) | 240 | 58.2 |
| Stems removed | 4 oz. | 61 | 14.9 |
| Red and white: | | | |
| Whole | 1 lb. (weighed with stems) | 220 | 53.2 |
| Stems removed | 1 cup (3.9 oz.) | 55 | 13.3 |
| Dried (Del Monte) Zante | ½ cup (2.4 oz.) | 204 | 47.8 |
| **CURRANT JELLY** (Smucker's) | 1 T. (.7 oz.) | 53 | 13.5 |
| **CURRANT PRESERVE or JAM** (Smucker's) | 1 T. | 53 | 13.5 |
| **CUSTARD:** | | | |
| Home recipe (USDA) baked | ½ cup (4.7 oz.) | 152 | 14.7 |
| Chilled, *Swiss Miss:* | | | |
| Custard flavor | 4 oz. | 160 | 24.0 |
| Egg flavor | 4 oz. | 160 | 22.0 |
| **CUSTARD APPLE,** bullock's-heart, raw (USDA): | | | |
| Whole | 1 lb. (weighed with skin & seeds) | 266 | 66.3 |
| Flesh only | 4 oz. | 115 | 28.6 |
| **CUSTARD PIE** (See PIE, Custard) | | | |
| **C.W. POST,** cereal: | | | |
| Family style | ¼ cup (1 oz.) | 131 | 20.3 |
| Family style with raisins | ¼ cup (1 oz.) | 128 | 20.4 |

| Food and Description | Measure or Quantity | Calories | Carbo- hydrates (grams) |
|---|---|---|---|

# D

**DAIQUIRI COCKTAIL:**
| | | | |
|---|---|---|---|
| (Hiram Walker) 52.5 proof | 3 fl. oz. | 177 | 12.0 |
| (Mr. Boston) 12½% alcohol | 3 fl. oz. | 99 | 9.0 |
| Mr. Boston) strawberry, 12½% alcohol | 3 fl. oz. | 111 | 12.0 |
| (National Distillers) *Duet,* 12% alcohol | 8-fl.-oz. can | 280 | 24.0 |
| (Party Tyme) banana, 12.5% alcohol | 2 fl. oz. | 66 | 5.7 |
| Dry Mix: | | | |
| (Bar-Tender's) | ⅝-oz. serving | 70 | 17.2 |
| (Holland House) | .6-oz. pkg. | 69 | 7.0 |
| (Holland House) banana | .6-oz. pkg. | 66 | 16.0 |

**DAMSON PLUM (See PLUM)**

**DANDELION GREENS, raw (USDA):**
| | | | |
|---|---|---|---|
| Trimmed | 1 lb. | 204 | 41.7 |
| Boiled, drained | ½ cup (3.2 oz.) | 30 | 5.8 |

**DANISH RINGS (Kellogg's):**
| | | | |
|---|---|---|---|
| Blueberry | 1½-oz. piece | 180 | 32.0 |
| Cherry | 1½-oz. piece | 180 | 31.0 |
| Dutch apple | 1½-oz. piece | 180 | 31.0 |
| Strawberry | 1½-oz. piece | 180 | 31.0 |

**DATE, dry:**
Domestic:
(USDA):
| | | | |
|---|---|---|---|
| With pits | 1 lb. (weighed with pits) | 1081 | 287.7 |
| Without pits | 4 oz. | 311 | 82.7 |
| Without pits, chopped | 1 cup (6.1 oz.) | 477 | 126.8 |

(USDA): United States Department of Agriculture
(HEW/FAO): Health, Education and Welfare/Food and Agriculture Organization
* Prepared as Package Directs

| Food and Description | Measure or Quantity | Calories | Carbo-hydrates (grams) |
|---|---|---|---|
| (Cal-Date): | | | |
| Whole | 1 date (.8 oz.) | 62 | 16.4 |
| Diced | 2 oz. | 161 | 42.8 |
| (Dromedary): | | | |
| Chopped | ½ cup (2.5 oz.) | 260 | 62.0 |
| Pitted | 1 date | 20 | 4.6 |
| Imported (Bordo) Iraq: | | | |
| Diced | ½ cup (2 oz.) | 159 | 39.8 |
| Whole | 4 average dates (.9 oz.) | 73 | 18.2 |
| DE CHAUNAC WINE (Great Western) 12% alcohol | 3 fl. oz. | 71 | 2.4 |
| DEVIL'S FOOD CAKE (See CAKE, Devil's Food) | | | |
| DEWBERRY, fresh (See BLACKBERRY, fresh) | | | |
| DILL SEED (French's) | 1 tsp. (2.1 grams) | 9 | 1.2 |
| *DING DONG* (Hostess) | 1.3-oz. cake | 170 | 21.1 |
| DIP: | | | |
| Avocado (Nalley's) | ½ oz. | 57 | .4 |
| Bacon & onion (Nalley's) | ½ oz. | 57 | .5 |
| Barbecue (Nalley's) | ½ oz. | 57 | .5 |
| Blue cheese: | | | |
| (Dean) tang | 1 oz. | 61 | 2.3 |
| (Nalley's) | 1 oz. | 110 | .9 |
| Cheese-bacon (Nalley's) | 1 oz. | 119 | .8 |
| Clam (Nalley's) | 1 oz. | 101 | 1.1 |
| Dill pickle (Nalley's) | 1 oz. | 86 | .9 |
| Enchilada, *Fritos* | 1 oz. | 37 | 3.9 |
| Garlic: | | | |
| (Dean) | 1 oz. | 58 | 2.0 |
| (Nalley's) | 1 oz. | 120 | .9 |
| Guacamole (Nalley's) | 1 oz. | 114 | .9 |
| Jalapeno: | | | |
| *Fritos* | 1 oz. | 34 | 3.7 |
| (Nalley's) | 1 oz. | 109 | .8 |
| Onion: | | | |
| (Breakstone) | 1 T. (.5 oz.) | 29 | 1.0 |

| Food and Description | Measure or Quantity | Calories | Carbo-hydrates (grams) |
|---|---|---|---|
| (Dean) French | 1 oz. | 58 | 2.0 |
| (Nalley's) French | 1 oz. | 106 | 1.4 |
| (Sealtest) | 1 oz. | 60 | 1.5 |
| Ranch house (Nalley's) | 1 oz. | 121 | .6 |
| **DISTILLED LIQUOR.** The values below would apply to unflavored bourbon whiskey, brandy, Canadian whiskey, gin, Irish whiskey, rum, rye, whiskey, Scotch whiskey, tequila and vodka. The caloric content of distilled liquors depends on the percentage of alcohol. The proof is twice the alcohol percent and the following values apply to all brands (USDA): | | | |
| 80 proof | 1 fl. oz. | 65 | Tr. |
| 86 proof | 1 fl. oz. | 70 | Tr. |
| 90 proof | 1 fl. oz. | 74 | Tr. |
| 94 proof | 1 fl. oz. | 77 | Tr. |
| 100 proof | 1 fl. oz. | 83 | Tr. |
| **DOCK,** including **SHEEP SORREL** (USDA): | | | |
| Raw, whole | 1 lb. (weighed untrimmed) | 89 | 17.8 |
| Boiled, drained | 4 oz. | 22 | 4.4 |
| **DOLLY VARDEN,** raw, meat & skin (USDA) | 4 oz. | 163 | 0. |
| **DOUGHNUT:** (USDA): | | | |
| Cake type | 1.1-oz. piece | 125 | 16.4 |

(USDA): United States Department of Agriculture
(HEW/FAO): Health, Education and Welfare/Food and Agriculture
Organization
* Prepared as Package Directs

| Food and Description | Measure or Quantity | Calories | Carbo-hydrates (grams) |
|---|---|---|---|
| Yeast-leavened (Hostess): | .6-oz. piece | 83 | 8.6 |
| Cinnamon | 1-oz. piece | 111 | 14.5 |
| Enrobed | 1-oz. piece | 136 | 13.6 |
| Krunch | 1-oz. piece | 105 | 16.5 |
| Old fashioned | 1½-oz. piece | 177 | 19.6 |
| Plain | 1-oz. piece | 120 | 12.8 |
| Powdered | 1-oz. piece | 117 | 15.1 |
| Frozen (Morton): | | | |
| Bavarian creme | 2-oz. piece | 180 | 22.1 |
| Boston creme | 2.3-oz. piece | 208 | 28.5 |
| Chocolate iced | 1.5-oz. piece | 148 | 19.6 |
| Glazed | 1.5-oz. piece | 150 | 19.2 |
| Jelly | 1.8-oz. piece | 175 | 22.9 |
| Mini | 1.1-oz. piece | 122 | 16.0 |
| **DRAMBUIE LIQUEUR** (Hiram Walker) 80 proof | 1 fl. oz. | 110 | 11.0 |
| **DREAMSICLE** (Popsicle Industries) | 2½ fl. oz. | 70 | 13.1 |
| **DRUM,** raw (USDA): | | | |
| Freshwater: | | | |
| Whole | 1 lb. (weighed whole) | 143 | 0. |
| Meat only | 4 oz. | 137 | 0. |
| Red: | | | |
| Whole | 1 lb. (weighed whole) | 149 | 0. |
| Meat only | 4 oz. | 91 | 0. |
| **DUCK,** raw (USDA): | | | |
| Domesticated: | | | |
| Ready-to-cook | 1 lb. (weighed with bone) | 1213 | 0. |
| Meat only | 4 oz. | 187 | 0. |
| Wild: | | | |
| Dressed | 1 lb. (weighed dressed) | 613 | 0. |
| Meat only | 4 oz. | 156 | 0. |

| Food and Description | Measure or Quantity | Calories | Carbo-hydrates (grams) |
|---|---|---|---|
| **DUMPLINGS**, canned, dietetic: | | | |
| (Dia-Mel) stuffed with | | | |
| chicken | 8-oz. can | 200 | 28.0 |
| (Featherweight) with | | | |
| chicken | 8-oz. can | 170 | 18.0 |

E

| | | | |
|---|---|---|---|
| **ECLAIR:** | | | |
| Home recipe (USDA) with custard filling & chocolate icing | 4 oz. | 271 | 26.3 |
| Frozen (Rich's) chocolate | 2.6-oz. piece | 234 | 30.0 |
| **EEL** (USDA): | | | |
| Raw, meat only | 4 oz. | 264 | 0. |
| Smoked, meat only | 4 oz. | 374 | 0. |
| **EGG** (USDA) (See also **EGG SUBSTITUTE**): | | | |
| Chicken: | | | |
| Raw: | | | |
| White only | 1 large egg (1.2 oz.) | 17 | .3 |
| White only | 1 cup (9 oz.) | 130 | 2.0 |
| Yolk only | 1 large egg (.6 oz.) | 59 | .1 |
| Yolk only | 1 cup (8.5 oz.) | 835 | 1.4 |
| Whole, small | 1 egg (1.3 oz.) | 60 | .3 |
| Whole, medium | 1 egg (1.5 oz.) | 71 | .4 |
| Whole, large | 1 egg (1.8 oz.) | 81 | .4 |
| Whole | 1 cup (8.8 oz.) | 409 | 2.3 |
| Whole, extra large | 1 egg (2 oz.) | 94 | .5 |
| Whole, jumbo | 1 egg (2.3 oz.) | 105 | .6 |
| Cooked: | | | |
| Boiled | 1 large egg (1.8 oz.) | 81 | .4 |

(USDA): United States Department of Agriculture
(HEW/FAO): Health, Education and Welfare/Food and Agriculture
         Organization
* Prepared as Package Directs

| Food and Description | Measure or Quantity | Calories | Carbo-hydrates (grams) |
|---|---|---|---|
| Fried in butter | 1 large egg | 99 | .1 |
| Omelet, mixed with milk & cooked in fat | 1 large egg | 107 | 1.5 |
| Poached | 1 large egg | 78 | .4 |
| Scrambled, mixed with milk & cooked in fat | 1 large egg | 111 | 1.5 |
| Scrambled, mixed with milk & cooked in fat | 1 cup (7.8 oz.) | 381 | 5.3 |
| Dried: | | | |
| Whole | 1 cup (3.8 oz.) | 639 | 4.4 |
| White, powder | 1 oz. | 105 | 1.6 |
| Yolk | 1 cup (3.4 oz.) | 637 | 2.4 |
| Duck, raw | 1 egg (2.8 oz.) | 153 | .6 |
| Goose, raw | 1 egg (5.8 oz.) | 303 | 2.1 |
| Turkey, raw | 1 egg (3.1 oz.) | 150 | 1.5 |
| *EGG FOO YOUNG, frozen (Chun King) stir fry | ⅙ of pkg. | 45 | 3.0 |
| EGG MIX (Durkee): | | | |
| Omelet: | | | |
| With bacon | 1.3-oz. pkg. | 128 | 18.0 |
| *With bacon | ½ pkg. | 210 | 10.0 |
| Puffy | 1.3-oz. pkg. | 113 | 19.0 |
| *Puffy | ½ of pkg. | 302 | 10.5 |
| Western | 1.1-oz. pkg. | 110 | 20.0 |
| *Western | ½ of pkg. | 302 | 11.0 |
| Scrambled: | | | |
| With bacon | 1.3-oz. pkg. | 181 | 6.0 |
| Plain | .8-oz. pkg. | 124 | 4.0 |
| EGG NOG, dairy: | | | |
| (Meadow Gold) | ½ cup | 164 | 25.5 |
| (Sealtest): | | | |
| 6% fat | ½ cup (4.6 oz.) | 174 | 18.0 |
| 8% fat | ½ cup (4.6 oz.) | 192 | 17.3 |
| EGG NOG COCKTAIL (Mr. Boston) 15% alcohol | 3 fl. oz. | 180 | 18.9 |
| EGG NOG ICE CREAM (Breyer's) | ¼ pt. | 150 | 16.0 |

| Food and Description | Measure or Quantity | Calories | Carbo-hydrates (grams) |
|---|---|---|---|
| **EGGPLANT:** | | | |
| Raw (USDA) whole | 1 lb. (weighed untrimmed) | 92 | 20.6 |
| Boiled (USDA) drained, diced | 1 cup (7.1 oz.) | 38 | 8.2 |
| Frozen: | | | |
| (Mrs. Paul's): | | | |
| Parmigiana | ½ of 11-oz. pkg. | 259 | 21.5 |
| Slices, breaded and fried | ⅓ of 9-oz. pkg. | 199 | 21.3 |
| Sticks, breaded and fried | ½ of 7-oz. pkg. | 262 | 27.3 |
| (Weight Watchers) parmigiana | 13-oz. meal | 251 | 25.1 |
| **EGG ROLL, frozen:** | | | |
| (Chun King): | | | |
| Chicken | ½-oz. egg roll | 23 | 3.0 |
| Meat & shrimp | ½-oz. egg roll | 25 | 3.5 |
| Meat & shrimp | 2½-oz. egg roll | 65 | 10.0 |
| Shrimp | ½-oz. egg roll | 23 | 3.8 |
| (La Choy): | | | |
| Chicken | .4-oz. egg roll | 30 | 3.6 |
| Lobster | .4-oz. egg roll | 27 | 3.6 |
| Meat & shrimp | .2-oz. egg roll | 17 | 2.3 |
| Meat & shrimp | .4-oz. egg roll | 27 | 3.5 |
| Shrimp | .4-oz. egg roll | 26 | 3.7 |
| Shrimp | 2½-oz. egg roll | 108 | 14.9 |
| **EGG, SCRAMBLED, frozen** (Swanson) & sausage, with hashed brown potatoes | 6¼-oz. breakfast | 460 | 22.0 |
| **EGG SUBSTITUTE:** | | | |
| *Egg Beaters* (Fleischmann) | ¼ cup (2.1 oz.) | 40 | 3.0 |
| *Eggstra* (Tillie Lewis) | 1 large egg substitute | 54 | 4.0 |
| *Scramblers* (Morningstar Farms) | ¼ cup | 72 | 2.7 |
| *Second Nature* (Avoset) chilled | 3 T. (1½ fl. oz.) | 38 | 1.8 |

(USDA): United States Department of Agriculture
(HEW/FAO): Health, Education and Welfare/Food and Agriculture
          Organization
* Prepared as Package Directs

| Food and Description | Measure or Quantity | Calories | Carbo-hydrates (grams) |
|---|---|---|---|
| **ELDERBERRY, fresh (USDA):** | | | |
| Whole | 1 lb. (weighed with stems) | 307 | 69.9 |
| Stems removed | 4 oz. | 82 | 18.6 |
| **ELDERBERRY JELLY** (Smucker's) | 1 T. (.7 oz.) | 53 | 13.5 |
| **ELDERBERRY PRESERVE or JAM** (Smucker's) | 1 T. | 53 | 13.5 |
| **ENCHILADA, frozen:** | | | |
| Beef: | | | |
| (Banquet) with sauce, cooking bag | 2 enchiladas with sauce | 207 | 28.9 |
| (Banquet) with cheese and chili gravy, buffet | 2-lb. pkg. | 1118 | 118.2 |
| Cheese (Van de Kamp's) with sauce | 7½-oz. pkg. | 330 | 19.0 |
| Chicken (Van de Kamp's) with sauce | 7½-oz. pkg. | 270 | 21.0 |
| **ENCHILADA DINNER,** frozen: | | | |
| Beef: | | | |
| (Banquet) | 12-oz. dinner | 479 | 63.8 |
| (Morton) | 12-oz. dinner | 351 | 47.7 |
| (Swanson) | 15-oz. dinner | 570 | 72.0 |
| (Van de Kamp's) | 12-oz. dinner | 420 | 41.0 |
| Cheese: | | | |
| (Banquet) | 12-oz. dinner | 459 | 58.8 |
| (Van de Kamp's) | 12-oz. dinner | 430 | 38.0 |
| **ENDIVE, BELGIAN or FRENCH (See CHICORY, WITLOOF)** | | | |
| **ENDIVE, CURLY,** raw (USDA): | | | |
| Untrimmed | 1 lb. (weighed untrimmed) | 80 | 16.4 |
| Trimmed | ½ lb. | 45 | 9.3 |
| Cut up or shredded | 1 cup (2.5 oz.) | 14 | 2.9 |

| Food and Description | Measure or Quantity | Calories | Carbohydrates (grams) |
|---|---|---|---|
| **ESCAROLE, raw (USDA):** | | | |
| Untrimmed | 1 lb. (weighed untrimmed) | 80 | 16.4 |
| Trimmed | ½ lb. | 46 | 9.2 |
| Cut up or shredded | 1 cup (2.5 oz.) | 14 | 2.9 |
| **ESCAROLE SOUP,** canned (Progresso) in chicken broth | 1 cup | 25 | 1.0 |
| **EULACHON or SMELT,** raw (USDA) meat only | 4 oz. | 134 | 0. |
| ***EXPRESSO COFFEE LIQUEUR*** | 1 fl. oz. | 104 | 15.0 |
| **EXTRACT** (See individual listings) | | | |

**F**

| | | | |
|---|---|---|---|
| **FARINA** (See also **CREAM OF WHEAT**): | | | |
| Regular: | | | |
| Dry: | | | |
| (USDA) | 1 cup (6 oz.) | 627 | 130.1 |
| (H-O) cream, enriched | 1 cup (6.1 oz.) | 625 | 133.8 |
| (H-O) cream, enriched | 1 T. | 41 | 8.8 |
| *Malt-O-Meal* | 1 oz. | 97 | 21.0 |
| Cooked: | | | |
| *(USDA) | 1 cup (8.4 oz.) | 100 | 20.7 |
| *(USDA) | 4 oz. | 48 | 9.9 |
| *(Pillsbury): | | | |
| Made with milk and salt | ⅔ cup | 200 | 26.0 |
| Made with water and salt | ⅔ cup | 80 | 2.0 |

(USDA): United States Department of Agriculture
(HEW/FAO): Health, Education and Welfare/Food and Agriculture Organization
* Prepared as Package Directs

| Food and Description | Measure or Quantity | Calories | Carbo-hydrates (grams) |
|---|---|---|---|
| Quick-cooking: | | | |
| Dry (USDA) | 1 oz. | 103 | 21.2 |
| Dry, *Malt-O-Meal* | 1 oz. | 101 | 22.2 |
| Cooked (USDA) | 1 cup (8.6 oz.) | 105 | 21.8 |
| Instant-cooking (USDA): | | | |
| Dry | 1 oz. | 103 | 21.2 |
| Cooked | 4 oz. | 62 | 12.9 |
| **FAT, COOKING,** vegetable: | | | |
| (USDA) | 1 cup (7.1 oz.) | 1768 | 0. |
| (USDA) | 1 T. (.4 oz.) | 106 | 0. |
| *Crisco* | 1 T. (.4 oz.) | 110 | 0. |
| *Fluffo* | 1 T. (.4 oz.) | 110 | 0. |
| *Mrs. Tucker's* | 1 T. | 120 | 0. |
| *Snowdrift* | 1 T. | 110 | 0. |
| *Spry* | 1 T. (.4 oz.) | 95 | 0. |
| **FENNEL LEAVES,** raw (USDA): | | | |
| Untrimmed | 1 lb. (weighed untrimmed) | 118 | 21.5 |
| Trimmed | 4 oz. | 32 | 5.8 |
| **FENNEL SEED** (French's) | 1 tsp. (2.1 grams) | 8 | 1.3 |
| **FIG:** | | | |
| Fresh (USDA): | | | |
| Regular size | 1 lb. | 363 | 92.1 |
| Small | 1.3-oz. fig (1½" dia.) | 30 | 7.7 |
| Candied (Bama) | 1 T. (.7 oz.) | 37 | 9.6 |
| Canned, regular pack, solids & liq.: | | | |
| (USDA): | | | |
| Light syrup | 4 oz. | 74 | 19.1 |
| Heavy syrup | 3 figs & 2 T. syrup (4 oz.) | 96 | 24.9 |
| Heavy syrup | ½ cup (4.4 oz.) | 106 | 27.5 |
| Extra heavy syrup | 4 oz. | 117 | 30.3 |
| (Del Monte) whole | ½ cup (4.3 oz.) | 114 | 28.1 |
| Canned, unsweetened or dietetic pack: | | | |
| (USDA) water pack, solids & liq. | 4 oz. | 54 | 14.1 |

| Food and Description | Measure or Quantity | Calories | Carbo-hydrates (grams) |
|---|---|---|---|
| (Diet Delight) Kadota, solids & liq. | ½ cup (4.4 oz.) | 76 | 18.2 |
| (Featherweight) Kadota, water pack, solids & liq. | ½ cup | 60 | 15.0 |
| Dried (USDA): | | | |
| Chopped | 1 cup (6 oz.) | 469 | 118.2 |
| Whole | .7-oz. fig (2" x 1") | 58 | 14.5 |
| **FIG JUICE,** *Real Fig* | ½ cup (4.5 oz.) | 61 | 15.8 |
| **FIGURINES** (Pillsbury) all flavors | 1 bar | 138 | 10.5 |
| **FILBERT or HAZELNUT** (USDA): | | | |
| Whole | 4 oz. (weighed in shell) | 331 | 8.7 |
| Shelled | 1 oz. | 180 | 4.7 |
| **FISH** (See individual listing) | | | |
| **FISH AU GRATIN,** frozen (Mrs. Paul's) | ½ of 10-oz. pkg. | 248 | 19.5 |
| **FISH CAKE:** | | | |
| Home recipe (USDA) fried | 2 oz. | 98 | 5.3 |
| Frozen (Mrs. Paul's): | | | |
| Breaded and fried | 2-oz. cake | 105 | 11.9 |
| Thins, breaded and fried | ½ of 10-oz. pkg. | 326 | 30.7 |
| **FISH & CHIPS,** frozen: | | | |
| (Mrs. Paul's) batter fried | ½ of 14-oz. pkg. | 366 | 43.4 |
| (Swanson): | | | |
| Dinner | 10¼-oz. dinner | 450 | 40.0 |
| Dinner, *Hungry Man* | 15¾-oz. dinner | 760 | 68.0 |
| Entree | 5-oz. entree | 290 | 25.0 |
| (Van de Kamp's) batter dipped, french-fried | 8-oz. serving | 500 | 45.0 |

(USDA): United States Department of Agriculture
(HEW/FAO): Health, Education and Welfare/Food and Agriculture Organization
* Prepared as Package Directs

| Food and Description | Measure or Quantity | Calories | Carbo- hydrates (grams) |
|---|---|---|---|
| **FISH DINNER,** frozen: | | | |
| (Banquet) | 8¾-oz. dinner | 382 | 43.6 |
| (Morton) | 9-oz. dinner | 253 | 20.5 |
| (Van de Kamp's) batter dipped, french-fried | 11-oz. dinner | 540 | 39.0 |
| **FISH FILLET,** frozen: | | | |
| (Mrs. Paul's): | | | |
| Batter fried | 2½-oz. piece | 142 | 14.1 |
| Breaded and fried | ½ of 8-oz. pkg. | 227 | 24.1 |
| Buttered | 2½-oz. piece | 155 | .9 |
| Miniature, light batter fried | ⅓ of 9-oz. pkg. | 154 | 15.3 |
| Parmesan | ½ of 10-oz. pkg. | 230 | 20.9 |
| (Van de Kamp's): | | | |
| Batter dipped, french- fried | 3-oz. piece | 220 | 12.5 |
| Country seasoned | 2.4-oz. piece | 180 | 10.5 |
| **FISH FILLET DINNER,** frozen (Van de Kamp's) batter dipped, french-fried | 13-oz. dinner | 300 | 25.0 |
| **FISH FLAKES,** canned (USDA) | 4 oz. | 126 | 0. |
| **FISH KABOBS,** frozen: | | | |
| (Mrs. Paul's) supreme light batter | ⅓ of 10-oz. pkg. | 200 | 18.0 |
| (Van de Kamp's) batter dipped, french-fried | .4-oz. piece | 26 | 1.6 |
| (Van de Kamp's) country seasoned | .4-oz. piece | 29 | 1.9 |
| **FISH LOAF,** home recipe (USDA) | 4 oz. | 141 | 8.3 |
| **FISH STICK,** frozen: | | | |
| (USDA) cooked, commercial, 3¾" x 1" x ½" sticks | 10 sticks (8-oz. pkg.) | 400 | 14.8 |

| Food and Description | Measure or Quantity | Calories | Carbo- hydrates (grams) |
|---|---|---|---|
| (Mrs. Paul's): | | | |
| Batter-fried | 1 stick (.9 oz.) | 55 | 5.5 |
| Breaded and fried | 1 stick (.75 oz.) | 43 | 4.1 |
| (Van de Kamp's) batter dipped, french-fried | 1-oz. piece | 62 | 3.2 |
| **FIT 'N FROSTY** (Alba '77), instant milk shake mix: | | | |
| Chocolate | .75-oz. envelope | 74 | 11.5 |
| Chocolate and marshmallow | 1 envelope | 70 | 11.0 |
| Strawberry | 1 envelope | 74 | 12.0 |
| Vanilla | 1 envelope | 69 | 11.3 |
| **\*FIVE ALIVE,** drink, chilled or frozen (Snow Crop) | 6 fl. oz. | 85 | 20.8 |
| **FLAN PUDDING** (See PUDDING, FLAN) | | | |
| **FLOUNDER:** | | | |
| Raw (USDA): | | | |
| Whole | 1 lb. (weighed whole) | 118 | 0. |
| Meat only | 4 oz. | 90 | 0. |
| Baked (USDA) | 4 oz. | 229 | 0. |
| Frozen: | | | |
| (Mrs. Paul's): | | | |
| Fillets, breaded and fried | 2-oz. fillet | 137 | 11.6 |
| Fillets, with lemon butter | ½ of 8½-oz. pkg. | 154 | 9.4 |
| (Weight Watchers): | | | |
| 2-compartment meal | 8½ oz. | 169 | 13.0 |
| 3-compartment meal | 16 oz. | 261 | 14.1 |
| **FLOUR:** | | | |
| (USDA): | | | |
| Buckwheat, dark, sifted | 1 cup (3.5 oz.) | 326 | 70.6 |

(USDA): United States Department of Agriculture
(HEW/FAO): Health, Education and Welfare/Food and Agriculture Organization
\* Prepared as Package Directs

| Food and Description | Measure or Quantity | Calories | Carbo-hydrates (grams) |
|---|---|---|---|
| Buckwheat, light, sifted | 1 cup (3.5 oz.) | 340 | 77.9 |
| Carob or St. John's-bread | 1 oz. | 51 | 22.9 |
| Chestnut | 1 oz. | 103 | 21.6 |
| Corn | 1 cup (3.9) | 405 | 84.5 |
| Cottonseed | 1 oz. | 101 | 9.4 |
| Fish, from whole fish | 1 oz. | 95 | 0. |
| Lima bean | 1 oz. | 97 | 17.9 |
| Potato | 1 oz. | 100 | 22.7 |
| Rice, stirred, spooned | 1 cup (5.6 oz.) | 574 | 125.6 |
| Rye: | | | |
|   Light: | | | |
|     Unsifted, spooned | 1 cup (3.6 oz.) | 361 | 78.7 |
|     Sifted, spooned | 1 cup (3.1 oz.) | 314 | 68.6 |
|   Medium: | 1 oz. | 99 | 21.2 |
|   Dark: | | | |
|     Unstirred | 1 cup (4.5 oz.) | 419 | 87.2 |
|     Stirred | 1 cup (4.5 oz.) | 415 | 86.5 |
| Soybean, defatted, stirred | 1 cup (3.6 oz.) | 329 | 38.5 |
| Soybean, high fat | 1 oz. | 108 | 9.4 |
| Sunflower seed, partially defatted | 1 oz. | 96 | 10.7 |
| Wheat: | | | |
|   All-purpose: | | | |
|     Unsifted, dipped | 1 cup (5 oz.) | 521 | 108.8 |
|     Unsifted, spooned | 1 cup (4.4 oz.) | 459 | 95.9 |
|     Sifted, spooned | 1 cup (4.1 oz.) | 422 | 88.3 |
|   Bread: | | | |
|     Unsifted, dipped | 1 cup (4.8 oz.) | 496 | 101.6 |
|     Unsifted, spooned | 1 cup (4.3 oz.) | 449 | 91.9 |
|     Sifted, spooned | 1 cup (4.1 oz.) | 427 | 87.4 |
|   Cake: | | | |
|     Unsifted, dipped | 1 cup (4.2 oz.) | 433 | 94.5 |
|     Unsifted, spooned | 1 cup (3.9 oz.) | 404 | 88.1 |
|     Sifted, spooned | 1 cup (3.5 oz.) | 360 | 78.6 |
|   Gluten: | | | |
|     Unsifted, dipped | 1 cup (5 oz.) | 537 | 67.0 |
|     Unsifted, spooned | 1 cup (4.8 oz.) | 510 | 63.7 |
|     Sifted, spooned | 1 cup (4.8 oz.) | 514 | 64.2 |
|   Self-rising: | | | |
|     Unsifted, dipped | 1 cup (4.6 oz.) | 458 | 96.5 |
|     Unsifted, spooned | 1 cup (4.5 oz.) | 447 | 94.2 |
|     Sifted, spooned | 1 cup (3.7 oz.) | 373 | 78.7 |
| Whole wheat | 1 oz. | 94 | 20.1 |

| Food and Description | Measure or Quantity | Calories | Carbo-hydrates (grams) |
|---|---|---|---|
| (Aunt Jemima) self-rising | ¼ cup (1 oz.) | 109 | 23.6 |
| *Ballard*, all-purpose | 1 cup | 400 | 87.0 |
| *Ballard*, self-rising | 1 cup | 380 | 84.0 |
| *Bisquick* (Betty Crocker) | ½ cup | 240 | 38.0 |
| *Gold Medal* (Betty Crocker) all-purpose | 1 cup | 483 | 100.7 |
| *Gold Medal* (Betty Crocker) self-rising | 1 cup | 476 | 100.5 |
| (Pillsbury) | | | |
| All-purpose | 1 cup | 400 | 87.0 |
| Instant blending | 1 cup | 50 | 11.0 |
| Medium rye | 1 cup | 420 | 89 |
| Self-rising | 1 cup | 380 | 84.0 |
| Unbleached | 1 cup | 400 | 86.0 |
| Whole wheat | 1 cup | 400 | 86.0 |
| *Presto*, self-rising | 1 cup (3.9 oz.) | 399 | 87.8 |
| *Robin Hood*, all-purpose | 1 cup (4 oz.) | 400 | 85.0 |
| *Robin Hood*, self-rising | 1 cup (4 oz.) | 380 | 81.0 |
| (Swans Down) cake | ¼ cup | 100 | 22.0 |
| (Swans Down) cake, self-rising | ¼ cup | 90 | 20.0 |
| **FOOD STICKS** (Pillsbury) all flavors | 1 stick | 45 | 6.8 |
| **FOUR FRUIT PRESERVE** (Smucker's) | 1 T. | 53 | 13.5 |
| **FRANKEN*BERRY**, cereal General Mills | 1 cup | 110 | 24.0 |
| **FRANKFURTER**, raw or cooked: (USDA): | | | |
| Raw, all kinds | 1 frankfurter (10 per lb.) | 140 | .8 |
| Raw, meat | 1 frankfurter (10 per lb.) | 134 | 1.1 |

(USDA): United States Department of Agriculture
(HEW/FAO): Health, Education and Welfare/Food and Agriculture Organization
* Prepared as Package Directs

| Food and Description | Measure or Quantity | Calories | Carbohydrates (grams) |
|---|---|---|---|
| Raw, with cereal | 1 frankfurter (10 per lb.) | 112 | <.1 |
| Cooked, all kinds | 1 frankfurter (10 per lb.) | 136 | .7 |
| (Eckrich): | | | |
| Beef or meat | 1.6-oz. frankfurter | 150 | 3.0 |
| Beef or meat, jumbo | 2-oz. frankfurter | 190 | 3.0 |
| Meat | 1.2-oz. frankfurter | 120 | 2.0 |
| (Hormel): | | | |
| Beef | 1.2-oz. frankfurter | 104 | .5 |
| Beef, smoked, *Range Brand Wranglers* | 1 frankfurter | 175 | 2.0 |
| Meat | 1.2-oz. frankfurter | 104 | .5 |
| Smoked, *Range Brand Wranglers* | 1.6-oz. frankfurter | 180 | 1.0 |
| (Hygrade): | | | |
| Beef | 1.6-oz. frankfurter | 146 | 1.4 |
| Beef, *Ball Park* | 2-oz. frankfurter | 169 | <.1 |
| Meat | 1.6-oz. frankfurter | 147 | 1.5 |
| Meat, *Ball Park* | 2-oz. frankfurter | 175 | <.1 |
| (Oscar Mayer): | | | |
| Beef | 1.6-oz. frankfurter | 144 | 1.4 |
| Beef | 2-oz. frankfurter | 180 | 1.8 |
| Little wiener | .3-oz. weiner | 30 | .2 |
| *Machiach* Brand | 2-oz. frankfurter | 179 | 1.8 |
| Wiener | 1.6-oz. frankfurter | 145 | 1.3 |
| Wiener | 2-oz. frankfurter | 184 | 1.6 |
| (Swift) | 1.6-oz. frankfurter | 150 | 1.2 |
| (Vienna) beef | 1 frankfurter | 132 | 1.0 |
| Canned (USDA) | 2 oz. | 125 | .1 |

**FRANKS AND BEANS (See BEANS & FRANKFURTERS**

| Food and Description | Measure or Quantity | Calories | Carbohydrates (grams) |
|---|---|---|---|
| **FRANKS-IN-BLANKETS,** frozen (Durkee) | 1 piece | 45 | 1.0 |
| **FRENCH TOAST,** frozen: (Aunt Jemima): | | | |
| Regular | 1.5-oz. slice | 85 | 13.2 |
| Cinnamon swirl | 1.5-oz. slice | 97 | 13.7 |
| (Eggo) | 1.5-oz. slice | 80 | 12.0 |
| (Swanson) with sausage | 4½-oz. breakfast | 300 | 22.0 |
| **FRITTER:** Clam: | | | |
| Home recipe (USDA) | 2″ x 1¾″ fritter (1.4 oz.) | 124 | 12.4 |
| Frozen (Mrs. Paul's) light batter fried | ½ of 7¾-oz. pkg. | 260 | 28.0 |
| Corn, frozen (Mrs. Paul's) | 2-oz. fritter | 130 | 15.4 |
| Crab, frozen (Mrs. Paul's) light batter fried | ½ of 7¾-oz. pkg. | 250 | 30.0 |
| Shrimp, frozen (Mrs. Paul's) light batter fried | ½ of 7¾-oz. pkg. | 240 | 26.0 |
| Tuna, frozen (Mrs. Paul's) light batter fried | ½ of 7¾-oz. pkg. | 270 | 27.0 |
| **FROG LEGS,** raw (USDA): | | | |
| Bone in | 1 lb. (weighed with bone) | 215 | 0. |
| Meat only | 4 oz. | 83 | 0. |
| **FROOT LOOPS,** cereal (Kellogg's) | 1 cup (1 oz.) | 110 | 25.0 |
| **FROSTED RICE,** cereal (Kellogg's) | 1 cup (1 oz.) | 110 | 26.0 |
| **FROSTING (See CAKE ICING)** | | | |

(USDA): United States Department of Agriculture
(HEW/FAO): Health, Education and Welfare/Food and Agriculture
    Organization
* Prepared as Package Directs

| Food and Description | Measure or Quantity | Calories | Carbo-hydrates (grams) |
|---|---|---|---|
| **FROSTY O's,** cereal (General Mills) | 1 cup (1 oz.) | 110 | 24.0 |
| **FROZEN CUSTARD** (See **ICE CREAM**) | | | |
| **FRUIT BITS,** dried (Sun-Maid) | 2-oz. serving | 150 | 40.0 |
| **FRUIT BRUTE,** cereal (General Mills) | 1 cup (1 oz.) | 110 | 24.0 |
| **FRUIT CAKE** (See **CAKE, Fruit**) | | | |
| **FRUIT COCKTAIL:** | | | |
| Canned, regular pack, solids & liq.: | | | |
| (USDA): | | | |
| Light syrup | 4 oz. | 68 | 17.8 |
| Heavy syrup | ½ cup (4.5 oz.) | 97 | 25.2 |
| Extra heavy syrup | 4 oz. | 104 | 26.9 |
| (Del Monte) heavy syrup, regular or chunky fruit | ½ cup | 95 | 23.1 |
| (Libby's) heavy syrup | ½ cup (4.5 oz.) | 101 | 24.7 |
| (Stokely-Van Camp) | ½ cup (4.5 oz.) | 95 | 23.0 |
| Canned, unsweetened or dietetic pack, solids & liq.: | | | |
| (USDA) water pack | 4 oz. | 42 | 11.0 |
| (Del Monte) *Lite* | ½ cup | 58 | 14.1 |
| (Diet Delight) syrup pack | ½ cup | 60 | 14.4 |
| (Diet Delight) water pack | ½ cup | 40 | 10.0 |
| (Featherweight) juice pack | ½ cup | 50 | 12.0 |
| (Libby's) water pack | ½ cup (4.3 oz.) | 44 | 10.4 |
| (Tillie Lewis) *Tasti Diet* | ½ cup (4.3 oz.) | 54 | 13.5 |
| **\*FRUIT COUNTRY** (Comstock): | | | |
| Apple | ¼ pkg. | 160 | 36.0 |

| Food and Description | Measure or Quantity | Calories | Carbo-hydrates (grams) |
|---|---|---|---|
| Blueberry | ¼ pkg. | 160 | 33.0 |
| Cherry | ¼ pkg. | 180 | 38.0 |
| Peach | ¼ pkg. | 130 | 28.0 |
| **FRUIT CUP** (Del Monte): | | | |
| Mixed, solids & liq. | 5-oz. container | 110 | 26.7 |
| Peaches, cling, diced, solids & liq. | 5-oz. container | 116 | 27.8 |
| **FRUIT JAM**, mixed (Smucker's) | 1 T. | 53 | 13.5 |
| **FRUIT, MIXED:** | | | |
| Canned, dietetic or low calorie (Del Monte) *Lite*, solids & liq. | ½ cup | 57 | 13.6 |
| Frozen (Birds Eye) quick thaw | ½ of 10-oz. pkg. | 143 | 34.5 |
| **FRUIT PUNCH:** | | | |
| Canned: | | | |
| (Ann Page) tropical | 1 cup (8.7 oz.) | 122 | 30.4 |
| (Hi-C) | 8 fl. oz. | 124 | 30.7 |
| (Lincoln) party | 8 fl. oz. | 139 | 34.8 |
| Chilled (Minute Maid) | 6 fl. oz. | 93 | 23.0 |
| **FRUIT ROLL**, frozen (La Choy) apple cinnamon | .5-oz. roll | 38 | 6.4 |
| **FRUIT SALAD:** | | | |
| Canned, regular pack, solids & liq.: | | | |
| (USDA): | | | |
| Light syrup | 4 oz. | 67 | 17.6 |
| Heavy syrup | ½ cup (4.3 oz.) | 85 | 22.0 |
| Extra heavy syrup | 4 oz. | 102 | 26.5 |
| (Del Monte): | | | |
| Fruit for salad | ½ cup (4.3 oz.) | 94 | 23.0 |

(USDA): United States Department of Agriculture
(HEW/FAO): Health, Education and Welfare/Food and Agriculture
　　　　　　　Organization
* Prepared as Package Directs

| Food and Description | Measure or Quantity | Calories | Carbo-hydrates (grams) |
|---|---|---|---|
| Tropical | ½ cup (4.4 oz.) | 107 | 26.0 |
| (Libby's) heavy syrup | ½ cup (4.4 oz.) | 99 | 24.0 |
| (Stokely-Van Camp) | ½ cup (4.5 oz.) | 95 | 22.0 |
| Canned, unsweetened or dietetic pack, solids & liq.: | | | |
| (USDA) water pack | 4 oz. | 40 | 10.3 |
| (Diet Delight) | ½ cup (4.4 oz.) | 68 | 16.3 |
| (Featherweight) juice | ½ cup | 50 | 12.0 |
| (Featherweight) water pack | ½ cup | 35 | 10.0 |
| **FUDGE ICE BAR** (Sealtest) | 2½ fl. oz. | 90 | 19.0 |
| **FUDGSICLE** (Popsicle Industries): | | | |
| Banana | 2½ fl. oz. | 102 | 23.5 |
| Chocolate | 2½ fl. oz. | 153 | 20.0 |
| ***FUNNY FACE** (Pillsbury) all flavors | 8 fl. oz. | 80 | 20.0 |

# G

| Food and Description | Measure or Quantity | Calories | Carbo-hydrates (grams) |
|---|---|---|---|
| **GARLIC,** raw (USDA): | | | |
| Whole | 2 oz. (weighed with skin) | 68 | 15.4 |
| Peeled | 1 oz. | 39 | 8.7 |
| **GARLIC FLAKES** (Gilroy) | 1 tsp. (1.5 grams) | 13 | 2.6 |
| **GARLIC POWDER** (Gilroy) | 1 tsp. | 10 | 2.0 |
| **GAZPACHO SOUP,** canned (Crosse & Blackwell) | ½ of 13-oz. can | 30 | 1.0 |
| **GELFILTE FISH,** canned (Manischewitz): | | | |
| 4-portion can | 3.8-oz. piece | 87 | 3.3 |
| 2-lb. jar | 3.5-oz. piece | 81 | 3.1 |
| Fish balls | 1.5-oz. piece | 40 | 1.6 |
| Fishlet | 7-gram piece | 6 | .2 |

| Food and Description | Measure or Quantity | Calories | Carbo- hydrates (grams) |
|---|---|---|---|
| **GELATIN,** unflavored, dry: | | | |
| (USDA) | 7-gram envelope | 23 | 0. |
| (Ann Page) | 7-gram envelope | 24 | 0. |
| **GELATIN DESSERT:** | | | |
| Powder: | | | |
| Regular: | | | |
| (USDA) | 3-oz. pkg. | 315 | 74.8 |
| *(USDA) | ½ cup (4.2 oz.) | 71 | 16.9 |
| *(USDA) with fruit added | ½ cup (4.2 oz.) | 81 | 19.8 |
| (Ann Page) all flavors | ¼ of 3-oz. pkg. | 82 | 19.0 |
| *(Jell-O) all fruit flavors | ½ cup (4.9 oz.) | 80 | 18.5 |
| *(Royal) all flavors | ½ cup (4.9 oz.) | 80 | 19.0 |
| Dietetic or low calorie: | | | |
| *(D-Zerta) all flavors | ½ cup (4.3 oz.) | 8 | .2 |
| *(Dia-Mel) *Gel-a-Thin,* all flavors | 4-oz. serving | 10 | 1.0 |
| *(Estee) all flavors | ½ cup | 40 | 9.0 |
| *(Featherweight) all flavors | 4-oz. serving | 35 | 7.0 |
| *(Featherweight) all flavors, artificially sweetened | 4-oz. serving | 10 | 0. |
| *(Louis Sherry) *Shimmer,* all flavors | ½ cup (4.4 oz.) | 10 | 1.0 |
| Canned, dietetic pack: | | | |
| (Dia-Mel) *Gel-a-Thin,* all flavors | 4-oz. container | 1 | .2 |
| **GELATIN DRINK** (Knox) orange | 1 envelope | 70 | 10.0 |
| **GERMAN DINNER,** frozen (Swanson) | 11¾-oz. dinner | 430 | 40.0 |
| **GIN,** unflavored (See **DISTILLED LIQUOR**) | | | |

(USDA): United States Department of Agriculture
(HEW/FAO): Health, Education and Welfare/Food and Agriculture Organization
* Prepared as Package Directs

| Food and Description | Measure or Quantity | Calories | Carbo-hydrates (grams) |
|---|---|---|---|
| **GINGERBREAD:** | | | |
| Home recipe (USDA) | 1.9-oz. piece (2" x 2" x 2") | 174 | 28.6 |
| Mix: | | | |
| (USDA) dry | 4 oz. | 482 | 88.7 |
| *(USDA) | ⅑ of 8" sq. (2.2 oz.) | 174 | 32.2 |
| *(Betty Crocker) | ⅑ of cake | 210 | 36.0 |
| *(Dromedary) | 2" x 2" sq. | 100 | 20.0 |
| *(Pillsbury) | 3" sq. | 190 | 36.0 |
| **GINGER, CANDIED** (USDA) | 1 oz. | 96 | 24.7 |
| **GINGER ROOT,** fresh (USDA): | | | |
| With skin | 1 oz. | 13 | 2.5 |
| (Without skin) | 1 oz. | 14 | 2.7 |
| **GIN, SLOE:** | | | |
| (DeKuyper) | 1 fl. oz. | 70 | 5.2 |
| (Garnier) | 1 fl. oz. | 83 | 8.5 |
| (Hiram Walker) | 1 fl. oz. | 68 | 4.8 |
| (Mr. Boston) | 1 fl. oz. | 68 | 4.7 |
| **GOLDEN GRAHAMS,** cereal (General Mills) | 1 cup (1 oz.) | 110 | 24.0 |
| **GOOBER GRAPE** (Smucker's) | 1-oz. serving | 125 | 14.0 |
| **GOOD HUMOR:** | | | |
| Chocolate eclair | 3-oz. piece | 220 | 25.0 |
| Sandwich | 2.5-oz. piece | 200 | 34.0 |
| Strawberry shortcake | 3-oz. piece | 200 | 21.0 |
| Toasted almond bar | 3-oz. piece | 170 | 25.0 |
| Vanilla, chocolate coated bar | 3-oz. piece | 170 | 12.0 |
| Whammy: | | | |
| Assorted | 1.6-oz. piece | 100 | 9.0 |
| Crisp crunch | 1.6-oz. piece | 110 | 10.0 |
| Vanilla | 1.4-oz. piece | 137 | 11.2 |
| Ice | 1.5-oz. piece | 50 | 13.0 |

| Food and Description | Measure or Quantity | Calories | Carbohydrates (grams) |
|---|---|---|---|
| **GOOSE**, domesticated (USDA): | | | |
| Raw | 1 lb. (weighed ready-to-cook) | 1172 | 0. |
| Roasted, meat & skin | 4 oz. | 500 | 0. |
| Roasted, meat only | 4 oz. | 264 | 0. |
| **GOOSEBERRY** (USDA): | | | |
| Fresh | 1 lb. | 177 | 44.0 |
| Fresh | 1 cup (5.3 oz.) | 58 | 14.6 |
| Canned, water pack, solids & liq. | 4 oz. | 29 | 7.5 |
| **GOOSE GIZZARD**, raw (USDA) | 4 oz. | 158 | 0. |
| **GRAHAM CRACKER** (See **CRACKER**) | | | |
| *GRAHAM CRAKOS*, cereal (Kellogg's) | 1-oz. serving | 110 | 24.0 |
| **GRANOLA:** | | | |
| *Heartland:* | | | |
| Coconut | ¼ cup (1 oz.) | 130 | 18.0 |
| Plain or raisin | ¼ cup (1 oz.) | 120 | 18.0 |
| Puffs, regular or cinnamon spice | ½ cup (1 oz.) | 120 | 20.0 |
| *Nature Valley:* | | | |
| Cinnamon & raisin | ⅓ cup (1 oz.) | 130 | 19.0 |
| Coconut & honey | ⅓ cup (1 oz.) | 150 | 18.0 |
| Fruit & nut | ⅓ cup (1 oz.) | 130 | 20.0 |
| Toasted oat mixture | ⅓ cup (1 oz.) | 130 | 19.0 |
| *Sun Country:* | | | |
| Almonds | ½ cup (2 oz.) | 250 | 34.0 |
| Raisin | ½ cup (2 oz.) | 240 | 37.0 |

(USDA): United States Department of Agriculture
(HEW/FAO): Health, Education and Welfare/Food and Agriculture Organization
* Prepared as Package Directs

| Food and Description | Measure or Quantity | Calories | Carbo- hydrates (grams) |
|---|---|---|---|
| **GRANOLA BARS,** *Nature Valley:* | | | |
| Almond | .8-oz. bar | 110 | 15.0 |
| Cinnamon | .8-oz. bar | 110 | 16.0 |
| Coconut | .8-oz. bar | 120 | 15.0 |
| Oats'n Honey | .8-oz. bar | 110 | 16.0 |
| Peanut | .8-oz. bar | 120 | 15.0 |
| **GRANOLA CLUSTERS,** *Nature Valley:* | | | |
| Almond | 1 roll | 140 | 25.0 |
| Caramel | 1 roll | 140 | 25.0 |
| Raisin | 1 roll | 140 | 26.0 |
| **GRAPE:** | | | |
| Fresh: | | | |
| American type (slip skin), Concord, Delaware, Niagara, Catawba and Scuppernong: | | | |
| (USDA) | ½ lb. (weighed with stem, skin & seeds) | 98 | 22.4 |
| (USDA) | ½ cup (2.7 oz.) | 33 | 7.5 |
| (USDA) | 3½" x 3" bunch (3.5 oz.) | 43 | 9.9 |
| European type (adherent skin), Malaga, Muscat, Thompson seedless, Emperor & Flame Tokay: | | | |
| (USDA) | ½ lb. (weighed with stem & seeds) | 139 | 34.9 |
| (USDA) whole | 20 grapes (¾" dia.) | 52 | 13.5 |
| (USDA) whole | ½ cup (.3 oz.) | 56 | 14.5 |
| (USDA) halves | ½ cup (.3 oz.) | 56 | 14.4 |
| Canned, solids & liq.: | | | |
| (USDA) Thompson, seedless, heavy syrup | 4 oz. | 87 | 22.7 |

| Food and Description | Measure or Quantity | Calories | Carbo-hydrates (grams) |
|---|---|---|---|
| (USDA) Thompson, seedless, water pack | 4 oz. | 58 | 15.4 |
| (Featherweight) water pack, seedless | ½ cup | 50 | 13.0 |
| **GRAPEADE,** chilled (Sealtest) | 6 fl. oz. | 96 | 24.2 |
| **GRAPE DRINK:** Canned: | | | |
| (Ann Page) | 1 cup (8.7 oz.) | 125 | 31.1 |
| (Hi-C) | 6 fl. oz. | 89 | 22.0 |
| (Lincoln) | 6 fl. oz. | 96 | 23.9 |
| *Mix (Hi-C) | 6 fl. oz. | 76 | 19.0 |
| **GRAPEFRUIT:** Fresh: White (USDA): | | | |
| Seeded type | 1 lb. (weighed with seeds & skin) | 86 | 22.4 |
| Seedless type | 1 lb. (weighed with skin) | 87 | 22.6 |
| Seeded type | ½ med. grapefruit (3¾" dia., 8.5 oz.) | 54 | 14.1 |
| Pink and red (USDA): | | | |
| Seeded type | 1 lb. (weighed with seeds & skin) | 87 | 22.6 |
| Seedless type | 1 lb. (weighed with skin) | 93 | 24.1 |
| Seeded type | ½ med. grapefruit (3¾" dia., 8.5 oz.) | 46 | 12.0 |
| Canned, syrup pack (Del Monte) solids & liq. | ½ cup | 74 | 17.5 |
| Canned, unsweetened or dietetic pack, solids & liq.: | | | |
| (USDA) water pack | ½ cup (4.2 oz.) | 36 | 9.1 |
| (Del Monte) sections | ½ cup | 46 | 10.5 |

(USDA): United States Department of Agriculture
(HEW/FAO): Health, Education and Welfare/Food and Agriculture Organization
* Prepared as Package Directs

| Food and Description | Measure or Quantity | Calories | Carbohydrates (grams) |
|---|---|---|---|
| (Diet Delight) sections | ½ cup (4.3 oz.) | 47 | 11.1 |
| (Featherweight) sections | ½ cup | 40 | 9.0 |
| (Tillie Lewis) *Tasti Diet* | ½ cup (4.4 oz.) | 44 | 11.0 |
| **GRAPEFRUIT DRINK,** canned: | | | |
| (Ann Page) natural | 6 fl. oz. (6.5 oz.) | 83 | 20.7 |
| (Lincoln) | 6 fl. oz. | 104 | 26.1 |
| **GRAPEFRUIT JUICE:** | | | |
| Fresh (USDA) pink, red or white, all varieties | ½ cup (4.3 oz.) | 48 | 11.3 |
| Canned: | | | |
| Sweetened: | | | |
| (USDA) | ½ cup (4.4 oz.) | 66 | 16.0 |
| (Del Monte) | 6 fl. oz. | 89 | 20.8 |
| Unsweetened: | | | |
| (USDA) | ½ cup (4.4 oz.) | 51 | 12.2 |
| (Del Monte) | 6 fl. oz. | 72 | 16.6 |
| (Ocean Spray) | 6 fl. oz. (6.5 oz.) | 64 | 14.6 |
| Chilled (Minute Maid) | 6 fl. oz. | 75 | 18.1 |
| Frozen, concentrate: | | | |
| Sweetened: | | | |
| (USDA) | 6-fl.-oz. can | 348 | 84.8 |
| *(USDA) diluted with 3 parts water | ½ cup (4.4 oz.) | 58 | 14.1 |
| Unsweetened: | | | |
| (USDA) | 6-fl.-oz. can | 300 | 71.6 |
| *(USDA) diluted with 3 parts water | ½ cup (4.4 oz.) | 51 | 12.2 |
| *(Minute Maid) | 6 fl. oz. | 75 | 18.3 |
| Dehydrated, crystals: | | | |
| (USDA) | 4-oz. can | 429 | 102.4 |
| *(USDA) reconstituted | ½ cup (4.4 oz.) | 50 | 11.9 |
| **GRAPEFRUIT PEEL, CANDIED** (USDA) | 1 oz. | 90 | 22.9 |
| **GRAPE JAM** (Smucker's) | 1 T. | 53 | 13.7 |
| **GRAPE JELLY:** | | | |
| Sweetened (Smucker's) | 1 T. | 53 | 13.5 |

| Food and Description | Measure or Quantity | Calories | Carbo- hydrates (grams) |
|---|---|---|---|
| Dietetic or low calorie: | | | |
| (Dia-Mel) | 1 tsp. | 2 | 0. |
| (Diet Delight) | 1 T. (.6 oz.) | 13 | 3.2 |
| (Featherweight) | 1 T. | 16 | 4.0 |
| (Featherweight) artificially sweetened | 1 T. | 6 | 1.0 |
| (Slenderella) | 1 T. (.6 oz.) | 24 | 6.0 |
| (Smucker's) artificially sweetened | 1 T. | 3 | 3.0 |
| (Tillie Lewis) *Tasti Diet* | 1 T. | 11 | 2.7 |
| **GRAPE JUICE:** | | | |
| Canned (USDA) | ½ cup (4.4 oz.) | 83 | 20.9 |
| Frozen, concentrate, sweetened: | | | |
| (USDA) | 6-fl.-oz. can | 395 | 100.0 |
| *(USDA) diluted | ½ cup (4.4 oz.) | 66 | 16.6 |
| *(Minute Maid) | 6 fl. oz. | 99 | 25.0 |
| **GRAPE JUICE DRINK,** canned (USDA) approximately 30% grape juice | 1 cup (8.8 oz.) | 135 | 34.5 |
| *GRAPE NUTS,* cereal (Post) | ¾ cup (1 oz.) | 107 | 23.4 |
| *GRAPE NUTS FLAKES,* Cereal (Post) | ⅞ cup (1 oz.) | 108 | 23.4 |
| **GRAPE SPREAD** (Smucker's) low sugar | 1 T. | 24 | 6.0 |
| **GRAVES WINE** (See also individual regional, vineyard or brand names): | | | |
| (Barton & Guestier) 12½% alcohol | 3 fl. oz. | 65 | .6 |
| (Cruse) 11½% alcohol | 3 fl. oz. | 69 | DNA |

(USDA): United States Department of Agriculture
(HEW/FAO): Health, Education and Welfare/Food and Agriculture
        Organization
* Prepared as Package Directs

| Food and Description | Measure or Quantity | Calories | Carbo-hydrates (grams) |
|---|---|---|---|
| **GRAVY:** | | | |
| Canned: | | | |
| Beef: | | | |
| (Ann Page) | 10½-oz. can | 118 | 18.3 |
| (Franco-American) | 10¼-oz. can | 154 | 15.4 |
| Brown: | | | |
| (Dawn Fresh) with mushroom broth | 2-oz. serving | 18 | 3.2 |
| (Franco-American) with onion | 10½-oz. can | 131 | 21.0 |
| (La Choy) | 5-oz. can | 417 | 101.3 |
| *Ready Gravy* | ¼-cup serving | 44 | 7.4 |
| Chicken (Franco-American) | 10½-oz. can | 263 | 15.8 |
| Chicken giblet (Franco-American) | 10½-oz. can | 184 | 15.8 |
| Mushroom (Franco-American) | 10½-oz. can | 184 | 21.0 |
| Mix, regular: | | | |
| Au jus: | | | |
| (Ann Page) | ¾-oz. pkg. | 52 | 10.9 |
| (Durkee) | 1-oz. pkg. | 62 | 13.0 |
| (Durkee) *Roastin' Bag* | 1-oz. pkg. | 64 | 14.0 |
| (French's) *Gravy Makins* | ¾-oz. pkg. | 63 | 12.0 |
| Brown: | | | |
| (Ann Page) | ¾-oz. pkg. | 78 | 12.0 |
| (Durkee) | .8-oz. pkg. | 59 | 10.0 |
| (Durkee) with mushrooms | .7-oz. pkg. | 59 | 11.0 |
| (Durkee) with onions | .8-oz. pkg. | 66 | 13.0 |
| *(Ehler's) | ¼-cup serving | 22 | 3.5 |
| (French's *Gravy Makins* | ¾-oz. pkg. | 78 | 13.7 |
| *(Spatini) | 1-oz. serving | 10 | 3.0 |
| Chicken: | | | |
| (Ann Page) | 1-oz. pkg. | 107 | 16.7 |
| (Durkee) | 1-oz. pkg. | 87 | 14.0 |
| (Durkee) creamy | 1.2-oz. pkg. | 156 | 14.0 |
| (Durkee) *Roastin' Bag* | 1.5-oz. pkg. | 122 | 24.0 |
| (Durkee) *Roastin' Bag,* creamy | 2-oz. pkg. | 242 | 22.0 |

| Food and Description | Measure or Quantity | Calories | Carbohydrates (grams) |
|---|---|---|---|
| (Durkee) *Roastin' Bag,* Italian style | 1.5-oz. pkg. | 144 | 31.0 |
| *(Ehler's) | ¼-cup serving | 21 | 4.0 |
| (French's) *Gravy Makins* | .9-oz. pkg. | 94 | 14.8 |
| *(Pillsbury) | ¼-cup serving | 15 | 3.0 |
| Homestyle: | | | |
| (Durkee) | .8-oz. pkg. | 70 | 11.0 |
| (French's) *Gravy Makins* | .9-oz. pkg. | 89 | 14.5 |
| *(Pillsbury) | ¼-cup serving | 15 | 3.0 |
| Meatloaf (Durkee) *Roastin' Bag* | 1.5-oz. pkg. | 129 | 18.0 |
| Mushroom: | | | |
| (Ann Page) | ⅜-oz. pkg. | 76 | 12.1 |
| (Durkee) | .8-oz. pkg. | 60 | 11.0 |
| (French's) *Gravy Makins* | ⅜-oz. pkg. | 70 | 13.7 |
| Onion: | | | |
| (Ann Page) | 1-oz. pkg. | 106 | 17.7 |
| (Durkee) | 1-oz. pkg. | 84 | 15.0 |
| (French's) *Gravy Makins* | 1-oz. pkg. | 84 | 17.3 |
| Pork: | | | |
| (Durkee) | 1-oz. pkg. | 70 | 14.0 |
| (Durkee) *Roastin' Bag* | 1.5-oz. pkg. | 130 | 26.0 |
| (French's) *Gravy Makins* | .7-oz. pkg. | 77 | 13.4 |
| Pot Roast (Durkee): | | | |
| *Roastin' Bag* | 1.5-oz. pkg. | 125 | 25.0 |
| *Roastin' Bag,* & onion | 1.5-oz. pkg. | 125 | 24.0 |
| Swiss steak (Durkee): | | | |
| Regular | 1-oz. pkg. | 68 | 16.0 |
| *Roastin' Bag* | 1.5-oz. pkg. | 115 | 28.0 |
| Turkey: | | | |
| (Durkee) | 1-oz. pkg. | 93 | 14.0 |
| (French's) *Gravy Makins* | .9-oz. pkg. | 89 | 14.0 |

(USDA): United States Department of Agriculture
(HEW/FAO): Health, Education and Welfare/Food and Agriculture Organization
* Prepared as Package Directs

| Food and Description | Measure or Quantity | Calories | Carbohydrates (grams) |
|---|---|---|---|
| *Mix, dietetic (Weight Watchers): | | | |
| Brown | ¼-cup serving | 8 | 1.0 |
| Brown, with mushroom | ¼-cup serving | 12 | 2.0 |
| Brown, with onion | ¼-cup serving | 13 | 2.0 |
| Chicken | ¼-cup serving | 10 | 2.0 |
| *GRAVY MASTER* | 1 fl. oz. (1.3 oz.) | 68 | 14.2 |
| **GRAVY WITH MEAT OR TURKEY:** | | | |
| Canned (Morton House): | | | |
| Sliced beef | ½ of 12½-oz. can | 190 | 8.0 |
| Sliced pork | ½ of 12½-oz. can | 190 | 9.0 |
| Sliced turkey | ½ of 12½-oz. can | 140 | 7.0 |
| Frozen: | | | |
| (Banquet): | | | |
| Giblet gravy and sliced turkey | 5-oz. cooking bag | 98 | 5.3 |
| Giblet gravy and sliced turkey | 2-lb. pkg. | 564 | 28.2 |
| Sliced beef | 5-oz. cooking bag | 116 | 4.8 |
| Sliced beef | 2-lb. pkg. | 782 | 34.5 |
| (Green Giant) *Toast Topper:* | | | |
| Sliced beef | 5-oz. serving | 122 | 5.7 |
| Sliced turkey | 5-oz. serving | 92 | 6.7 |
| **GREEN PEA (See PEA, GREEN)** | | | |
| **GRENADINE SYRUP:** | | | |
| (Gariner) nonalcoholic | 1 fl. oz. | 103 | 26.0 |
| (Giroux) nonalcoholic | 1 fl. oz. | 100 | 25.0 |
| (Leroux) 25 proof | 1 fl. oz. | 81 | 15.2 |
| **GRITS (See HOMINY GRITS)** | | | |
| **GROUND-CHERRY,** Poha or Cape Gooseberry (USDA): | | | |
| Whole | 1 lb. (weighed with husks & stems) | 221 | 46.7 |

| Food and Description | Measure or Quantity | Calories | Carbohydrates (grams) |
|---|---|---|---|
| Flesh only | 4 oz. | 60 | 12.7 |
| **GROUPER, raw (USDA):** | | | |
| Whole | 1 lb. (weighed whole) | 170 | 0. |
| Meat only | 4 oz. | 99 | 0. |
| **GUAVA, COMMON, fresh (USDA):** | | | |
| Whole | 1 lb. (weighed untrimmed) | 273 | 66.0 |
| Whole | 1 guava (2.8 oz.) | 48 | 11.7 |
| Flesh only | 4 oz. | 70 | 17.0 |
| **GUAVA JAM (Smucker's)** | 1 T. | 53 | 13.5 |
| **GUAVA JELLY (Smucker's)** | 1 T. | 53 | 13.5 |
| **GUAVA, STRAWBERRY, fresh (USDA):** | | | |
| Whole | 1 lb. (weighed untrimmed) | 289 | 70.2 |
| Flesh only | 4 oz. | 74 | 17.9 |
| **GUINEA HEN, raw (USDA):** | | | |
| Ready-to-cook | 1 lb. (weighed ready-to-cook) | 594 | 0. |
| Meat & skin | 4 oz. | 179 | 0. |

# H

| | | | |
|---|---|---|---|
| **HADDOCK:** | | | |
| Raw (USDA): | | | |
| Whole | 1 lb. (weighed whole) | 172 | 0. |
| Meat only | 4 oz. | 90 | 0. |

(USDA): United States Department of Agriculture
(HEW/FAO): Health, Education and Welfare/Food and Agriculture Organization
* Prepared as Package Directs

| Food and Description | Measure or Quantity | Calories | Carbo-hydrates (grams) |
|---|---|---|---|
| Fried, breaded (USDA) | 4" x 3" x ½" fillet (3.5 oz.) | 165 | 5.8 |
| Frozen: | | | |
| (Banquet) | 8¾-oz. dinner | 419 | 45.4 |
| (Mrs. Paul's): | | | |
| Breaded & fried | 2-oz. fillet | 114 | 11.8 |
| Buttered fillets | ½ of 10-oz. pkg. | 200 | 1.2 |
| (Van de Kamp's) batter dipped, french-fried | 2.4-oz. piece | 165 | 8.0 |
| (Weight Watchers): | | | |
| 2-compartment meal | 8¾-oz. meal | 169 | 13.9 |
| 3-compartment meal | 16-oz. meal | 261 | 13.2 |
| Smoked, canned or not (USDA) | 4 oz. | 117 | 0. |
| **HAKE, raw (USDA):** | | | |
| Whole | 1 lb. (weighed whole) | 144 | 0. |
| Meat only | 4 oz. | 84 | 0. |
| **HALF & HALF (milk & cream) (See CREAM)** | | | |
| **HALF & HALF WINE:** | | | |
| (Gallo) 20% alcohol | 3 fl. oz. | 100 | 5.7 |
| (Lejon) 18.5% alcohol | 3 fl. oz. | 116 | 6.7 |
| **HALIBUT:** | | | |
| Atlantic & Pacific: | | | |
| Raw (USDA): | | | |
| Whole | 1 lb. (weighed whole) | 268 | 0. |
| Meat only | 4 oz. | 113 | 0. |
| Broiled (USDA) | 4.4 oz. | 214 | 0. |
| Smoked (USDA) | 4 oz. | 254 | 0. |
| California, raw (USDA) meat only | 4 oz. | 110 | 0. |
| Greenland (See TURBOT) | | | |
| Frozen (Van de Kamp's) batter dipped, french-fried | 1.3-oz. piece | 90 | 5.7 |

| Food and Description | Measure or Quantity | Calories | Carbohydrates (grams) |
|---|---|---|---|
| **HAM** (See also **PORK**): | | | |
| Cooked: | | | |
| (Eckrich) sliced | 1.2-oz. slice | 37 | .9 |
| (Hormel) | .8-oz. slice | 26 | Tr. |
| Canned: | | | |
| (Hormel) *Tender Chunk* | 1 oz. | 49 | .2 |
| (Oscar Mayer) *Jubilee*, | | | |
| extra lean, cooked | ¹⁄₁₂ of 3-lb. ham | | |
| | (4 oz.) | 133 | .5 |
| (Swift) *Hostess* | ¼″ slice (3.5 oz.) | 141 | .8 |
| (Swift) *Premium* | 1¾-oz. slice | | |
| | (5″ x 2″ x ¼″) | 111 | .3 |
| Canned, chopped or | | | |
| minced: | | | |
| (USDA) | 1 oz. | 65 | 1.2 |
| (Hormel) | 1 oz. (8-lb. can) | 89 | .4 |
| Canned, deviled: | | | |
| (USDA) | 1 T. (.5 oz.) | 46 | 0. |
| (Hormel) | 1 T. (.5 oz.) | 35 | .1 |
| Canned, deviled: | | | |
| (Libby's) | 1 T. (.5 oz.) | 40 | .1 |
| (Underwood) | 1-oz. serving | 97 | Tr. |
| Packaged: | | | |
| (Eckrich) | 1-oz. slice | 40 | .7 |
| (Oscar Mayer): | | | |
| Chopped | 1 oz. | 62 | .3 |
| Sliced, *Jubilee* | 2-oz. slice | 69 | .5 |
| Steak, *Jubilee* | 8-oz. steak | 257 | 0. |
| **HAMBURGER** (See **BEEF,** Ground; *MC DONALD'S* and *BURGER KING*): | | | |
| **HAMBURGER MIX:** | | | |
| (Ann Page): | | | |
| Beef noodle | ⅛ of 7-oz. pkg. | 146 | 48.2 |
| Cheeseburger macaroni | ⅛ of 8-oz. pkg. | 175 | 29.1 |
| Chili tomato | ⅛ of 8-oz. pkg. | 156 | 32.5 |

(USDA): United States Department of Agriculture
(HEW/FAO): Health, Education and Welfare/Food and Agriculture Organization
* Prepared as Package Directs

| Food and Description | Measure or Quantity | Calories | Carbohydrates (grams) |
|---|---|---|---|
| Hash | ⅙ of 6-oz. pkg. | 121 | 27.7 |
| Potato stroganoff | ⅙ of 7-oz. pkg. | 141 | 28.2 |
| *Hamburger Helper (General Mills): | | | |
| Beef noodle | ⅕ of pkg. | 320 | 26.0 |
| Beef Romanoff | ⅕ of pkg. | 340 | 28.0 |
| Cheeseburger macaroni | ⅕ of pkg. | 360 | 28.0 |
| Chili tomato | ⅕ of pkg. | 320 | 29.0 |
| Hamburger hash | ⅕ of pkg. | 300 | 24.0 |
| Hamburger stew | ⅕ of pkg. | 290 | 23.0 |
| Lasagne | ⅕ of pkg. | 330 | 32.0 |
| Pizza dish | ⅕ of pkg. | 340 | 33.0 |
| Potato stroganoff | ⅕ of pkg. | 330 | 29.0 |
| Potatoes au gratin | ⅕ of pkg. | 320 | 27.0 |
| Rice oriental | ⅕ of 8-oz. pkg. | 340 | 35.0 |
| Spaghetti | ⅕ of pkg. | 330 | 31.0 |
| Make-a-Better Burger (Lipton) mildly seasoned or onion | ⅛ of pkg. | 30 | 3.0 |
| **HAMBURGER SEASONING MIX:** | | | |
| (Durkee) | 1-oz. pkg. | 110 | 15.0 |
| *(Durkee) | 1 cup | 663 | 7.5 |
| (French's) | 1-oz. pkg. | 100 | 20.0 |
| **HAM & BUTTER BEAN SOUP, canned (Campbell)** | | | |
| Chunky | 10¾-oz. can | 290 | 31.0 |
| **HAM & CHEESE (Oscar Mayer):** | | | |
| Loaf | 1-oz. slice | 75 | .3 |
| Spread | 1-oz. serving | 67 | .7 |
| **HAM DINNER, frozen:** | | | |
| (Banquet) | 10-oz. dinner | 369 | 47.7 |
| (Morton) | 10-oz. dinner | 449 | 56.9 |
| (Swanson) | 10¼-oz. dinner | 380 | 47.0 |
| **HAM SALAD SPREAD:** | | | |
| (Carnation) spreadable | 1½-oz. serving | 78 | 3.4 |
| (Oscar Mayer) | 1-oz. serving | 62 | 3.0 |

| Food and Description | Measure or Quantity | Calories | Carbo- hydrates (grams) |
|---|---|---|---|
| **HAWAIIAN PUNCH:** | | | |
| Canned: | | | |
| Cherry | 6 fl. oz. | 87 | 22.8 |
| Grape | 6 fl. oz. | 93 | 23.4 |
| Orange | 6 fl. oz. | 97 | 24.4 |
| Red | 6 fl. oz. | 84 | 21.3 |
| *Very Berry* | 6 fl. oz. | 87 | 21.6 |
| *Mix, red punch | 8 fl. oz. | 100 | 25.0 |
| **HAWS, SCARLET,** raw (USDA): | | | |
| Whole | 1 lb. (weighed with core) | 316 | 75.5 |
| Flesh & Skin | 4 oz. | 99 | 23.6 |
| **HAZELNUT** (See **FILBERT**) | | | |
| **HEADCHEESE:** | | | |
| (USDA) | 1-oz. serving | 76 | .3 |
| (Oscar Mayer) | 1-oz. serving | 64 | .6 |
| **HERRING:** | | | |
| Raw (USDA): | | | |
| Atlantic, whole | 1 lb. (weighed whole) | 407 | 0. |
| Atlantic, meat only | 4 oz. | 200 | 0. |
| Pacific, meat only | 4 oz. | 111 | 0. |
| Canned: | | | |
| (USDA) in tomato sauce, solids & liq. | 4-oz. serving | 200 | 4.2 |
| (Vita): | | | |
| Bismarck, drained | 5-oz. jar | 273 | 6.9 |
| Cocktail, drained | 8-oz. jar | 342 | 24.8 |
| In cream sauce, drained | 8-oz. jar | 397 | 18.1 |
| Lunch, drained | 8-oz. jar | 483 | 13.1 |
| Matjis, drained | 8-oz. jar | 304 | 26.2 |
| Party snacks, drained | 8-oz. jar | 401 | 16.6 |

(USDA): United States Department of Agriculture
(HEW/FAO): Health, Education and Welfare/Food and Agriculture
Organization
* Prepared as Package Directs

| Food and Description | Measure or Quantity | Calories | Carbo-hydrates (grams) |
|---|---|---|---|
| Tastee Bits, drained | 8-oz. jar | 361 | 24.7 |
| In wine sauce, drained | 8-oz. jar | 401 | 16.6 |
| Pickled (USDA) Bismarck type | 4-oz. serving | 253 | 0. |
| Salted or brined (USDA) | 4-oz. serving | 247 | 0. |
| Smoked (USDA): | | | |
| Bloaters | 4-oz. serving | 222 | 0. |
| Hard | 4-oz. serving | 340 | 0. |
| Kippered | 4-oz. serving | 239 | 0. |
| **HICKORY NUT** (USDA): | | | |
| Whole | 1 lb. (weighed in shell) | 1068 | 20.3 |
| Shelled | 4 oz. | 763 | 14.5 |
| ***HO-HOS*** (Hostess) | 1-oz. cake | 124 | 16.5 |
| **HOMINY GRITS:** | | | |
| Dry: | | | |
| (USDA): | | | |
| Degermed | 1 oz. | 103 | 22.1 |
| Degermed | ½ cup (2.8 oz.) | 282 | 60.9 |
| (Albers) quick, degermed | 1½ oz. | 150 | 33.0 |
| (Aunt Jemima/Quaker) | 3 T. (1 oz.) | 101 | 22.4 |
| (Pocono) creamy | 1 oz. | 101 | 23.6 |
| (Quaker): | | | |
| Instant | .8-oz. packet | 79 | 17.7 |
| Instant, with imitation bacon bits | 1-oz. packet | 101 | 21.6 |
| Instant, with imitation ham | 1-oz. packet | 99 | 21.3 |
| (3-Minute-Brand) quick, enriched | ⅛ cup (1 oz.) | 98 | 22.2 |
| Cooked (USDA) degermed | ⅔ cup (5.6 oz.) | 84 | 18.0 |
| **HONEY,** strained: | | | |
| (USDA) | ½ cup (5.7 oz.) | 496 | 134.1 |
| (USDA) | 1 T. (.7 oz.) | 61 | 16.5 |
| ***HONEYCOMB,*** cereal | | | |
| (Post) | 1⅓ cup (1 oz.) | 113 | 25.1 |

| Food and Description | Measure or Quantity | Calories | Carbohydrates (grams) |
|---|---|---|---|
| **HONEYDEW**, fresh (USDA): | | | |
| Whole | 1 lb. (weighed whole) | 94 | 22.0 |
| Wedge | 2" x 7" wedge (5.3 oz.) | 31 | 7.2 |
| Flesh only | 4 oz. | 37 | 8.7 |
| Flesh only, diced | 1 cup (5.9 oz.) | 55 | 12.9 |
| **HOPPING JOHN**, frozen (Green Giant) Southern recipe | ⅓ of 10-oz. pkg. | 116 | 16.7 |
| **HORSERADISH:** | | | |
| Raw (USDA): | | | |
| Whole | 1 lb. (weighed unpared) | 288 | 65.2 |
| Pared | 1 oz. | 25 | 5.6 |
| Prepared (Nalley's) sauce | 1 oz. | 106 | 3.1 |
| **HYACINTH BEAN** (USDA): | | | |
| Young pod, raw | | | |
| Whole | 1 lb. (weighed untrimmed) | 140 | 29.1 |
| Trimmed | 4 oz. | 40 | 8.3 |
| Dry seeds | 4 oz. | 383 | 69.2 |
| **ICE CREAM** and **FROZEN CUSTARD** (See also listing by flavor or brand name, e.g., **CHOCOLATE ICE CREAM,** *DREAMSICLE* or *GOOD HUMOR*): | | | |
| Sweetened: | | | |
| (USDA): | | | |
| 10% fat | 1 cup (4.7 oz.) | 257 | 27.7 |

(USDA): United States Department of Agriculture
(HEW/FAO): Health, Education and Welfare/Food and Agriculture Organization
* Prepared as Package Directs

| Food and Description | Measure or Quantity | Calories | Carbo-hydrates (grams) |
|---|---|---|---|
| 12% fat | 1 cup (5 oz.) | 294 | 29.3 |
| 12% fat, brick-type | 2½-oz. slice | 147 | 14.6 |
| 12% fat | small container (3½ fl. oz.) | 128 | 12.8 |
| 16% fat | 1 cup (5.2 oz.) | 329 | 26.6 |
| (Dean) fruit, 10.4% fat | 1 cup (5.6 oz.) | 336 | 41.1 |
| Dietetic (See **FROZEN DESSERT**) | | | |
| **ICE CREAM BAR**, chocolate-coated (Sealtest) | 1 bar (2½ fl. oz.) | 150 | 12.0 |
| **ICE CREAM CONE** (Comet) cone only: | | | |
| Any color | 1 piece (4 grams) | 20 | 4.0 |
| Rolled sugar, any color | 1 piece (.4 oz.) | 40 | 9.0 |
| **ICE CREAM CUP**, cup only (Comet) any color | 1 piece (5 grams) | 20 | 4.0 |
| **ICE CREAM SANDWICH** (Sealtest) | 1 sandwich (3 fl. oz.) | 170 | 26.0 |
| **ICE MILK:** | | | |
| (USDA): | | | |
| Hardened | 1 cup (4.6 oz.) | 199 | 29.3 |
| Soft-serve | 1 cup (6.3 oz.) | 266 | 39.2 |
| (Dean): | | | |
| *Count Calorie,* 2.1% fat | 1 cup (4.8 oz.) | 155 | 17.1 |
| 5% fat | 1 cup (4.9 oz.) | 227 | 35.0 |
| *Light'n Easy:* | | | |
| Chocolate | ½ cup (2¼ oz.) | 108 | 17.7 |
| Strawberry | ½ cup (2¼ oz.) | 104 | 17.7 |
| Vanilla | ½ cup (2¼ oz.) | 105 | 17.2 |
| (Meadow Gold): | | | |
| Chocolate, *Viva* | 1 cup | 200 | 36.0 |
| Vanilla, *Viva* | 1 cup | 200 | 34.0 |
| (Sealtest) *Light'n Lively:* | | | |
| Banana | 1 cup (4.8 oz.) | 206 | 39.4 |
| Banana strawberry twirl | 1 cup (5 oz.) | 220 | 40.0 |
| Buttered almond | 1 cup (4.8 oz.) | 240 | 36.0 |
| Caramel nut | 1 cup (4.8 oz.) | 240 | 37.4 |

| Food and Description | Measure or Quantity | Calories | Carbo-hydrates (grams) |
|---|---|---|---|
| Cherry pineapple | 1 cup (4.8 oz.) | 200 | 36.0 |
| Chocolate | 1 cup (4.8 oz.) | 220 | 40.0 |
| Coffee | 1 cup (4.8 oz.) | 200 | 36.0 |
| Lemon Chiffon | 1 cup (4.8 oz.) | 236 | 48.6 |
| Orange-pineapple | 1 cup | 200 | 36.0 |
| Peach | 1 cup | 200 | 36.0 |
| Raspberry | 1 cup (4.8 oz.) | 198 | 35.6 |
| Strawberry | 1 cup (4.8 oz.) | 200 | 36.0 |
| Strawberry royale | 1 cup (5 oz.) | 224 | 43.2 |
| Toffee | 1 cup (4.8 oz.) | 220 | 38.2 |
| Toffee crunch | 1 cup (4.8 oz.) | 238 | 40.4 |
| Vanilla | 1 cup (4.8 oz.) | 200 | 36.0 |
| Vanilla, with chocolate and strawberry | 1 cup | 200 | 36.0 |
| Vanilla fudge royale | 1 cup (5 oz.) | 220 | 42.0 |
| **ICE MILK BAR** (Sealtest) chocolate-coated | 1 bar (2½ fl. oz.) | 130 | 14.0 |
| **ICE STICK** (Sealtest) twin pop | 3 fl. oz. | 70 | 18.0 |

**ICES** (See individual fruit ice flavors)

**ICING** (See **CAKE ICING**)

**INSTANT BREAKFAST** (See individual brand name or company listings)

| *INTERNATIONAL DESSERTS,* frozen (Sara Lee): | | | |
|---|---|---|---|
| Chocolate Bavarian | ⅛ of pkg. | 285 | 22.6 |
| French cream cheese | ⅛ of pkg. | 274 | 24.9 |
| Lemon Bavarian | ⅛ of pkg. | 258 | 27.5 |

(USDA): United States Department of Agriculture
(HEW/FAO): Health, Education and Welfare/Food and Agriculture Organization
* Prepared as Package Directs

| Food and Description | Measure or Quantity | Calories | Carbohydrates (grams) |
|---|---|---|---|
| Strawberry French cream cheese | ⅛ of pkg. | 258 | 27.5 |
| **IRISH WHISKEY** (See **DISTILLED LIQUORS**) | | | |
| **ITALIAN DINNER**, frozen (Banquet) | 11-oz. dinner | 446 | 44.6 |

# J

| Food and Description | Measure or Quantity | Calories | Carbohydrates (grams) |
|---|---|---|---|
| **JACKFRUIT**, fresh (USDA): | | | |
| Whole | 1 lb. (weighed with seeds & skin) | 124 | 32.3 |
| Flesh only | 4 oz. | 111 | 28.8 |
| **JACK MACKERAL**, raw (USDA) meat only | 4 oz. | 162 | 0. |
| **JACK ROSE MIX** (Bar-Tender's) | ⅝-oz. serving | 70 | 17.2 |
| **JAM**, sweetened (See also individual listings by flavor): | | | |
| (USDA) | 1 oz. | 77 | 19.8 |
| (USDA) | 1 T. (.7 oz.) | 54 | 14.0 |
| (Ann·Page) all flavors | 1 tsp. (6.8 grams) | 19 | 4.8 |
| **JELLY**, sweetened (See also individual listings by flavor): | | | |
| (USDA) | 1 T. (.6 oz.) | 49 | 12.7 |
| (Ann Page) all flavors | 1 tsp. | 19 | 4.6 |
| (Crosse & Blackwell) | 1 T. (.7 oz.) | 51 | 12.8 |
| **JERUSALEM ARTICHOKE** (USDA): | | | |
| Unpared | 1 lb. (weighed with skin) | 207 | 52.3 |
| Pared | 4 oz. | 75 | 18.9 |

| Food and Description | Measure or Quantity | Calories | Carbo-hydrates (grams) |
|---|---|---|---|
| **JOHANNISBERGER RIESLING WINE:** | | | |
| (Deinhard) 11% alcohol | 3 fl. oz. | 72 | 4.5 |
| (Inglenook) Estate, 12% alcohol | 3 fl. oz. | 61 | .9 |
| (Louis M. Martini) 12.5% alcohol | 2 fl. oz. | 90 | .2 |
| **JORDAN ALMOND** (See CANDY) | | | |
| **JUICE** (See individual flavors) | | | |
| **JUJUBE or CHINESE DATE** (USDA): | | | |
| Fresh, whole | 1 lb. (weighed with seeds) | 443 | 116.4 |
| Fresh, flesh only | 4 oz. | 119 | 31.3 |
| Dried, whole | 1 lb. (weighed with seeds) | 1159 | 297.1 |
| Dried, flesh only | 4 oz. | 325 | 83.5 |
| **JUNIOR FOOD** (See BABY FOOD) | | | |
| **JUNIORS** (Tastykake): | | | |
| Chocolate | 2¾-oz. pkg. | 307 | DNA |
| Coconut | 2¾-oz. pkg. | 330 | DNA |
| Coconut devil food | 2¾-oz. pkg. | 318 | DNA |
| Koffee Kake | 2½-oz. pkg. | 313 | DNA |
| Lemon | 2¾-oz. pkg. | 297 | DNA |

# K

| Food and Description | Measure or Quantity | Calories | Carbo-hydrates (grams) |
|---|---|---|---|
| **KABOOM,** cereal (General Mills) | 1 cup (1 oz.) | 110 | 24.0 |

(USDA): United States Department of Agriculture
(HEW/FAO): Health, Education and Welfare/Food and Agriculture
Organization

* Prepared as Package Directs

| Food and Description | Measure or Quantity | Calories | Carbo-hydrates (grams) |
|---|---|---|---|
| **KAFE VIN** (Lejon) | | | |
| 19.7% alcohol | 3 fl. oz. | 183 | 22.8 |
| **KALE:** | | | |
| Raw (USDA) leaves only | 1 lb. (weighed untrimmed) | 154 | 26.1 |
| Boiled (USDA) leaves, including stems | ½ cup (1.9 oz.) | 15 | 2.2 |
| Frozen | | | |
| (Birds Eye) chopped | ⅓ of pkg. | 25 | 5.0 |
| (McKenzie) chopped | 3.3-oz. serving | 32 | 4.5 |
| (Seabrook Farms) chopped | ⅓ of 10-oz. pkg. | 32 | 4.5 |
| **KANDY KAKES** (Tastykake): | | | |
| Chocolate | 1.3-oz. pkg. | 181 | DNA |
| Peanut butter | 1.3-oz. pkg. | 190 | DNA |
| **KARO SYRUP:** | | | |
| Dark corn | 1 T. (.7 oz.) | 60 | 15.0 |
| Imitation maple | 1 T. (.1 oz.) | 59 | 14.6 |
| Light corn | 1 T. (.7 oz.) | 60 | 14.9 |
| Pancake & waffle | 1 T. (.7 oz.) | 60 | 14.9 |
| **KEFIR** (Alta-Dena Dairy): | | | |
| Plain | 1 cup (8.6 oz.) | 180 | 13.0 |
| Flavored | 1 cup (7.3 oz.) | 190 | 24.0 |
| **KETCHUP** (See **CATSUP**) | | | |
| **KIDNEY** (USDA): | | | |
| Beef, raw | 4 oz. | 147 | 1.0 |
| Beef, braised | 4 oz. | 286 | .9 |
| Calf, raw | 4 oz. | 128 | .1 |
| Hog, raw | 4 oz. | 120 | 1.2 |
| Lamb, raw | 4 oz. | 119 | 1.0 |
| **KIELBASA:** | | | |
| (Eckrich) skinless | 2-oz. link | 190 | 2.0 |
| (Vienna) | 2½-oz. serving | 206 | 1.1 |
| **KINGFISH**, raw (USDA): | | | |
| Whole | 1 lb. (weighed whole) | 210 | 0. |
| Meat only | 4 oz. | 119 | 0. |

| Food and Description | Measure or Quantity | Calories | Carbo-hydrates (grams) |
|---|---|---|---|
| **KING VITAMAN**, cereal (Quaker) | ¾ cup (1 oz.) | 120 | 23.3 |
| **KIPPERS** (See **HERRING**) | | | |
| **KIRSCH LIQUEUR** (Garnier) 96 proof | 1 fl. oz. | 83 | 8.8 |
| **KIRSCHWASSER** (Leroux) 96 proof | 1 fl. oz. | 80 | 0. |
| **KIX**, cereal | 1½ cups (1 oz.) | 110 | 24.0 |
| **KNOCKWURST** (USDA) | 1 oz. | 79 | .6 |
| **KOHLARBI** (USDA): | | | |
| Raw, whole | 1 lb. (weighed with skin, without leaves) | 96 | 21.9 |
| Raw, diced | 1 cup (4.8 oz.) | 40 | 9.1 |
| Boiled, drained | 4 oz. | 27 | 6.0 |
| Boiled, drained | 1 cup (5.5 oz.) | 37 | 8.2 |
| *****KOOL-AID** (General Foods): | | | |
| Unsweetened | 8 fl. oz. | 100 | 25.0 |
| Sweetened | 8 fl. oz. | 93 | 23.2 |
| Sweetened, tropical punch | 8 fl. oz. | 98 | 24.5 |
| **KRIMPETS** (Tastykake): | | | |
| Butterscotch | .9-oz. cake | 96 | DNA |
| Chocolate, creme filled | 1.2-oz. cake | 126 | DNA |
| Jelly | .9-oz. cake | 84 | DNA |
| **KRIMPIE** (Tastykake) Vanilla | 1 piece | 239 | DNA |
| **KUMMEL LIQUEUR:** | | | |
| (Garnier) 70 proof | 1 fl. oz. | 75 | 4.3 |
| (Hiram Walker) 70 proof | 1 fl. oz. | 71 | 3.2 |
| (Leroux) 70 proof | 1 fl. oz. | 75 | 4.1 |

(USDA): United States Department of Agriculture
(HEW/FAO): Health, Education and Welfare/Food and Agriculture Organization
* Prepared as Package Directs

| Food and Description | Measure or Quantity | Calories | Carbo-hydrates (grams) |
|---|---|---|---|
| **KUMQUAT,** fresh (USDA): | | | |
| Whole | 1 lb. (weighed with seeds) | 274 | 72.1 |
| Flesh & skin | 4 oz. | 74 | 19.4 |
| Flesh only | 5-6 med. kumquats | 65 | 17.1 |

# L

| | | | |
|---|---|---|---|
| **LAKE COUNTRY WINE** (Taylor): | | | |
| Gold, 12% alcohol | 3 fl. oz. | 78 | 5.4 |
| Pink, 12½% alcohol | 3 fl. oz. | 78 | 4.8 |
| Red, 12½% alcohol | 3 fl. oz. | 81 | 4.8 |
| White, 12½% alcohol | 3 fl. oz. | 81 | 4.2 |
| **LAKE HERRING,** raw (USDA): | | | |
| Whole | 1 lb. | 226 | 0. |
| Meat only | 4 oz. | 109 | 0. |
| **LAKE TROUT,** raw (USDA): | | | |
| Drawn | 1 lb. (weighed with head, fins & bones) | 282 | 0. |
| Meat only | 4 oz. | 191 | 0. |
| **LAKE TROUT or SISCOWET,** raw (USDA): | | | |
| Less than 6.5 lb. whole | 1 lb. (weighed whole) | 404 | 0. |
| Less than 6.5 lb. whole | 4 oz. (meat only) | 273 | 0. |
| More than 6.5 lb. whole | 1 lb. (weighed whole) | 856 | 0. |
| More than 6.5 lb. whole | 4 oz. (meat only) | 594 | 0. |
| **LAMB,** choice grade (USDA): Chop, broiled: Loin. One 5-oz. chop (weighed before cooking with bone) will give you: | | | |
| Lean & fat | 2.8 oz. | 280 | 0. |

| Food and Description | Measure or Quantity | Calories | Carbo-hydrates (grams) |
|---|---|---|---|
| Lean only | 2.3 oz. | 122 | 0. |
| Rib. One 5-oz. chop (weighed before cooking with bone) will give you: | | | |
| Lean & fat | 2.9 oz. | 334 | 0. |
| Lean only | 2 oz. | 118 | 0. |
| Fat, separable, cooked | 1 oz. | 201 | 0. |
| Leg: | | | |
| Raw, lean & fat | 1 lb. (weighed with bone) | 845 | 0. |
| Roasted, lean & fat | 4 oz. | 316 | 0. |
| Roasted, lean only | 4 oz. | 211 | 0. |
| Shoulder: | | | |
| Raw, lean & fat | 1 lb. (weighed with bone) | 1082 | 0. |
| Roasted, lean & fat | 4 oz. | 383 | 0. |
| Roasted, lean only | 4 oz. | 232 | 0. |
| **LAMB'S-QUARTERS** (USDA): | | | |
| Raw, trimmed | 1 lb. | 195 | 33.1 |
| Boiled, drained | 4 oz. | 36 | 5.7 |
| **LAMB STEW,** canned, dietetic (Featherweight) | 7¼-oz. can | 230 | 23.0 |
| **LARD:** | | | |
| (USDA) | 1 cup (7.2 oz.) | 1849 | 0. |
| (USDA) | 1 T. (.5 oz.) | 117 | 0. |
| **LASAGNE:** | | | |
| Canned: | | | |
| (Hormel) *Short Orders* | 7½-oz. can | 260 | 24.0 |
| (Nalley's) | 8-oz. serving | 239 | 25.0 |
| Frozen: | | | |
| (Green Giant): | | | |
| With meat sauce, boil-in-bag | 9-oz. serving | 294 | 32.2 |

(USDA): United States Department of Agriculture
(HEW/FAO): Health, Education and Welfare/Food and Agriculture Organization
* Prepared as Package Directs

| Food and Description | Measure or Quantity | Calories | Carbo-hydrates (grams) |
|---|---|---|---|
| With meat sauce, oven bake | ⅓ of 21-oz. pkg. | 295 | 27.8 |
| (Ronzoni) | ⅙ of 26-oz. pkg. | 160 | 22.0 |
| (Stouffer's) | ½ of 21-oz. pkg. | 380 | 35.8 |
| (Swanson): | | | |
| Dinner | 13-oz. dinner | 390 | 54.0 |
| Dinner, *Hungry Man*, with meat | 17¾-oz. dinner | 790 | 91.0 |
| Entree, *Hungry Man*, with meat | 12¾-oz. entree | 540 | 51.0 |
| Entree, with meat in tomato sauce | 11¾-oz. entree | 450 | 46.0 |
| (Weight Watchers) 1-compartment casserole | 13-oz. meal | 368 | 35.1 |
| Mix (Golden Grain) | | | |
| *Stir-n-Serve* | ⅛ of 7-oz. pkg. | 140 | 26.3 |
| **LEEKS**, raw (USDA): | | | |
| Whole | 1 lb. (weighed untrimmed) | 123 | 26.4 |
| Trimmed | 4 oz. | 59 | 12.7 |
| **LEMON**, fresh (USDA) peeled | 1 med. (2⅛″ dia.) | 20 | 6.1 |
| **LEMONADE:** | | | |
| Chilled (Minute Maid): | | | |
| Regular | 6 fl. oz. | 79 | 18.0 |
| Pink | 6 fl. oz. | 78 | 18.0 |
| Canned, *Country Time* | 12-fl.-oz. can | 134 | 33.5 |
| Frozen, concentrate, sweetened: | | | |
| (USDA) | 6-fl.-oz. can | 427 | 112.0 |
| *(USDA) diluted | ½ cup (4.4 oz.) | 55 | 14.1 |
| *Country Time*, regular or pink | 8 fl. oz. | 91 | 22.7 |
| *(Minute Maid) | 6 fl. oz. | 74 | 19.6 |
| *(Sunkist) regular or pink | 6 fl. oz. | 81 | 21.1 |
| Mix: | | | |
| *Country Time*, regular or pink | 8 fl. oz. | 90 | 22.0 |
| *(Hi-C) | 6 fl. oz. | 76 | 19.0 |

| Food and Description | Measure or Quantity | Calories | Carbohydrates (grams) |
|---|---|---|---|
| *(Kool-Aid) unsweetened, regular or pink | 8 fl. oz. | 100 | 25.0 |
| *(Kool-Aid) sweetened, regular or pink | 8 fl. oz. | 89 | 22.2 |
| *Lemon Tree (Lipton) | 8 fl. oz. | 90 | 22.0 |
| **LEMON EXTRACT:** | | | |
| (Durkee) imitation | 1 tsp. | 17 | DNA |
| (Ehlers) pure | 1 tsp. | 30 | DNA |
| (Virginia Dare) 77% alcohol | 1 tsp. | 22 | 0. |
| **LEMON JUICE:** | | | |
| Fresh (USDA) | 1 cup (8.6 oz.) | 61 | 19.5 |
| Fresh (USDA) | 1 T. (.5 oz.) | 4 | 1.2 |
| Canned, unsweetened: | | | |
| (USDA) | 1 cup (8.6 oz.) | 56 | 18.6 |
| (USDA) | 1 T. (.5 oz.) | 3 | 1.1 |
| (Sunkist) | 1 T. | 3 | 1.2 |
| Plastic container: | | | |
| (USDA) | ¼ cup (2 oz.) | 13 | 4.3 |
| *ReaLemon* | 1 T. (.5 oz.) | 3 | .8 |
| Frozen, unsweetened: | | | |
| (USDA): | | | |
| Concentrate | ½ cup (5.1 oz.) | 169 | 54.6 |
| Single strength | ½ cup (4.3 oz.) | 27 | 8.8 |
| (Minute Maid) full strength, already reconstituted | 6 fl. oz. | 74 | 19.6 |
| **LEMON PEEL, CANDIED** | | | |
| (USDA) | 1 oz. | 90 | 22.9 |
| **LENTIL:** | | | |
| Whole: | | | |
| Dry: | | | |
| (USDA) | ½ lb. | 771 | 136.3 |

(USDA): United States Department of Agriculture
(HEW/FAO): Health, Education and Welfare/Food and Agriculture Organization
* Prepared as Package Directs

| Food and Description | Measure or Quantity | Calories | Carbo-hydrates (grams) |
|---|---|---|---|
| (USDA) | 1 cup (6.7 oz.) | 649 | 114.8 |
| (Sinsheimer) | 1 oz. | 95 | 17.0 |
| Cooked (USDA) drained | ½ cup (3.6 oz.) | 107 | 19.5 |
| Split (USDA) dry | ½ lb. | 782 | 140.2 |
| **LENTIL SOUP,** canned (Crosse & Blackwell) with ham | ½ of 13-oz. can | 80 | 13.0 |
| **LETTUCE** (USDA): | | | |
| Bibb, untrimmed | 1 lb. (weighed untrimmed) | 47 | 8.4 |
| Bibb, untrimmed | 7.8-oz. head (4″ dia.) | 23 | 4.1 |
| Boston, untrimmed | 1 lb. (weighed untrimmed) | 47 | 8.4 |
| Boston, untrimmed | 7.8-oz. head (4″ dia.) | 23 | 4.1 |
| Butterhead varieties (See Bibb & Boston) | | | |
| Cos (See Romaine) | | | |
| Dark green (See Romaine) | | | |
| Grand Rapids | 1 lb. (weighed untrimmed) | 52 | 10.2 |
| Grand Rapids | 2 large leaves (1.8 oz.) | 9 | 1.8 |
| Great Lakes | 1 lb. (weighed untrimmed) | 56 | 12.5 |
| Great Lakes, trimmed | 1-lb. head (4¾″ dia.) | 59 | 13.2 |
| Iceberg: | | | |
| Untrimmed | 1 lb. (weighed untrimmed) | 56 | 12.5 |
| Trimmed | 1-lb. head (4¾″ dia.) | 59 | 13.2 |
| Leaves | 1 cup (2.3 oz.) | 9 | 1.9 |
| Chopped | 1 cup (2 oz.) | 8 | 1.7 |
| Chunks | 1 cup (2.6 oz.) | 10 | 2.1 |
| Looseleaf varieties (See Salad Bowl) | | | |
| New York | 1 lb. (weighed untrimmed) | 56 | 12.5 |

| Food and Description | Measure or Quantity | Calories | Carbohydrates (grams) |
|---|---|---|---|
| New York | 1-lb. head (4¾″ dia.) | 59 | 13.2 |
| Romaine: | | | |
| Untrimmed | 1 lb. (weighed untrimmed) | 52 | 10.2 |
| Trimmed, shredded & broken into pieces | ½ cup (.8 oz.) | 4 | .8 |
| Salad Bowl | 1 lb. (weighed untrimmed) | 52 | 10.2 |
| Salad Bowl | 2 large leaves (1.8 oz.) | 9 | 1.8 |
| Simpson | 1 lb. (weighed untrimmed) | 52 | 10.2 |
| Simpson | 2 large leaves (1.8 oz.) | 9 | 1.8 |
| White Paris (See Romaine) | | | |
| LIFE, cereal (Quaker) | ⅔ cup (1 oz.) | 105 | 19.7 |
| LIMA BEAN (See BEAN, LIMA) | | | |
| LIME, fresh (USDA): | | | |
| Whole | 1 lb. (weighed with skin & seeds) | 107 | 36.2 |
| Whole | 1 med. (2″ dia., 2.4 oz.) | 15 | 4.9 |
| LIMEADE, frozen, concentrate, sweetened: | | | |
| (USDA) | 6-fl.-oz. can | 408 | 107.9 |
| *(USDA) diluted with 4⅓ parts water | ½ cup (4.4 oz.) | 51 | 13.6 |
| *(Minute Maid) | 6 fl. oz. | 75 | 20.1 |
| LIME JUICE: | | | |
| Fresh (USDA) | 1 cup (8.7 oz.) | 64 | 22.1 |

(USDA): United States Department of Agriculture
(HEW/FAO): Health, Education and Welfare/Food and Agriculture Organization
* Prepared as Package Directs

| Food and Description | Measure or Quantity | Calories | Carbo-hydrates (grams) |
|---|---|---|---|
| Canned or bottled, unsweetened: | | | |
| (USDA) | 1 cup (8.7 oz.) | 64 | 22.1 |
| (USDA) | 1 fl. oz. (1.1 oz.) | 8 | 2.8 |
| Plastic container, *ReaLime* | 1 T. (.5 oz.) | 2 | .5 |
| **LINGCOD**, raw (USDA): | | | |
| Whole | 1 lb. (weighed whole) | 130 | 0. |
| Meat only | 4 oz. | 95 | 0. |
| **LINGUINI IN CLAM SAUCE**, frozen: | | | |
| (Ronzoni) | 4-oz. serving | 120 | 16.0 |
| (Stouffer's) | 10½-oz. pkg. | 284 | 35.8 |
| **LIQUEUR** (See individual kinds) | | | |
| **LITCHI NUT** (USDA): | | | |
| Fresh: | | | |
| Whole | 4 oz. (weighed in shell with seeds) | 44 | 11.2 |
| Flesh only | 4 oz. | 73 | 18.6 |
| Dried: | | | |
| Whole | 4 oz. (weighed in shell with seeds) | 145 | 36.9 |
| Flesh only | 2 oz. | 157 | 40.1 |
| **LIVER:** | | | |
| Beef: | | | |
| (USDA): | | | |
| Raw | 1 lb. | 635 | 24.0 |
| Fried | 4 oz. | 260 | 6.0 |
| (Swift) packaged, True-Tender, sliced, cooked | ⅛ of 1-lb. pkg. | 141 | 3.1 |
| Calf (USDA): | | | |
| Raw | 1 lb. | 635 | 18.6 |
| Fried | 4 oz. | 296 | 4.5 |
| Chicken: | | | |
| Raw | 1 lb. | 585 | 13.2 |

| Food and Description | Measure or Quantity | Calories | Carbohydrates (grams) |
|---|---|---|---|
| Simmered | 4 oz. | 187 | 3.5 |
| Goose, raw (USDA) | 1 lb. | 826 | 24.5 |
| Hog (USDA): | | | |
| Raw | 1 lb. | 594 | 11.8 |
| Fried | 4 oz. | 273 | 2.8 |
| Lamb (USDA): | | | |
| Raw | 1 lb. | 617 | 13.2 |
| Broiled | 4 oz. | 296 | 3.2 |
| Turkey, raw (USDA) | 1 lb. | 626 | 13.2 |
| **LIVER PÂTÉ** (See PÂTÉ) | | | |
| **LIVER SAUSAGE** or **LIVERWURST,** spread (Underwood) | 1 oz. | 92 | 1.1 |
| **LOBSTER:** | | | |
| Raw (USDA): | | | |
| Whole | 1 lb. (weighed whole) | 107 | .6 |
| Meat only | 4 oz. | 103 | .6 |
| Cooked, meat only (USDA) | 4 oz. | 108 | .3 |
| Canned (USDA) meat only | 4 oz. | 108 | .3 |
| Frozen, South African rock lobster tail | 2-oz. tail | 65 | .1 |
| **LOBSTER NEWBURG,** home recipe (USDA) | 4 oz. | 220 | 5.8 |
| **LOBSTER PASTE,** canned (USDA) | 1 oz. | 51 | .4 |
| **LOBSTER SALAD,** home recipe (USDA) | 4 oz. | 125 | 2.6 |
| *LOCHON ORA,* Scottish liqueur (Leroux) 70 proof | 1 fl. oz. | 89 | 7.4 |

(USDA): United States Department of Agriculture
(HEW/FAO): Health, Education and Welfare/Food and Agriculture
        Organization
* Prepared as Package Directs

| Food and Description | Measure or Quantity | Calories | Carbo-hydrates (grams) |
|---|---|---|---|
| **LOGANBERRY** (USDA): | | | |
| Fresh: | | | |
| Untrimmed | 1 lb. (weighed with caps) | 267 | 64.2 |
| Trimmed | 1 cup (5.1 oz.) | 89 | 21.5 |
| Canned, solids & liq.: | | | |
| Extra heavy syrup | 4 oz. | 101 | 25.2 |
| Heavy syrup | 4 oz. | 101 | 25.2 |
| Juice pack | 4 oz. | 61 | 14.4 |
| Light syrup | 4 oz. | 79 | 19.5 |
| Water pack | 4 oz. | 45 | 10.7 |
| **LOG CABIN,** syrup: | | | |
| Regular | 1 T. (.7 oz.) | 52 | 13.1 |
| Buttered | 1 T. (.7 oz.) | 55 | 13.0 |
| Maple-honey | 1 T. | 56 | 13.9 |
| **LONGAN** (USDA): | | | |
| Fresh: | | | |
| Whole | 1 lb. (weighed with shell & seeds) | 147 | 38.0 |
| Flesh only | 4 oz. | 69 | 17.9 |
| Dried: | | | |
| Whole | 1 lb. (weighed with shell & seeds) | 467 | 120.8 |
| Flesh only | 4 oz. | 324 | 83.9 |
| **LOQUAT,** fresh (USDA): | | | |
| Whole | 1 lb. (weighed with seeds) | 168 | 43.3 |
| Flesh only | 4 oz. | 54 | 14.1 |
| **LOVE BIRD COCKTAIL,** dry mix (Holland House) | .6-oz. pkg. | 69 | 17.0 |
| **LUCKY CHARMS,** cereal | 1 cup (1 oz.) | 110 | 24.0 |
| **LUNCHEON MEAT** (See also individual listings, e.g., **BOLOGNA**): | | | |
| All meat (Oscar Meyer) | 1-oz. slice | 98 | .7 |

| Food and Description | Measure or Quantity | Calories | Carbo-hydrates (grams) |
|---|---|---|---|
| Banquet loaf (Eckrich) | ¾-oz. slice | 55 | 1.0 |
| Banquet loaf (Eckrich) | 1-oz. slice | 75 | 1.5 |
| *Bar-B-Q-Loaf* (Oscar Mayer) | 1-oz. slice | 47 | 1.7 |
| BBQ Loaf (Hormel) | 1-oz. slice | 50 | .5 |
| Buffet loaf (Hormel) | 1-oz. slice | 50 | .5 |
| Gourmet loaf (Eckrich) | 1-oz. slice | 32 | 1.7 |
| Ham & cheese (See **HAM & CHEESE**) | | | |
| Honey loaf: | | | |
| (Eckrich) | 1-oz. slice | 40 | 1.8 |
| (Oscar Mayer) | 1-oz. slice | 35 | 1.1 |
| Liver cheese (Oscar Mayer) | 1.3-oz. slice | 112 | .5 |
| Meat loaf (USDA) | 1-oz. serving | 57 | .9 |
| *New England Brand* sliced sausage (Oscar Mayer) | .8-oz. slice | 33 | .3 |
| New England (Hormel) | 1-oz. slice | 49 | .2 |
| Old fashioned loaf: | | | |
| (Eckrich) | 1-oz. slice | 75 | 2.0 |
| (Oscar Mayer) | 1-oz. slice | 66 | 2.3 |
| Olive loaf: | | | |
| (Hormel) | 1-oz. slice | 59 | 1.5 |
| (Oscar Mayer) | 1-oz. slice | 65 | 2.6 |
| Peppered beef (Vienna) | 1 oz. | 50 | .4 |
| Peppered loaf (Oscar Mayer) | 1-oz. slice | 41 | 1.3 |
| Pickle loaf: | | | |
| (Eckrich) | 1-oz. slice | 85 | 1.5 |
| (Hormel) | 1-oz. slice | 59 | 1.3 |
| Pickle & pimiento (Oscar Mayer) | 1-oz. slice | 65 | 2.9 |
| Picnic loaf (Oscar Mayer) | 1-oz. slice | 64 | 1.4 |
| Sandwich spread (Oscar Mayer) | 1-oz. serving | 69 | 4.0 |
| Spiced (Hormel) | 1 oz. | 77 | .4 |
| **LUNG, raw** (USDA): | | | |
| Beef | 1 lb. | 435 | 0. |

(USDA): United States Department of Agriculture
(HEW/FAO): Health, Education and Welfare/Food and Agriculture
        Organization
* Prepared as Package Directs

| Food and Description | Measure or Quantity | Calories | Carbo-hydrates (grams) |
|---|---|---|---|
| Calf | 1 lb. | 481 | 0. |
| Lamb | 1 lb. | 467 | 0. |

# M

**MACADAMIA NUT:**

| | | | |
|---|---|---|---|
| Whole (USDA) | 1 lb. (weighed in shell) | 972 | 22.4 |
| Shelled (Royal Hawaiian) | ¼ cup (2 oz.) | 394 | 9.0 |

**MACARONI.** Plain macaroni products are essentially the same in caloric value and carbohydrate content on the same weight basis. The longer they are cooked, the more water is absorbed and this affects the nutritive values. (USDA):

| | | | |
|---|---|---|---|
| Dry: | | | |
| Elbow-type | 1 cup (4.8 oz.) | 502 | 102.3 |
| 1-inch pieces | 1 cup (3.8 oz.) | 406 | 82.7 |
| 2-inch pieces | 1 cup (3 oz.) | 317 | 64.7 |
| Cooked: | | | |
| 8-10 minutes, firm | 1 cup (4.6 oz.) | 192 | 39.1 |
| 8-10 minutes, firm | 4 oz. | 168 | 34.1 |
| 14-20 minutes, tender | 1 cup (4.9 oz.) | 155 | 32.2 |
| 14-20 minutes, tender | 4 oz. | 126 | 26.1 |

**MACARONI & BEEF:**

| | | | |
|---|---|---|---|
| Canned: | | | |
| (Bounty) in tomato sauce, *Chili Mac* | 7¾-oz. can | 255 | 29.7 |
| (Franco-American) in tomato sauce, *Beefy Mac* | 7½-oz. can | 220 | 28.0 |
| (Nalley's) | 8-oz. serving | 236 | 29.5 |
| Frozen: | | | |
| (Banquet): | | | |
| Buffet | 2-lb. pkg. | 1000 | 106.4 |
| Dinner | 12-oz. dinner | 394 | 55.1 |

| Food and Description | Measure or Quantity | Calories | Carbo-hydrates (grams) |
|---|---|---|---|
| (Green Giant) with tomato sauce | 9-oz. entree | 233 | 30.7 |
| (Morton) | 10-oz. dinner | 267 | 45.5 |
| (Stouffer's) with tomatoes | 11½-oz. pkg. | 384 | 39.8 |
| (Swanson) | 12-oz. dinner | 400 | 56.0 |
| **MACARONI & CHEESE:** | | | |
| Home recipe (USDA) baked | 1 cup (7.1 oz.) | 430 | 40.2 |
| Canned: | | | |
| (USDA) | 1 cup | 228 | 25.7 |
| (Franco-American) | ½ of 14¾-oz. can | 184 | 23.5 |
| (Franco-American) elbow | 7½-oz. can | 186 | 23.8 |
| (Hormel) *Short Orders* | 7½-oz. can | 170 | 22.0 |
| Frozen: | | | |
| (Banquet): | | | |
| Buffet | 2-lb. pkg. | 1027 | 110.9 |
| Cooking bag | 8-oz. bag | 261 | 28.6 |
| Dinner | 12-oz. dinner | 326 | 45.6 |
| Entree | 8-oz. entree | 279 | 35.9 |
| (Green Giant): | | | |
| Boil-in-bag | 9-oz. entree | 304 | 35.8 |
| Oven bake | 12-oz. serving | 432 | 47.4 |
| (Morton): | | | |
| Casserole | 8-oz. casserole | 227 | 36.4 |
| Dinner | 11-oz. dinner | 306 | 53.1 |
| (Stouffer's) | 12-oz. pkg. | 502 | 47.8 |
| (Swanson): | | | |
| Dinner | 12½-oz. dinner | 390 | 55.0 |
| Entree | 12-oz. entree | 420 | 40.0 |
| (Van de Kamp's) | 10-oz. pkg. | 300 | 46.0 |
| **MACARONI & CHEESE MIX:** | | | |
| (USDA) dry | 1 oz. | 113 | 17.8 |
| (Ann Page) dinner | ¼ of 7¼-oz. pkg. | 189 | 37.5 |
| (Betty Crocker) | ¼ of pkg. | 200 | 37.0 |
| *(Betty Crocker) | ¼ of pkg. | 310 | 38.0 |

(USDA): United States Department of Agriculture
(HEW/FAO): Health, Education and Welfare/Food and Agriculture
 Organization

* Prepared as Package Directs

| Food and Description | Measure or Quantity | Calories | Carbohydrates (grams) |
|---|---|---|---|
| (Golden Grain) dinner, deluxe | ¼ of 7½-oz. pkg. | 200 | 38.1 |
| *(Kraft) | ¾ cup | 290 | 32.0 |
| *(Pennsylvania Dutch Brand) | ½ cup serving | 160 | 25.0 |
| *(Prince) | ¾ cup serving | 268 | 34.6 |
| *Tuna Helper (General Mills) | ¼ pkg. | 310 | 38.0 |
| **MACARONI DINNER or ENTREE,** frozen (Weight Watchers) ziti | 13-oz. meal | 363 | 39.1 |
| **MACARONI SALAD,** canned (Nalley's) | 4-oz. serving | 206 | 15.9 |
| **MACE** (French's) | 1 tsp. (1.8 grams) | 10 | .8 |
| **MACKEREL** (USDA): | | | |
| Atlantic: | | | |
| Raw: | | | |
| Whole | 1 lb. (weighed whole) | 468 | 0. |
| Meat only | 4 oz. | 217 | 0. |
| Broiled with butter | 4 oz. | 268 | 0. |
| Canned, solids & liq. | 4 oz. | 208 | 0. |
| Pacific: | | | |
| Raw: | | | |
| Dressed | 1 lb. (weighed with bones & skin) | 519 | 0. |
| Meat only | 4 oz. | 180 | 0. |
| Canned, solids & liq. | 4 oz. | 204 | 0. |
| Salted | 4 oz. | 346 | 0. |
| Smoked | 4 oz. | 248 | 0. |
| **MACKEREL, JACK** (See JACK MACKEREL) | | | |
| **MADEIRA WINE** (Leacock) 19% alcohol | 3 fl. oz. | 120 | 6.3 |
| **MAI TAI COCKTAIL:** | | | |
| (Lemon Hart) 48 proof | 3 fl. oz. | 180 | 15.6 |
| (Mr. Boston) 12½% alcohol | 3 fl. oz. | 111 | 12.3 |

| Food and Description | Measure or Quantity | Calories | Carbo-hydrates (grams) |
|---|---|---|---|
| (National Distillers) *Duet*, 12.5% alcohol | 8-fl.-oz. can | 288 | 28.8 |
| (Party Tyme) 12.5% alcohol | 2 fl. oz. | 65 | 5.7 |
| Dry mix (Bar-Tender's) | 1 serving (5.8 oz.) | 69 | 17.0 |
| Dry mix (Holland House) | 1 serving (.6-oz. pkg.) | 69 | 17.0 |
| Dry mix (Party Tyme) | 1 serving (½ oz.) | 50 | 11.8 |
| Liquid mix (Holland House) | 1½ fl. oz. | 50 | 12.0 |
| Liquid mix (Party Tyme) | 2 fl. oz. | 44 | 11.2 |
| **MALT, dry (USDA)** | 1 oz. | 104 | 21.9 |
| **MALTED MILK MIX:** | | | |
| (USDA) Dry powder | 1 oz. | 116 | 20.1 |
| (Carnation): | | | |
| Chocolate | 3 heaping tsps. (.7 oz.) | 85 | 18.0 |
| Natural | 3 heaping tsps. (.7 oz.) | 90 | 15.6 |
| (Horlicks): | | | |
| Chocolate | 3 heaping tsps. (1.1 oz.) | 124 | 26.0 |
| Natural | 3 heaping tsps. (1.1 oz.) | 127 | 22.3 |
| **MALT EXTRACT, dried (USDA)** | 1 oz. | 104 | 25.3 |
| **MALT LIQUOR:** | | | |
| *Champale*, 6.25% alcohol | 12 fl. oz. | 173 | 11.5 |
| *Country Club*, 6.8% alcohol | 12 fl. oz. | 183 | 2.8 |
| **MAMEY or MAMMEE APPLE, fresh (USDA)** | 1 lb. (weighed with skin & seeds) | 143 | 35.2 |
| **MANDARIN ORANGE (See TANGERINE)** | | | |

(USDA): United States Department of Agriculture
(HEW/FAO): Health, Education and Welfare/Food and Agriculture Organization
* Prepared as Package Directs

| Food and Description | Measure or Quantity | Calories | Carbo-hydrates (grams) |
|---|---|---|---|
| **MANGO, fresh (USDA):** | | | |
| Whole | 1 lb. (weighed with seeds & skin) | 201 | 51.1 |
| Whole | 1 med. (7 oz.) | 88 | 22.5 |
| Flesh only, diced or sliced | ½ cup (2.9 oz.) | 54 | 13.8 |
| **MANHATTAN COCKTAIL:** | | | |
| (Hiram Walker) 55 proof | 3 fl. oz. | 147 | 3.0 |
| (Mr. Boston) 20% alcohol | 3 fl. oz. | 123 | 6.3 |
| (National Distillers) | | | |
|    *Duet*, 20% alcohol | 8-fl.-oz. can | 576 | 11.2 |
| (Party Tyme) 20% alcohol | 2 fl. oz. | 74 | 1.5 |
| Dry mix (Bar-Tender's) | 1 serving (⅛ oz.) | 24 | 5.6 |
| **MAPLE SYRUP (See also individual brand names):** | | | |
| (USDA) | 1 T. (.7 oz.) | 50 | 13.0 |
| (Cary's) | 1 T. (.8 oz.) | 63 | 15.7 |
| **MARGARINE, salted or unsalted:** | | | |
| (USDA) | 1 lb. | 3266 | 1.8 |
| (USDA) | 1 cup (8 oz.) | 1633 | .9 |
| (USDA) | 1 T. (.5 oz.) | 101 | <.1 |
| *Autumn*, soft or stick | 1 T. | 102 | Tr. |
| (Blue Bonnet) regular or soft | 1 T. (.5 oz.) | 100 | 0. |
| *Chiffon*, soft | 1 T. | 90 | 0. |
| *Chiffon*, stick | 1 T. | 100 | 0. |
| (Fleishmann's) regular or soft | 1 T. (.5 oz.) | 101 | 0. |
| *Golden Mist* | 1 T. | 100 | 0. |
| (Holiday) | 1 T. (.5 oz.) | 103 | 0. |
| (Imperial) soft or stick | 1 T. (.5 oz.) | 102 | <.1 |
| (Mazola) | 1 T. (.5 oz.) | 104 | .1 |
| (Miracle) corn oil | 1 T. (9 grams) | 67 | <.1 |
| (Nucoa) | 1 T. (.5 oz.) | 103 | 0. |
| (Nucoa) soft | 1 T. (.4 oz.) | 82 | 0. |
| (Parkay) regular | 1 T. (.5 oz.) | 102 | .1 |
| (Parkay) soft | 1 T. (.5 oz.) | 101 | .2 |
| (Parkay) *Squeeze* | 1 T. (.5 oz.) | 101 | .2 |
| (Phenix) | 1 T. (.5 oz.) | 101 | .1 |
| (Promise) soft or stick | 1 T. (.5 oz.) | 102 | <.1 |

| Food and Description | Measure or Quantity | Calories | Carbohydrates (grams) |
|---|---|---|---|
| (Saffola) regular or soft | 1 T. (.5 oz.) | 101 | <.1 |
| Imitation or dietetic: | | | |
| (Fleishmann's) | 1 T. (.5 oz.) | 50 | 0. |
| (Imperial) soft | 1 T. (.5 oz.) | 50 | 0. |
| (Mazola) | 1 T. (.5 oz.) | 50 | 0. |
| (Parkay) soft | 1 T. | 50 | 0. |
| (Weight Watchers) | 1 T. | 50 | 0. |
| Whipped: | | | |
| (Blue Bonnet) | 1 T. (9 grams) | 67 | <.1 |
| *Chiffon* | 1 T. | 70 | 0. |
| *Fleischmann's*, soft | 1 T. | 70 | 0. |
| *Imperial* | 1 T. (9 grams) | 65 | 0. |
| (Parkay) cup | 1 T. | 67 | <.1 |
| **MARGARITA COCKTAIL:** | | | |
| (Mr. Boston) 12½% alcohol | 3 fl. oz. | 105 | 10.8 |
| (Mr. Boston) strawberry, 12½% alcohol | 3 fl. oz. | 138 | 18.9 |
| (National Distillers) | | | |
| *Duet*, 12½% alcohol | 8-fl.-oz. can | 248 | 20.0 |
| (Party Tyme) 12½% alcohol | 2 fl. oz. | 66 | 5.7 |
| Dry mix (Bar-Tender's) | ⅝-oz. serving | 70 | 17.3 |
| **MARINADE MIX:** | | | |
| (Adolph's): | | | |
| Chicken | 1-oz. pkg. | 64 | 14.4 |
| Meat | .8-oz. pkg. | 38 | 8.5 |
| (Durkee) meat | 1-oz. pkg. | 47 | 9.0 |
| (French's) meat | 1-oz. pkg. | 80 | 16.0 |
| **MARJORAM** (French's) | 1 tsp. (1.2 grams) | 4 | .8 |
| **MARMALADE:** | | | |
| Sweetened: | | | |
| (USDA) | 1 T. (.7 oz.) | 51 | 14.0 |
| (Ann Page) | 1 T. (.7 oz.) | 59 | 14.8 |
| (Crosse & Blackwell) all flavors | 1 T. (.6 oz.) | 60 | 14.9 |

(USDA): United States Department of Agriculture
(HEW/FAO): Health, Education and Welfare/Food and Agriculture Organization
* Prepared as Package Directs

| Food and Description | Measure or Quantity | Calories | Carbo-hydrates (grams) |
|---|---|---|---|
| (Keiller) all flavors | 1 T. | 60 | 15.0 |
| (Ma Brown) | 1 oz. | 73 | 17.0 |
| (Smucker's) English style or sweet | 1 T. (.7 oz.) | 53 | 13.5 |
| Dietetic or low calorie: | | | |
| (Dia-Mel) | 1 tsp. | 6 | 0. |
| (Featherweight) | 1 T. | 16 | 4.0 |
| (Louis Sherry) | 1 tsp. | 2 | 0. |
| (Tillie Lewis) | 1 T. (.5 oz.) | 12 | 3.0 |
| **MARSHMALLOW FLUFF** | 1 heaping tsp. (.7 oz.) | 66 | 15.6 |
| **MARTINI COCKTAIL:** | | | |
| Gin: | | | |
| Canned: | | | |
| (Hiram Walker) 65.5 proof | 3 fl. oz. | 168 | .6 |
| (Mr. Boston) extra dry, 20% alcohol | 3 fl. oz. | 99 | 0. |
| (National Distillers) *Duet,* 21% alcohol | 8-fl.-oz. can | 560 | 1.6 |
| (Party Tyme) 24% alcohol | 2 fl. oz. | 82 | 0. |
| Liquid mix: | | | |
| (Holland House) | 1½ fl. oz. | 15 | 3.8 |
| (Party Tyme) | 2 fl. oz. | 12 | 3.2 |
| Vodka: | | | |
| Canned: | | | |
| (Hiram Walker) 60 proof | 3 fl. oz. | 147 | Tr. |
| (Mr. Boston) 20% alcohol | 3 fl. oz. | 102 | .9 |
| (National Distillers) *Duet,* 20% alcohol | 8-fl.-oz. can | 536 | 1.6 |
| (Party Tyme) 21% alcohol | 2 fl. oz. | 72 | 0. |
| **MASA HARINA** (Quaker) | ⅛ cup | 137 | 27.4 |
| **MATZO:** | | | |
| (Goodman's): | | | |
| *Diet-10's* | 1 sq. | 109 | 23.0 |

| Food and Description | Measure or Quantity | Calories | Carbo-hydrates (grams) |
|---|---|---|---|
| *Midgetea* | 1 matzo (.4 oz.) | 40 | 7.4 |
| Round tea | 1 matzo (.6 oz.) | 70 | 12.9 |
| Unsalted | 1 matzo (1 oz.) | 109 | 23.0 |
| (Horowitz-Margareten) | | | |
| unsalted | 1 matzo (1.2 oz.) | 135 | 28.2 |
| (Manischewitz): | | | |
| Regular | 1 matzo (1.1 oz.) | 114 | 28.1 |
| American | 1 matzo (1 oz.) | 121 | 22.6 |
| Diet-thins | 1 matzo (1 oz.) | 113 | 24.5 |
| Egg | 1 matzo (1.2 oz.) | 133 | 26.6 |
| Egg'n onion | 1 matzo (1 oz.) | 116 | 24.6 |
| *Onion Tams* | 1 piece (3 grams) | 13 | 1.9 |
| *Tam Tams* | 1 piece (3 grams) | 14 | 1.7 |
| *Tasteas* | 1 matzo (1 oz.) | 119 | 24.2 |
| Thin tea | 1 matzo (1 oz.) | 114 | 24.8 |
| Whole wheat | 1 matzo (1.2 oz.) | 124 | 24.2 |
| **MATZO MEAL** | | | |
| (Manischewitz) | 1 cup (4.1 oz.) | 438 | 96.2 |
| **MAYONNAISE:** | | | |
| (USDA) | 1 cup (7.8 oz.) | 1587 | 4.9 |
| (USDA) | 1 T. (.5 oz.) | 101 | .3 |
| (Ann Page) | 1 T. (.5 oz.) | 105 | .1 |
| (Best Foods) *Real* | 1 T. (.5 oz.) | 103 | <.1 |
| (Dia-Mel) | 1 T. (.5 oz.) | 106 | .2 |
| (Diet Delight) *Mayo-Lite,* | | | |
| imitation | 1 T. | 26 | .7 |
| (Hellmann's) *Real* | 1 T. (.5 oz.) | 103 | <.1 |
| (Nalley's) | 1 T. | 103 | .3 |
| (Saffola) | 1 T. (.5 oz.) | 95 | .3 |
| (Sultana) | 1 T. (.5 oz.) | 103 | .2 |
| (Tillie Lewis) *Tasti Diet,* | | | |
| imitation | 1 T. | 25 | 1.0 |
| (Weight Watchers) imitation | 1 T. | 40 | 1.0 |
| ***MAYPO,*** cereal, dry: | | | |
| 30-second style | ¼ cup (.8 oz.) | 89 | 16.4 |
| Vermont style | ¼ cup | 121 | 22.0 |

(USDA): United States Department of Agriculture
(HEW/FAO): Health, Education and Welfare/Food and Agriculture
Organization
* Prepared as Package Directs

| Food and Description | Measure or Quantity | Calories | Carbohydrates (grams) |
|---|---|---|---|
| **MAY WINE** (Deinhard) 11% alcohol | 3 fl. oz. | 60 | 1.0 |
| ***McDONALD'S:*** | | | |
| *Big Mac* | 1 hamburger (7.2 oz.) | 563 | 40.6 |
| Cheeseburger | 1 cheeseburger (4.0 oz.) | 307 | 29.8 |
| Cookie, *McDonaldland* | 1 package (2.4 oz.) | 308 | 48.7 |
| *Egg McMuffin* | 1 serving | 327 | 31.0 |
| English muffin, buttered | 1 muffin (2.2 oz.) | 186 | 29.5 |
| *Filet-o-Fish* | 1 sandwich | 432 | 37.4 |
| French fries, regular | 1 serving | 220 | 26.1 |
| Hamburger | 1 hamburger | 255 | 29.5 |
| Hash Brown Potatoes | 1 serving (1.9 oz.) | 125 | 14.0 |
| Hot cakes with butter & syrup | 1 serving | 500 | 93.9 |
| Pie: | | | |
| Apple | 1 pie (3.0 oz.) | 253 | 29.3 |
| Cherry | 1 pie (3.1 oz.) | 260 | 32.1 |
| *Quarter Pounder*, regular | 1 burger | 454 | 32.7 |
| *Quarter Pounder*, with cheese | 1 burger with cheese | 524 | 32.2 |
| Sausage, pork | 1 serving (1.9 oz.) | 206 | .6 |
| Scrambled eggs | 1 serving | 180 | 2.5 |
| Shake: | | | |
| Chocolate | 1 serving (10.3 oz.) | 383 | 65.5 |
| Strawberry | 1 serving (10.2 oz.) | 362 | 62.1 |
| Vanilla | 1 serving (10.3 oz.) | 352 | 59.6 |
| Sundae: | | | |
| Hot caramel | 5.8-oz. serving | 328 | 52.5 |
| Hot fudge | 5.8-oz. serving | 310 | 46.2 |
| Strawberry | 5.8-oz. serving | 289 | 46.1 |
| **MEATBALL DINNER or ENTREE,** frozen (Swanson) with brown gravy & whipped potatoes | 9½-oz. entree | 330 | 26.0 |

| Food and Description | Measure or Quantity | Calories | Carbo-hydrates (grams) |
|---|---|---|---|
| **MEATBALL SEASONING MIX:** | | | |
| (Durkee) Italian | 1-oz. pkg. | 22 | 9.0 |
| *(Durkee) Italian | ¼ of 1-oz. pkg. | 285 | 2.3 |
| (French's) | 1½-oz. pkg. | 140 | 28.0 |
| **MEATBALL STEW, canned:** | | | |
| (Libby's) | ⅓ of 24-oz. can | 281 | 24.3 |
| (Morton House) | ⅓ of 24-oz. can | 290 | 18.0 |
| (Nalley's) | 8-oz. serving | 261 | 18.2 |
| **MEATBALL, SWEDISH,** frozen (Stouffer's) with parsley noodles | 11-oz. pkg. | 473 | 32.8 |
| **MEAT LOAF DINNER or ENTREE, frozen:** | | | |
| (Banquet): | | | |
| Buffet | 2-lb. pkg. | 1445 | 46.4 |
| Cooking bag | 5-oz. bag | 224 | 13.6 |
| Dinner | 11-oz. dinner | 412 | 29.0 |
| Dinner, *Man Pleaser* | 19-oz. dinner | 916 | 63.6 |
| (Morton) dinner | 11-oz. dinner | 341 | 28.1 |
| (Morton) *Country Table* | 15-oz. dinner | 477 | 59.7 |
| (Swanson): | | | |
| Dinner | 10¾-oz. dinner | 530 | 48.0 |
| Entree, with tomato sauce & whipped potatoes | 9-oz. entree | 330 | 27.0 |
| **MEAT LOAF SEASONING MIX:** | | | |
| (Contadina) | 3¾-oz. pkg. | 360 | 72.4 |
| (French's) | 1½-oz. pkg. | 160 | 40.0 |
| **MEAT, POTTED** (Libby's) | 1-oz. serving | 57 | .3 |
| **MEAT TENDERIZER:** | | | |
| (Adolph's): | | | |
| Unseasoned | 1 tsp. (5 grams) | 2 | .5 |

(USDA): United States Department of Agriculture
(HEW/FAO): Health, Education and Welfare/Food and Agriculture Organization
* Prepared as Package Directs

| Food and Description | Measure or Quantity | Calories | Carbo-hydrates (grams) |
|---|---|---|---|
| Seasoned | 1 tsp. (5 grams) | 1 | .3 |
| (French's) unseasoned or seasoned | 1 tsp. (5 grams) | 2 | <.5 |
| **MELBA TOAST** (Old London): | | | |
| Garlic, rounds | 1 piece (2 grams) | 10 | 1.8 |
| Onion, rounds | 1 piece (2 grams) | 10 | 1.8 |
| Pumpernickel | 1 piece (5 grams) | 17 | 3.4 |
| Rye: | | | |
| Regular | 1 piece (5 grams) | 17 | 3.4 |
| Unsalted | 1 piece (5 grams) | 18 | 3.5 |
| Sesame, rounds | 1 piece (2 grams) | 11 | 1.6 |
| Wheat: | | | |
| Regular | 1 piece (5 grams) | 17 | 3.4 |
| Unsalted | 1 piece (5 grams) | 18 | 3.5 |
| White: | | | |
| Regular | 1 piece (5 grams) | 17 | 3.4 |
| Rounds | 1 piece (2 grams) | 10 | 1.8 |
| Unsalted | 1 piece (5 grams) | 18 | 3.5 |
| **MELON** (See individual listings such as CANTA-LOUPE, WATERMELON, etc.) | | | |
| **MELON BALLS** (cantaloupe & honeydew) in syrup, frozen (USDA) | ½ cup (4.1 oz.) | 72 | 18.2 |
| **MENAHADEN**, Atlantic (USDA) canned, solids & liq. | 4 oz. | 195 | 0. |
| **MEXICAN DINNER,** frozen: | | | |
| (Banquet): | | | |
| Combination | 12-oz. dinner | 571 | 72.1 |
| Mexican style | 16-oz. dinner | 608 | 73.5 |
| (Swanson) combination | 16-oz. dinner | 600 | 72.0 |
| (Van de Kamp's): | | | |
| Regular | 12-oz. dinner | 480 | 47.0 |
| Combination | 11-oz. dinner | 420 | 37.0 |

| Food and Description | Measure or Quantity | Calories | Carbo- hydrates (grams) |
|---|---|---|---|
| **MILK, CONDENSED** | | | |
| (USDA) sweetened, canned | 1 cup (10.8 oz.) | 982 | 166.2 |
| **MILK, DRY:** | | | |
| Whole (USDA) packed cup | 1 cup (5.1 oz.) | 728 | 55.4 |
| Nonfat, instant: | | | |
| (USDA) ⅞ cup makes | | | |
| 1 quart | ⅞ cup (3.2 oz.) | 330 | 47.6 |
| *(Alba) | 8 fl. oz. | 81 | 11.6 |
| *(Alba) chocolate flavor | 8 fl. oz. | 80 | 12.9 |
| *(Carnation) | 8 fl. oz. | 80 | 12.0 |
| (Featherweight) low | | | |
| sodium | ⅔ oz. | 70 | 10.0 |
| *(Pet) | 1 cup | 80 | 12.0 |
| *(Sanalac) | 1 cup | 80 | 12.0 |
| **MILK, EVAPORATED,** | | | |
| canned: | | | |
| Regular: | | | |
| (USDA) unsweetened | 1 cup (8.9 oz.) | 345 | 24.4 |
| (Carnation) | 1 fl. oz. | 42 | 3.0 |
| (Pet) | ½ cup | 170 | 12.0 |
| Filled (Pet) | ½ cup (4 oz.) | 150 | 12.0 |
| Low fat (Carnation) | 1 fl. oz. | 28 | 3.0 |
| Skimmed: | | | |
| (Carnation) | 1 fl. oz. | 25 | 3.5 |
| (Pet) | ½ cup | 100 | 14.0 |
| **MILK, FRESH:** | | | |
| Whole: | | | |
| (Dean) 3.5% fat | 1 cup | 151 | 11.0 |
| (Meadow Gold) Vitamins | | | |
| A & D, 2% fat | 1 cup | 120 | 11.0 |
| (Meadow Gold) | | | |
| Vitamin D | 1 cup | 150 | 11.0 |
| (Sealtest): | | | |
| 3.25% fat | 1 cup (8.6 oz.) | 144 | 10.8 |
| 3.5% fat | 1 cup (8.6 oz.) | 151 | 11.0 |

(USDA): United States Department of Agriculture
(HEW/FAO): Health, Education and Welfare/Food and Agriculture
         Organization
* Prepared as Package Directs

| Food and Description | Measure or Quantity | Calories | Carbohydrates (grams) |
|---|---|---|---|
| 3.7% fat | 1 cup (8.6 oz.) | 157 | 11.1 |
| Extra rich, Vitamin D | 1 cup | 170 | 11.0 |
| Skim: | | | |
| (Dean): | | | |
| .5% fat | 1 cup (8.2 oz.) | 91 | 11.7 |
| 2% fat | 1 cup (8.7 oz.) | 133 | 12.5 |
| (Meadow Gold): | | | |
| Vitamins A & D | 1 cup | 90 | 11.0 |
| *Viva*, 2% fat, Vitamins A & D | 1 cup | 130 | 12.0 |
| (Sealtest): | | | |
| Regular | 1 cup (8.6 oz.) | 79 | 11.3 |
| Protein fortified, Vitamins A & D | 1 cup | 100 | 10.0 |
| Protein fortified, 1% fat, Vitamins A & D | 1 cup | 110 | 14.0 |
| Protein fortified, 1.5% fat, Vitamins A & D | 1 cup | 130 | 13.0 |
| Vitamins A & D | 1 cup | 90 | 11.0 |
| Buttermilk, cultured, fresh: | | | |
| (Dean) | 1 cup (8.6 oz.) | 95 | 11.5 |
| (Meadow Gold) .5% fat | 1 cup | 105 | 12.0 |
| (Sealtest): | | | |
| Regular | 1 cup | 90 | 11.0 |
| With golden nugget flakes | 1 cup | 90 | 11.0 |
| Protein fortified | 1 cup | 110 | 12.0 |
| Protein fortified, *Light 'n Lively* | 1 cup | 110 | 14.0 |
| Whole | 1 cup | 150 | 11.0 |
| Chocolate milk drink, fresh: | | | |
| With whole milk: | | | |
| (Dean) 1% fat | 1 cup (8.9 oz.) | 166 | 27.9 |
| (Dean) 3.5% fat | 1 cup | 212 | 25.5 |
| (Sealtest) 3.4% fat | 1 cup (8.6 oz.) | 207 | 25.9 |
| With skim milk (Sealtest): | | | |
| .5% fat | 1 cup (8.6 oz.) | 146 | 26.2 |
| 1% fat | 1 cup (8.6 oz.) | 180 | 28.0 |
| **MILK, HUMAN** (USDA) | 1 oz. (by wt.) | 22 | 2.7 |

| Food and Description | Measure or Quantity | Calories | Carbo-hydrates (grams) |
|---|---|---|---|
| **MILLET**, whole-grain (USDA) | 1 lb. | 1483 | 330.7 |
| **MINCEMEAT (See PIE FILLING)** | | | |
| **MINCE PIE (See PIE, Mince)** | | | |
| **MINESTRONE SOUP:** | | | |
| (USDA) Condensed | 8 oz. (by wt.) | 197 | 26.3 |
| *(USDA) prepared with equal volume water | 1 cup (8.6 oz.) | 105 | 14.2 |
| *(Ann Page) with beef stock | 1 cup | 82 | 12.8 |
| (Campbell): | | | |
| *Chunky* | 19-oz. can | 280 | 42.0 |
| Condensed | 10-oz. serving | 90 | 13.0 |
| (Crosse & Blackwell) | ½ of 13-oz. can | 90 | 18.0 |
| ***MINI-WHEATS**, cereal* | | | |
| (Kellogg's): | | | |
| Frosted | 4 biscuits (1 oz.) | 110 | 24.0 |
| Toasted | 5 biscuits (1 oz.) | 100 | 22.0 |
| **MOLASSES:** | | | |
| (USDA): | | | |
| Barbados | 1 T. (.7 oz.) | 51 | 13.3 |
| Blackstrap | 1 T. (.7 oz.) | 40 | 10.4 |
| Light | 1 T. (.7 oz.) | 48 | 12.4 |
| Dark | 1 T. (.7 oz.) | 48 | 12.4 |
| Medium | 1 T. (.7 oz.) | 44 | 11.4 |
| (Brer Rabbit) dark, Green Label | 1 T. | 33 | 10.6 |
| (Grandma's) unsulphured | 1 T. | 60 | 15.0 |
| **MORTADELLA (USDA)** sausage | 1 oz. | 89 | .2 |

(USDA): United States Department of Agriculture
(HEW/FAO): Health, Education and Welfare/Food and Agriculture Organization
* Prepared as Package Directs

| Food and Description | Measure or Quantity | Calories | Carbo- hydrates (grams) |
|---|---|---|---|
| **MOSELLE WINE** (Great Western) Delaware, 12% alcohol | 3 fl. oz. | 73 | 2.9 |
| **MOST**, cereal (Kellogg's) | 1-oz. serving | 110 | 22.0 |
| **MUFFIN** (See also **MUFFIN MIX**): | | | |
| Blueberry: | | | |
| Home recipe (USDA) | 3" muffin (1.4 oz.) | 112 | 16.8 |
| Frozen (Morton): | | | |
| Regular | 1.6-oz. muffin | 125 | 22.9 |
| Rounds | 1.6-oz. muffin round | 115 | 20.9 |
| Bran: | | | |
| Home recipe (USDA) | 3" muffin (1.4 oz.) | 104 | 17.2 |
| (Arnold) *Oroweat, Bran'nola* | 2.3-oz. muffin | 160 | 30.0 |
| Corn: | | | |
| Home recipe (USDA) prepared with whole-ground cornmeal | 1.4-oz. muffin | 115 | 17.0 |
| (Thomas') | 2-oz. muffin | 184 | 25.8 |
| Frozen (Morton): | | | |
| Regular | 1.7-oz. muffin | 129 | 20.3 |
| Rounds | 1.5-oz. muffin round | 127 | 20.9 |
| English: | | | |
| (Arnold) extra crisp | 2.3-oz. muffin | 150 | 30.0 |
| *Home Pride:* | | | |
| Regular | 2-oz. muffin | 136 | 25.0 |
| Wheat | 2-oz. muffin | 141 | 25.0 |
| (Pepperidge Farm): | | | |
| Regular | 1 muffin | 140 | 27.0 |
| Cinnamon raisin | 1 muffin | 140 | 28.0 |
| (Thomas'): | | | |
| Regular | 2-oz. muffin | 133 | 26.6 |
| Onion | 2-oz. muffin | 129 | 26.3 |
| (Wonder) | 2-oz. muffin | 130 | 26.0 |
| Plain, home recipe (USDA) | 1.4-oz. muffin (3" dia.) | 118 | 16.9 |

| Food and Description | Measure or Quantity | Calories | Carbo-hydrates (grams) |
|---|---|---|---|
| **Raisin:** | | | |
| (Arnold) *Oroweat* | 2.5-oz. muffin | 170 | 35.0 |
| (Wonder) rounds | 2-oz. muffin round | 150 | 27.8 |
| Sourdough (Wonder) | 2-oz. muffin | 135 | 27.3 |
| **MUFFIN MIX:** | | | |
| Blueberry: | | | |
| *(Betty Crocker) wild | 1 muffin | 120 | 19.0 |
| (Duncan Hines) | ½ pkg. | 99 | 17.0 |
| Corn: | | | |
| Home recipe (USDA) prepared with egg & milk | 1.4-oz. muffin | 92 | 14.2 |
| Home recipe (USDA) prepared with egg & water | 1.4-oz. muffin | 119 | 20.8 |
| *(Betty Crocker) | 1 muffin | 160 | 25.0 |
| *(Dromedary) | 1 muffin | 130 | 20.0 |
| *(Flako) | 1 muffin | 140 | 23.0 |
| **MUG-O-LUNCH** (General Mills): | | | |
| Chicken-flavored noodles & sauce | 1 pouch | 150 | 25.0 |
| Macaroni & cheese | 1 pouch | 230 | 40.0 |
| Noodles & beef-flavored sauce | 1 pouch | 170 | 30.0 |
| Oriental noodles & sauce | 1 pouch | 190 | 28.0 |
| Spaghetti & tomato sauce | 1 pouch | 160 | 31.0 |
| **MULLET,** raw (USDA): | | | |
| Whole | 1 lb. (weighed whole) | 351 | 0. |
| Meat only | 4 oz. | 166 | 0. |
| **MUNG BEAN SPROUT** (See **BEAN SPROUT**) | | | |

(USDA): United States Department of Agriculture
(HEW/FAO): Health, Education and Welfare/Food and Agriculture Organization
* Prepared as Package Directs

| Food and Description | Measure or Quantity | Calories | Carbo-hydrates (grams) |
|---|---|---|---|
| **MUSCATEL WINE:** | | | |
| (Gallo) 20% alcohol | 3 fl. oz. | 111 | 8.3 |
| (Gold Seal) 19% alcohol | 3 fl. oz. | 159 | 9.4 |
| **MUSHROOM:** | | | |
| Raw (USDA) whole | ½ lb. (weighed untrimmed) | 62 | 9.7 |
| Raw (USDA) trimmed, slices | ½ cup (1.2 oz.) | 10 | 1.5 |
| Canned, solids & liq.: | | | |
| (USDA) | ½ cup (4.3 oz.) | 21 | 2.9 |
| (Green Giant) | 2-oz. serving | 12 | 1.7 |
| (Shady Oak) | 4-oz. can | 19 | 2.0 |
| Dried (HEW/FAO) | 1 oz. | 72 | 10.5 |
| Frozen: | | | |
| (Green Giant) in butter sauce | ½ of 6-oz. pkg. | 42 | 2.6 |
| (McKenzie) chopped | 3.3-oz. serving | 25 | 3.4 |
| (Seabrook Farms) chopped | ⅛ of 10-oz. pkg. | 25 | 3.4 |
| **MUSHROOM, CHINESE:** | | | |
| Dried (HEW/FAO) | 1 oz. | 81 | 18.9 |
| Dried (HEW/FAO) soaked, drained | 1 oz. | 12 | 2.4 |
| **MUSHROOM SOUP:** | | | |
| Canned, regular pack: | | | |
| (USDA): | | | |
| Cream of, condensed | 8 oz. (by wt.) | 252 | 19.1 |
| *Cream of, condensed, prepared with equal volume water | 1 cup (8.5 oz.) | 134 | 10.1 |
| *Cream of, condensed, prepared with equal volume milk | 1 cup (8.6 oz.) | 216 | 16.2 |
| *(Ann Page) cream of, condensed | 1 cup | 126 | 10.2 |
| (Campbell): | | | |
| *Cream of, condensed | 10-oz. serving | 120 | 11.0 |
| Cream of, savory, *Soup For One* | 7½-oz. can | 140 | 13.0 |
| *Golden, condensed | 8-oz. serving | 88 | 8.8 |

| Food and Description | Measure or Quantity | Calories | Carbo- hydrates (grams) |
|---|---|---|---|
| (Crosse & Blackwell) cream of, bisque | ½ of 13-oz. can | 90 | 8.0 |
| Canned, dietetic or low calorie: | | | |
| (Campbell) cream of, low sodium | 7¼-oz. can | 140 | 10.0 |
| *(Dia-Mel) cream of, condensed | 8-oz. serving | 45 | 9.0 |
| (Featherweight) cream of, low sodium | 8-oz. can | 120 | 18.0 |
| Mix: | | | |
| *(Lipton): | | | |
| Beef mushroom | 1 cup | 45 | 7.0 |
| *Cream of, Cup-a-Soup | 6 fl. oz. | 80 | 11.0 |
| (Nestle) Souptime | 6 fl. oz. | 80 | 9.0 |
| **MUSKELLUNGE, raw (USDA):** | | | |
| Whole | 1 lb. (weighed whole) | 242 | 0. |
| Meat only | 4 oz. | 124 | 0. |
| **MUSKMELON (See CANTA- LOUPE, CASABA or HONEYDEW)** | | | |
| **MUSKRAT, roasted (USDA)** | 4 oz. | 174 | 0. |
| **MUSSEL (USDA):** | | | |
| Atlantic & Pacific, raw, in shell | 1 lb. (weighed in shell) | 153 | 7.2 |
| Atlantic & Pacific, raw, meat only | 4 oz. | 108 | 3.7 |
| Pacific, canned, drained | 4 oz. | 129 | 1.7 |
| **MUSTARD POWDER** (French's) | 1 tsp. | 9 | .3 |

(USDA): United States Department of Agriculture
(HEW/FAO): Health, Education and Welfare/Food and Agriculture Organization
* Prepared as Package Directs

| Food and Description | Measure or Quantity | Calories | Carbohydrates (grams) |
|---|---|---|---|
| **MUSTARD, PREPARED:** | | | |
| Brown: | | | |
| (USDA) | 1 tsp. | 8 | .5 |
| (French's) 'N Spicy | 1 tsp. | 5 | .3 |
| (Gulden's) | 1 scant tsp. | 6 | .4 |
| Cream salad (French's) | 1 tsp. | 3 | .3 |
| *Grey Poupon* | 1 tsp. | 5 | .2 |
| Horseradish: | | | |
| (French's) | 1 tsp. | 5 | .3 |
| (Nalley's) | 1 tsp. | 6 | .3 |
| Hot, *Mr. Mustard* | 1 tsp. | 11 | .4 |
| Medford (French's) | 1 tsp. | 5 | .3 |
| Onion (French's) | 1 tsp. | 8 | 1.7 |
| Yellow: | | | |
| (USDA) | 1 tsp. | 7 | .6 |
| (Gulden's) | 1 scant tsp. | 5 | .4 |
| **MUSTARD GREENS:** | | | |
| Raw (USDA) whole | 1 lb. (weighed untrimmed) | 98 | 17.8 |
| Boiled (USDA) drained | 1 cup (7.8 oz.) | 51 | 8.8 |
| Frozen: | | | |
| (USDA) boiled, drained | ½ cup (3.8 oz.) | 21 | 3.3 |
| (Birds Eye) chopped | ⅓ pkg. (3.3 oz.) | 20 | 3.0 |
| **MUSTARD SPINACH** (USDA): | | | |
| Raw | 1 lb. | 100 | 17.7 |
| Boiled, drained | 4 oz. | 18 | 3.2 |

**N**

| Food and Description | Measure or Quantity | Calories | Carbohydrates (grams) |
|---|---|---|---|
| **NATURAL CEREAL:** | | | |
| *Heartland:* | | | |
| Coconut | ½ cup (1 oz.) | 122 | 18.1 |
| Coconut, hot | ¼ cup (1 oz.) | 126 | 19.0 |
| Plain, oat | ¼ cup (1 oz.) | 122 | 18.7 |
| Raisin | ¼ cup (1 oz.) | 122 | 18.7 |
| Regular, hot | ¼ cup (1 oz.) | 121 | 19.0 |
| Spice, hot | ¼ cup (1 oz.) | 121 | 19.1 |
| Toasted corn | ¼ cup (1 oz.) | 115 | 21.1 |

| Food and Description | Measure or Quantity | Calories | Carbohydrates (grams) |
|---|---|---|---|
| Toasted wheat (Quaker): | ¼ cup (1 oz.) | 120 | 20.7 |
| 100% | ¼ cup (1 oz.) | 139 | 17.0 |
| 100%, with apples & cinnamon | ¼ cup (1 oz.) | 135 | 18.0 |
| 100%, with raisins & dates | ¼ cup (1 oz.) | 134 | 17.8 |
| Whole wheat, hot | ⅓ cup (1 oz.) | 100 | 20.6 |
| **NATURE SNACKS** (Sun-Maid): | | | |
| Carob crunch | 1-oz. serving | 150 | 13.0 |
| CoCo Banana | 1-oz. serving | 140 | 16.0 |
| Go-Bananas | 1-oz. serving | 280 | 36.0 |
| Nuts Galore | 1-oz. serving | 170 | 5.0 |
| Raisin Crunch | 1-oz. serving | 130 | 18.0 |
| Rocky Road | 1-oz. serving | 160 | 13.0 |
| Tahitian Treat | 1-oz. serving | 140 | 18.0 |
| **NEAR BEER** (See **BEER, NEAR**) | | | |
| **NECTARINE,** fresh (USDA): | | | |
| Whole | 1 lb. (weighed with pits) | 267 | 71.4 |
| Flesh only | 4 oz. | 73 | 19.4 |
| **NEAPOLITAN CREAM PIE,** frozen (Morton) | ⅙ of 16-oz. pie | 192 | 22.7 |
| **NEOPOLITAN ICE CREAM** (Sealtest) | ¼ pt. | 130 | 18.0 |
| **NEW ZEALAND SPINACH** (USDA): | | | |
| Raw | 1 lb. | 86 | 14.1 |
| Boiled, drained | 4 oz. | 15 | 2.4 |

(USDA): United States Department of Agriculture
(HEW/FAO): Health, Education and Welfare/Food and Agriculture Organization
* Prepared as Package Directs

| Food and Description | Measure or Quantity | Calories | Carbo-hydrates (grams) |
|---|---|---|---|
| **NOODLE.** Plain noodle products are essentially the same in caloric value and carbohydrate content on the same weight basis. The longer they are cooked, the more water is absorbed and this affects the nutritive values. (USDA): | | | |
| Dry, 1½" strips | 1 cup (2.6 oz.) | 283 | 52.6 |
| Dry | 1 oz. | 110 | 20.4 |
| Cooked | 1 cup (5.6 oz.) | 200 | 37.3 |
| Cooked | 1 oz. | 35 | 6.6 |
| **NOODLE & BEEF:** | | | |
| Canned (Hormel) *Short Orders* | 7½-oz. can | 230 | 15.0 |
| Frozen (Banquet) | 2-lb. pkg. | 754 | 83.6 |
| **NOODLE, CHOW MEIN,** canned: | | | |
| (USDA) | 1 cup (1.6 oz.) | 220 | 26.1 |
| (Chun King) | ⅛ of 5-oz. can | 100 | 13.0 |
| (La Choy) | ½ cup (1 oz.) | 153 | 15.8 |
| (La Choy) wide | ½ cup (1 oz.) | 149 | 16.0 |
| **NOODLE MIX:** | | | |
| *(Betty Crocker): | | | |
| Almondine | ¼ pkg. | 260 | 27.0 |
| Romanoff | ¼ pkg. | 230 | 23.0 |
| Stroganoff | ¼ pkg. | 230 | 26.0 |
| *Noodle Roni,* parmesano | ⅙ of 6-oz. pkg. | 130 | 23.2 |
| *(Pennsylvania Dutch Brand) *Noodles Plus Sauce:* | | | |
| Beef | ½ cup | 130 | 24.0 |
| Butter | ½ cup | 150 | 23.0 |
| Cheese | ½ cup | 150 | 24.0 |
| Chicken | ½ cup | 150 | 25.0 |
| *Tuna Helper* (General Mills): | | | |
| Almondine | ¼ pkg. | 240 | 27.0 |

| Food and Description | Measure or Quantity | Calories | Carbo-hydrates (grams) |
|---|---|---|---|
| Romanoff | ¼ pkg. | 230 | 23.0 |
| Stroganoff | ¼ pkg. | 230 | 26.0 |
| **\*NOODLE, RAMEN, canned** (La Choy): | | | |
| Beef | 1 cup | 225 | 33.4 |
| Chicken | 1 cup | 202 | 29.1 |
| Oriental | 1 cup | 207 | 30.7 |
| **NOODLE, RICE, canned** (La Choy) | ⅛ of 3-oz. can | 130 | 19.9 |
| **NOODLE ROMANOFF,** frozen (Stouffer's) | ⅓ of 12-oz. pkg. | 168 | 15.9 |
| **NUITS ST. GEORGE,** French red Burgundy (Barton & Guestier) 13½% alcohol | 3 fl. oz. | 70 | .5 |
| **NUT, MIX** (See also individual kinds): | | | |
| Dry roasted: | | | |
| (A&P) | 1 oz. | 179 | 6.6 |
| (Flavor House) salted | 1 oz. | 172 | 5.4 |
| (Planters) | 1 oz. | 160 | 7.0 |
| Oil roasted: | | | |
| (A&P) Fancy, without peanuts | 1 oz. | 190 | 5.9 |
| (Excel) with peanut | 1 oz. | 187 | 5.4 |
| (Planters): | | | |
| With peanuts | 1 oz. | 180 | 6.0 |
| Without peanuts | 1 oz. | 180 | 6.0 |
| **NUT ICE CREAM** (Dean) 14% fat | 1 cup (5.6 oz.) | 376 | 36.3 |
| **NUT LOAF** (See BREAD, CANNED) | | | |

(USDA): United States Department of Agriculture
(HEW/FAO): Health, Education and Welfare/Food and Agriculture Organization
\* Prepared as Package Directs

| Food and Description | Measure or Quantity | Calories | Carbo-hydrates (grams) |
|---|---|---|---|
| **NUTMEG** (French's) | 1 tsp. | 11 | .9 |
| *NUTRIMATO* (Mott's) | 6 fl. oz. | 70 | 17.0 |

| Food and Description | Measure or Quantity | Calories | Carbo-hydrates (grams) |
|---|---|---|---|
| **OAT FLAKES**, cereal (Post) | ⅔ cup (1 oz.) | 107 | 20.1 |
| **OATMEAL:** | | | |
| Instant, dry: | | | |
| (H-O): | | | |
| Regular | 1 T. (4 grams) | 16 | 2.8 |
| Regular | 1 cup (2.4 oz.) | 258 | 44.3 |
| With maple & brown sugar flavor | 1.5-oz. packet | 160 | 31.7 |
| Sweet & mellow | 1.4-oz. packet | 150 | 28.9 |
| (Quaker): | | | |
| Regular | 1-oz. packet | 105 | 18.1 |
| Apple & cinnamon | 1¼-oz. packet | 134 | 26.0 |
| Bran & raisins | 1½-oz. packet | 153 | 29.2 |
| Cinnamon & spice | 1⅝-oz. packet | 176 | 34.8 |
| Maple & brown sugar | 1½-oz. packet | 163 | 31.9 |
| Raisins & spice | 1½-oz. packet | 159 | 31.4 |
| (3-Minute Brand) *Stir'n Eat:* | | | |
| Dutch apple brown sugar | 1⅛-oz. packet | 120 | 23.3 |
| Natural flavor | 1-oz. packet | 106 | 18.0 |
| Quick, dry: | | | |
| (H-O) | 1 T. (4 grams) | 16 | 2.8 |
| (H-O) | 1 cup (2.5 oz.) | 269 | 46.3 |
| (Ralston Purina) | ⅓ cup (1 oz.) | 110 | 19.0 |
| (3-Minute Brand) | ⅓ cup (1 oz.) | 108 | 18.5 |
| Regular, dry: | | | |
| (USDA) | 1 T. | 18 | 3.1 |
| (H-O) old-fashioned | 1 T. (5 grams) | 17 | 3.0 |
| (H-O) old-fashioned | 1 cup (2.6 oz.) | 278 | 48.0 |
| (Ralston Purina) | ⅓ cup (1 oz.) | 110 | 19.0 |
| Regular, cooked (USDA) | 1 cup (8.5 oz.) | 132 | 23.3 |

| Food and Description | Measure or Quantity | Calories | Carbohydrates (grams) |
|---|---|---|---|
| **OCEAN PERCH:** | | | |
| Fresh (USDA): | | | |
| Atlantic: | | | |
| Raw, whole | 1 lb. (weighed whole) | 124 | 0. |
| Fried | 4 oz. | 257 | 7.7 |
| Pacific: | | | |
| Raw, whole | 1 lb. (weighed whole) | 116 | 0. |
| Meat only, raw | 4 oz. | 108 | 0. |
| Frozen: | | | |
| (USDA) Atlantic, breaded, fried, reheated | 4 oz. | 362 | 18.7 |
| (Banquet) | 8¾-oz. dinner | 434 | 49.8 |
| **OCTOPUS, raw (USDA)** | | | |
| meat only | 4 oz. | 83 | 0. |
| **OIL, SALAD or COOKING:** | | | |
| (USDA) all, including olive | 1 T. (.5 oz.) | 124 | 0. |
| (USDA) all, including olive | ½ cup (3.9 oz.) | 972 | 0. |
| Corn: | | | |
| (Fleischmann's) | 1 T. (.5 oz.) | 126 | 0. |
| (Mazola) | 1 T. | 128 | 0. |
| (Mazola) | ½ cup (3.9 oz.) | 997 | 0. |
| *Crisco* | 1 T. | 126 | 0. |
| *Mrs. Tucker's,* corn or soybean | 1 T. | 130 | 0. |
| Peanut (Planters) | 1 T. | 130 | 0. |
| *Puritan* | 1 T. | 126 | 0. |
| Safflower, *Golden Thistle* | 1 T. | 130 | 0. |
| *Saffola* | 1 T. (.5 oz.) | 124 | 0. |
| *Saffola* | ½ cup (3.9 oz.) | 972 | 0. |
| *Wesson* | 1 T. | 120 | 0. |
| **OKRA:** | | | |
| Raw (USDA) whole | 1 lb. (weighed untrimmed) | 140 | 29.6 |

(USDA): United States Department of Agriculture
(HEW/FAO): Health, Education and Welfare/Food and Agriculture Organization
* Prepared as Package Directs

| Food and Description | Measure or Quantity | Calories | Carbo-hydrates (grams) |
|---|---|---|---|
| Boiled (USDA) drained: | | | |
| Whole | ½ cup (3.1 oz.) | 26 | 5.3 |
| Pods | 8 pods, 3″ x ⅝″ (3 oz.) | 25 | 5.1 |
| Slices | ½ cup (2.8 oz.) | 23 | 4.8 |
| Canned (King Pharr) with tomatoes | ½ cup | 26 | 5.0 |
| Frozen: | | | |
| (USDA) cut, boiled, drained | ½ cup (3.2 oz.) | 35 | 8.1 |
| (USDA) whole, boiled, drained | ½ cup (2.4 oz.) | 26 | 6.1 |
| (Birds Eye): | | | |
| Cut | ⅓ of 10-oz. pkg. | 25 | 5.0 |
| Whole | ⅓ of 10-oz. pkg. | 30 | 7.0 |
| (Green Giant) gumbo | ⅓ of 10-oz. pkg. | 83 | 5.2 |
| (McKenzie or Seabrook Farms): | | | |
| Cut | ⅓ of 10-oz. pkg. | 32 | 6.1 |
| Whole | ⅓ of 10-oz. pkg. | 36 | 6.9 |
| **OLD-FASHIONED COCKTAIL:** | | | |
| Canned (Hiram Walker) 62 proof | 3 fl. oz. | 165 | 3.0 |
| Mix: | | | |
| Dry (Bar-Tender's) | ⅛-oz. serving | 20 | 4.7 |
| Liquid (Holland House) | 1 fl. oz. | 36 | 9.0 |
| **OLEOMARGARINE** (See MARGARINE) | | | |
| **OLIVE:** | | | |
| Green style (USDA): | | | |
| With pits, drained | 1 oz. | 77 | 2.0 |
| Pitted, drained | 1 oz. | 96 | 2.5 |
| Green (USDA) | 1 oz. | 33 | .4 |
| Ripe, by variety (USDA): | | | |
| Ascalano, any size, pitted & drained | 1 oz. | 37 | .7 |
| Manzanilla, any size | 1 oz. | 37 | .7 |
| Mission, any size | 1 oz. | 52 | .9 |
| Mission | 3 small or 2 large | 18 | .3 |

| Food and Description | Measure or Quantity | Calories | Carbo-hydrates (grams) |
|---|---|---|---|
| Mission, slices | ½ cup (2.2 oz.) | 114 | 2.0 |
| Sevillano, any size | 1 oz. | 26 | 6.1 |
| Ripe, by size (Lindsay): | | | |
| Colossal | 1 olive | 13 | .3 |
| Extra large | 1 olive | 5 | .1 |
| Giant | 1 olive | 8 | .2 |
| Jumbo | 1 olive | 10 | .2 |
| Large | 1 olive | 5 | .1 |
| Mammoth | 1 olive | 6 | .1 |
| Medium | 1 olive | 4 | .1 |
| Select | 1 olive | 3 | .1 |
| Supercolossal | 1 olive | 16 | .3 |
| Super supreme | 1 olive | 18 | .3 |
| ONION (See also ONION, GREEN and ONION, WELCH) | | | |
| Raw (USDA): | | | |
| Whole | 1 lb. (weighed untrimmed) | 157 | 35.9 |
| Whole | 3.9-oz. onion (2½" dia.) | 38 | 8.7 |
| Chopped | ½ cup (3 oz.) | 33 | 7.5 |
| Chopped | 1 T. (.4 oz.) | 4 | 1.0 |
| Grated | 1 T. (.5 oz.) | 5 | 1.2 |
| Slices | ½ cup (2 oz.) | 21 | 4.9 |
| Boiled, drained (USDA): | | | |
| Whole | ½ cup (3.7 oz.) | 30 | 6.8 |
| Whole, pearl onions | ½ cup (3.2 oz.) | 27 | 6.0 |
| Halves or pieces | ½ cup (3.2 oz.) | 26 | 5.8 |
| Canned, O & C: | | | |
| In cream sauce | ¼ of 15½-oz. can | 554 | 65.9 |
| French-fried | 3-oz. can | 534 | 30.6 |
| Dehydrated: | | | |
| Flakes: | | | |
| (USDA) | 1 tsp. (1.3 grams) | 5 | 1.1 |
| (Gilroy) | 1 tsp. | 5 | 1.2 |
| Powder (Gilroy) | 1 tsp. | 9 | 2.0 |

(USDA): United States Department of Agriculture
(HEW/FAO): Health, Education and Welfare/Food and Agriculture
              Organization
* Prepared as Package Directs

| Food and Description | Measure or Quantity | Calories | Carbo-hydrates (grams) |
|---|---|---|---|
| **Frozen:** | | | |
| (Birds Eye): | | | |
| Chopped | 1 oz. | 8 | 2.0 |
| Small, whole | ⅓ of 12-oz. pkg. | 40 | 10.0 |
| Small, with cream sauce | ⅓ of 9-oz. pkg. | 118 | 11.2 |
| (Green Giant) creamed | ⅓ of 10-oz. pkg. | 50 | 5.1 |
| (Mrs. Paul's) batter fried rings | ½ of 5-oz. pkg. | 156 | 21.2 |
| (Ore-Ida): | | | |
| Chopped | ½ of 12-oz. pkg. | 20 | 4.0 |
| *Onion Ringers* | ½ of 12-oz. pkg. | 160 | 17.0 |
| **ONION BOUILLON:** | | | |
| (Herb-Ox) | 1 cube | 10 | 1.3 |
| (Herb-Ox) instant | 1 packet | 14 | 1.9 |
| *MBT* | 1 packet | 16 | 2.0 |
| **ONION, GREEN, raw** | | | |
| (USDA): | | | |
| Whole | 1 lb. (weighed untrimmed) | 157 | 35.7 |
| Bulb & entire top | 1 oz. | 10 | 2.3 |
| Bulb without green top | 3 small onions (.9 oz.) | 11 | 2.6 |
| Slices, bulb & white portion of top | ½ cup (1.8 oz.) | 22 | 5.2 |
| Tops only | 1 oz. | 8 | 1.6 |
| **ONION SOUP:** | | | |
| Canned: | | | |
| (USDA) condensed | 8 oz. (by wt.) | 131 | 9.8 |
| *(USDA) condensed, prepared with equal volume water | 1 cup (8.5 oz.) | 65 | 5.3 |
| *(Campbell) condensed | 10-oz. serving | 80 | 10.0 |
| *(Campbell) cream of, condensed | 10-oz. serving | 180 | 20.0 |
| Mix: | | | |
| (USDA) | 1 cup (8.1 oz.) | 34 | 5.3 |
| (Ann Page) | 1¾-oz. pkg. | 115 | 21.1 |
| *(Lipton): | | | |
| Regular | 1 cup (8 oz.) | 40 | 6.0 |
| Beefy onion | 1 cup (8 oz.) | 30 | 4.0 |

| Food and Description | Measure or Quantity | Calories | Carbo-hydrates (grams) |
|---|---|---|---|
| Cup-a-Soup | 6 fl. oz. | 30 | 5.0 |
| Onion mushroom | 1 cup (8 oz.) | 35 | 5.0 |
| *(Nestle) Souptime, French onion | 6 fl. oz. | 20 | 4.0 |
| **ONION WELCH, raw (USDA):** | | | |
| Whole | 1 lb. (weighed untrimmed) | 100 | 19.2 |
| Trimmed | 4 oz. | 39 | 7.4 |
| **OPOSSUM (USDA) roasted, meat only** | 4 oz. | 251 | 0. |
| **ORANGE, fresh (USDA):** | | | |
| California Navel: | | | |
| Whole | 1 lb. (weighed with rind & seeds) | 157 | 39.2 |
| Whole | 6.3-oz. orange (2⅘" dia.) | 62 | 15.5 |
| Sections | 1 cup (8.5 oz.) | 123 | 30.6 |
| California Valencia: | | | |
| Whole | 1 lb. (weighed with rind & seeds) | 174 | 42.2 |
| Fruit including peel | 6.3-oz. orange (2⅝" dia.) | 72 | 27.9 |
| Sections | 1 cup (8.5 oz.) | 123 | 29.9 |
| Florida, all varieties: | | | |
| Whole | 1 lb. (weighed with rind & seeds) | 158 | 40.3 |
| Whole | 7.4-oz. orange (3" dia.) | 73 | 18.6 |
| Sections | 1 cup (8.5 oz.) | 113 | 28.9 |
| **ORANGEADE, chilled (Sealtest)** | ½ cup | 60 | 8.0 |

(USDA): United States Department of Agriculture
(HEW/FAO): Health, Education and Welfare/Food and Agriculture Organization
* Prepared as Package Directs

| Food and Description | Measure or Quantity | Calories | Carbo-hydrates (grams) |
|---|---|---|---|
| **ORANGE-APRICOT JUICE DRINK, canned:** | | | |
| (USDA) 40% fruit juices | 1 cup (8.8 oz.) | 123 | 31.6 |
| (Ann Page) | 1 cup (8.7 oz.) | 125 | 31.2 |
| **ORANGE CREAM BAR** (Sealtest) | 2½-fl.-oz. bar | 100 | 18.0 |
| **ORANGE DRINK:** | | | |
| Canned: | | | |
| (Ann Page) | 1 cup (8.7 oz.) | 121 | 30.2 |
| (Hi-C) | 6 fl. oz. | 92 | 23.0 |
| (Lincoln) | 6 fl. oz. | 96 | 23.9 |
| Chilled (Sealtest) | 6 fl. oz. | 87 | 21.3 |
| *Mix (Hi-C) | 6 fl. oz. | 76 | 19.0 |
| **ORANGE EXTRACT** (Virginia Dare) 79% alcohol | 1 tsp. | 22 | 0. |
| **ORANGE-GRAPEFRUIT JUICE:** | | | |
| Canned, unsweetened: | | | |
| (USDA) | 1 cup (8.7 oz.) | 106 | 24.8 |
| (Del Monte) | 6 fl. oz. | 79 | 18.3 |
| Canned, sweetened: | | | |
| (USDA) | 1 cup (8.9 oz.) | 126 | 30.6 |
| (Del Monte) | 6 fl. oz. (6.5 oz.) | 91 | 21.1 |
| Frozen: | | | |
| *(USDA) unsweetened | ½ cup (4.4 oz.) | 55 | 13.0 |
| *(Minute Maid) unsweetened | 6 fl. oz. | 76 | 19.1 |
| **ORANGE ICE** (Sealtest) | ¼ pt. (3.2 oz.) | 130 | 33.0 |
| **ORANGE JUICE:** | | | |
| Fresh (USDA): | | | |
| California Navel | ½ cup (4.4 oz.) | 60 | 14.0 |
| California Valencia | ½ cup (4.4 oz.) | 58 | 13.0 |
| Florida, early or midseason | ½ cup (4.4 oz.) | 50 | 11.5 |
| Florida Temple | ½ cup (4.4 oz.) | 67 | 16.0 |
| Florida Valencia | ½ cup (4.4 oz.) | 56 | 13.0 |

| Food and Description | Measure or Quantity | Calories | Carbo-hydrates (grams) |
|---|---|---|---|
| Canned, unsweetened: | | | |
| (USDA) | ½ cup (4.4 oz.) | 60 | 13.9 |
| (Del Monte) | 6 fl. oz. (6.5 oz.) | 82 | 18.5 |
| (Featherweight) low sodium | ½ cup | 53 | 12.0 |
| (Sunkist) | ½ cup (4.4 oz.) | 60 | 14.0 |
| Canned, sweetened: | | | |
| (USDA) | ½ cup (4.4 oz.) | 66 | 15.4 |
| (Del Monte) | 6 fl. oz. | 76 | 17.4 |
| Chilled (Minute Maid) | 6 fl. oz. | 83 | 19.7 |
| *Dehydrated crystals (USDA) | ½ cup (4.4 oz.) | 57 | 13.4 |
| Frozen: | | | |
| *(USDA) | ½ cup (4.4 oz.) | 56 | 13.3 |
| *(Minute Maid) unsweetened | 6 fl. oz. | 90 | 21.4 |
| *(Snow Crop) unsweetened | 6 fl. oz. | 90 | 21.4 |
| *(Sunkist) | 6 fl. oz. | 92 | 21.7 |

**ORANGE, MANDARIN (See TANGERINE)**

| | | | |
|---|---|---|---|
| **ORANGE PEEL, CANDIED** | | | |
| (USDA) | 1 oz. | 90 | 22.9 |
| **ORANGE-PINEAPPLE DRINK, canned:** | | | |
| (Ann Page) | 1 cup (8.7 oz.) | 126 | 31.5 |
| (Hi-C) | 6 fl. oz. | 94 | 23.0 |
| (Lincoln) | 6 fl. oz. | 97 | 24.3 |
| *_ORANGE PLUS_ (Birds Eye) frozen | 6 fl. oz. | 99 | 23.5 |

**ORANGE SHERBET (See SHERBET)**

(USDA): United States Department of Agriculture
(HEW/FAO): Health, Education and Welfare/Food and Agriculture Organization
* Prepared as Package Directs

| Food and Description | Measure or Quantity | Calories | Carbo-hydrates (grams) |
|---|---|---|---|
| **OREGANO,** dried (French's) | 1 tsp. | 6 | 1.0 |
| **OVALTINE,** dry: | | | |
| Chocolate flavor | ¾ oz. (4 heaping tsps.) | 80 | 16.0 |
| Malt flavor | ¾ oz. (4 heaping tsps.) | 80 | 17.0 |
| **OYSTER:** | | | |
| Raw, Eastern (USDA) meat only | 13-19 med. oysters (1 cup, 8.5 oz.) | 158 | 8.2 |
| Raw, Eastern (USDA) meat only | 4 oz. | 75 | 3.9 |
| Raw, Pacific (USDA) meat only | 4 oz. | 103 | 7.3 |
| Canned, solids & liq.: | | | |
| (USDA) | 4 oz. | 86 | 5.6 |
| (Bumble Bee) whole | ½ of 8-oz. can | 86 | 5.5 |
| Fried (USDA) dipped in egg, milk & breadcrumbs | 4 oz. | 271 | 21.1 |
| **OYSTER CRACKER (See CRACKER)** | | | |
| **OYSTER STEW:** | | | |
| Home recipe (USDA) 1 part oysters to 1 part milk by volume | 1 cup (8.5 oz., 6-8 oysters) | 245 | 14.2 |
| Home recipe (USDA) 1 part oysters to 2 parts milk by volume | 1 cup (8.5 oz.) | 233 | 10.8 |
| Home recipe (USDA) 1 part oysters to 3 parts milk by volume | 1 cup (8.5 oz.) | 206 | 11.3 |
| Frozen: | | | |
| *(USDA) prepared with equal volume water | 1 cup (8.5 oz.) | 122 | 8.2 |
| *(USDA) prepared with equal volume milk | 1 cup (8.5 oz.) | 201 | 14.2 |

| Food and Description | Measure or Quantity | Calories | Carbo-hydrates (grams) |
|---|---|---|---|
| *OYSTER STEW SOUP (Campbell) prepared with milk | 10-oz. serving | 70 | 5.0 |

# P

| Food and Description | Measure or Quantity | Calories | Carbo-hydrates (grams) |
|---|---|---|---|
| PAGAN PINK WINE (Gallo) 11% alcohol | 2 fl. oz. | 81 | 6.8 |
| *PAISANO WINE* (Gallo) 13% alcohol | 3 fl. oz. | 53 | 1.3 |
| PANCAKE, home recipe (USDA) | 4" pancake (1 oz.) | 62 | 9.2 |
| PANCAKE & SAUSAGE, frozen (Swanson) | 6-oz. breakfast | 500 | 50.0 |
| PANCAKE & WAFFLE BATTER, frozen: | | | |
| Plain: | | | |
| (Aunt Jemima) | 4" pancake | 70 | 14.1 |
| (Rich's) | 1 pancake | 113 | 17.9 |
| Blueberry: | | | |
| (Aunt Jemima) | 4" pancake | 68 | 13.8 |
| (Rich's) | 1.6-oz. pancake (1/10 of pkg.) | 102 | 16.5 |
| Buttermilk: | | | |
| (Aunt Jemima) | 4" pancake | 71 | 14.2 |
| (Rich's) | 1 pancake (1/10 of pkg.) | 109 | 16.9 |
| PANCAKE & WAFFLE MIX: | | | |
| Plain: | | | |
| (USDA) | 1 oz. | 101 | 21.5 |
| (USDA) | 1 cup (4.8 oz.) | 481 | 102.2 |

(USDA): United States Department of Agriculture
(HEW/FAO): Health, Education and Welfare/Food and Agriculture Organization
* Prepared as Package Directs

| Food and Description | Measure or Quantity | Calories | Carbo-hydrates (grams) |
|---|---|---|---|
| *(USDA) prepared with milk | 4″ pancake (1 oz.) | 55 | 8.6 |
| *(USDA) prepared with egg & milk | 4″ pancake | 61 | 8.7 |
| (Aunt Jemima): | | | |
| Complete | ⅓ cup (1.9 oz.) | 198 | 38.2 |
| *Complete | 4″ pancake | 66 | 12.7 |
| Original | 1¼ cups (1.1 oz.) | 108 | 22.5 |
| *Original | 4″ pancake | 73 | 8.7 |
| *(Log Cabin) complete | 4″ pancake | 58 | 11.2 |
| *(Pillsbury) *Hungry Jack:* | | | |
| Complete | 4″ pancake | 73 | 14.0 |
| *Extra Lights* | 4″ pancake | 60 | 8.7 |
| *Blueberry (Pillsbury) *Hungry Jack* | 4″ pancake | 113 | 14.3 |
| Buckwheat: | | | |
| (USDA) | 1 cup (4.8 oz.) | 443 | 94.9 |
| *(USDA) prepared with egg & milk | 4″ pancake | 54 | 6.4 |
| (Aunt Jemima) | ¼ cup (1.1 oz.) | 110 | 21.3 |
| *(Aunt Jemima) | 4″ pancake | 67 | 8.3 |
| Buttermilk: | | | |
| (USDA) | 1 cup (4.8 oz.) | 481 | 102.2 |
| *(USDA) prepared with egg & milk | 4″ pancake | 61 | 8.7 |
| (Aunt Jemima) | ⅓ cup (1.8 oz.) | 175 | 36.5 |
| *(Aunt Jemima) | 4″ pancake | 100 | 13.3 |
| (Aunt Jemima) complete | ⅓ cup (2.3 oz.) | 236 | 46.2 |
| *(Aunt Jemima) complete | 4″ pancake | 79 | 15.4 |
| *(Betty Crocker) | 4″ pancake | 93 | 13.0 |
| *(Betty Crocker) complete | 4″ pancake | 70 | 13.7 |
| *(Log Cabin) | 4″ pancake | 77 | 10.7 |
| *(Pillsbury) *Hungry Jack* | 4″ pancake | 80 | 9.7 |
| *(Pillsbury) *Hungry Jack,* complete | 4″ pancake | 113 | 11.3 |
| Whole wheat (Aunt Jemima) | ⅓ cup (1.5 oz.) | 142 | 28.5 |
| *Whole wheat (Aunt Jemima) | 4″ pancake | 83 | 10.7 |
| *Dietetic or low calorie (Tillie Lewis) complete | 4″ pancake (.5 oz. dry) | 45 | 8.6 |

| Food and Description | Measure or Quantity | Calories | Carbo-hydrates (grams) |
|---|---|---|---|
| **PANCAKE & WAFFLE SYRUP** (See also individual kinds such as **LOG CABIN,** etc.) | | | |
| Sweetened: | | | |
| (USDA) cane & maple | 1 T. (.7 oz.) | 50 | 13.0 |
| (USDA) chiefly corn, light & dark | 1 T. (.7 oz.) | 58 | 15.0 |
| (Golden Griddle) | 1 T. (.7 oz.) | 54 | 13.4 |
| *Mrs. Butterworth's* | 1 T. (.7 oz.) | 55 | 13.0 |
| Dietetic or low calorie: | | | |
| (Diet Delight) | 1 T. (.6 oz.) | 14 | 3.5 |
| (Featherweight) | 1 T. | 16 | 4.0 |
| (Tillie Lewis) *Tasti Diet* | 1 T. (.5 oz.) | 13 | .1 |
| **PANCREAS, raw (USDA):** | | | |
| Beef, lean only | 4 oz. | 160 | 0. |
| Calf | 4 oz. | 183 | 0. |
| Hog or hog sweetbread | 4 oz. | 274 | 0. |
| **PAPAW, fresh (USDA):** | | | |
| Whole | 1 lb. (weighed with rind & seeds) | 289 | 57.2 |
| Flesh only | 4 oz. | 96 | 19.1 |
| **PAPAYA, fresh (USDA):** | | | |
| Whole | 1 lb. (weighed with skin & seeds) | 119 | 30.4 |
| Cubed | 1 cup (6.4 oz.) | 71 | 18.2 |
| **PAPAYA JUICE, canned (HEW/FAO)** | 4 oz. | 77 | 19.6 |
| **PAPRIKA, domestic (French's)** | 1 tsp. | 7 | 1.1 |
| **PARSLEY, fresh (USDA):** | | | |
| Whole | ½ lb. | 100 | 19.3 |

(USDA): United States Department of Agriculture
(HEW/FAO): Health, Education and Welfare/Food and Agriculture Organization
\* Prepared as Package Directs

| Food and Description | Measure or Quantity | Calories | Carbo-hydrates (grams) |
|---|---|---|---|
| Chopped | 1 T. (4 grams) | 2 | .3 |
| **PARSLEY FLAKES,** dehydrated (French's) | 1 tsp. (1.1 grams) | 4 | .6 |
| **PARSNIP** (USDA): | | | |
| Raw, whole | 1 lb. (weighed unprepared) | 293 | 67.5 |
| Boiled, drained, cut in pieces | ½ cup (3.7 oz.) | 70 | 15.8 |
| *PARTY PUNCH WINE,* undiluted (Mogen David) 12% alcohol | 3 fl. oz. | 156 | 21.4 |
| *PASHA TURKISH COFFEE LIQUEUR* (Leroux) 53 proof | 1 fl. oz. | 97 | 13.3 |
| **PASSION FRUIT,** fresh (USDA): | | | |
| Whole | 1 lb. (weighed with shell) | 212 | 50.0 |
| Pulp & seeds | 4 oz. | 102 | 24.0 |
| **PASSION FRUIT JUICE,** fresh (HEW/FAO) | 4 oz. | 50 | 11.5 |
| **PASTINA,** dry: (USDA): | | | |
| Carrot | 1 oz. | 105 | 21.5 |
| Egg | 1 oz. | 109 | 20.4 |
| Spinach | 1 oz. | 104 | 21.2 |
| (Ann Page) regular | 1 oz. | 108 | 20.5 |
| *PASTOSO* (Petri) 12% alcohol | 3 fl. oz. | 71 | 1.2 |
| **PASTRAMI,** packaged: | | | |
| (Eckrich) sliced | 1-oz. slice | 47 | 1.3 |
| (Vienna) | 1 oz. | 86 | 0. |
| **PASTRY SHELL** (See also **PIE CRUST**) home recipe (USDA) baked | 1 shell (1.5 oz.) | 212 | 18.6 |

| Food and Description | Measure or Quantity | Calories | Carbo-hydrates (grams) |
|---|---|---|---|
| **PÂTÉ, canned:** | | | |
| (USDA) de foie gras | 1 T. (.5 oz.) | 69 | .7 |
| (USDA) de foie gras | 1 oz. | 131 | 1.4 |
| (Hormel) liver | 1 T. (.5 oz.) | 33 | .4 |
| **PDQ:** | | | |
| Chocolate flavor | 1 T. (.6 oz.) | 66 | 14.6 |
| Egg nog flavor | 2 heaping T. (.9 oz.) | 113 | 27.5 |
| Strawberry flavor | 1 T. (.5 oz.) | 60 | 15.1 |
| **PEA, GREEN:** | | | |
| Raw (USDA): | | | |
| In pod | 1 lb. (weighed in pod) | 145 | 24.8 |
| Shelled | 1 lb. | 381 | 65.3 |
| Shelled | ½ cup (2.4 oz.) | 58 | 9.9 |
| Boiled, drained (USDA) | ½ cup (2.9 oz.) | 58 | 9.9 |
| Canned, regular pack: | | | |
| (USDA): | | | |
| Alaska, early or June, solids & liq. | ½ cup (4.4 oz.) | 82 | 15.5 |
| Alaska, early or June, drained solids | ½ cup (3 oz.) | 76 | 14.4 |
| Sweet, solids & liq. | ½ cup (4.4 oz.) | 71 | 12.9 |
| Sweet, drained solids | ½ cup (3 oz.) | 69 | 12.9 |
| Sweet, drained liquid | 4 oz. | 25 | 4.9 |
| (April Showers) Early, solids & liq. | ½ of 8½-oz. can | 61 | 10.6 |
| (Del Monte): | | | |
| Early garden, solids & liq. | ½ cup (4 oz.) | 52 | 9.9 |
| Early garden, drained solids | ½ cup (4 oz.) | 72 | 12.5 |
| Seasoned, solids & liq. | ½ cup | 54 | 9.8 |
| Seasoned, drained solids | ½ cup | 53 | 9.2 |
| Sweet, tiny size, solids & liq. | ½ cup | 50 | 9.0 |

(USDA): United States Department of Agriculture
(HEW/FAO): Health, Education and Welfare/Food and Agriculture Organization
* Prepared as Package Directs

| Food and Description | Measure or Quantity | Calories | Carbohydrates (grams) |
|---|---|---|---|
| Sweet, tiny size, drained solids | ½ cup | 62 | 10.7 |
| (Green Giant): | | | |
| Early, with onion, solids & liq. | ¼ of 17-oz. can | 61 | 10.6 |
| Sweet, solids & liq. | ½ of 8½-oz. can | 52 | 8.5 |
| Sweet, small, *Sweetlets*, solids & liq. | ½ of 8½-oz. can | 49 | 8.2 |
| Sweet, with onion, solids & liq. | ¼ of 17-oz. can | 52 | 8.5 |
| (Kounty Kist): | | | |
| Early, solids & liq. | ½ of 8½-oz. can | 71 | 12.8 |
| Sweet, solids & liq. | ½ of 8½-oz. can | 64 | 10.5 |
| (Le Sueur) early, small, solids & liq. | ½ of 8½-oz. can | 52 | 9.2 |
| (Libby's) sweet, solids & liq. | ½ cup (4.2 oz.) | 66 | 11.6 |
| (Lindy): | | | |
| Early, solids & liq. | ½ of 8½-oz. can | 71 | 12.8 |
| Sweet, solids & liq. | ½ of 8½-oz. can | 64 | 10.5 |
| (Minnesota Valley) early, small, solids & liq. | ½ of 8½-oz. can | 53 | 9.4 |
| (Stokely-Van Camp): | | | |
| Early, solids & liq. | ½ cup (4.4 oz.) | 65 | 12.5 |
| Sweet, solids & liq. | ½ cup (4.4 oz.) | 65 | 12.0 |
| Canned, dietetic or low calorie pack: | | | |
| (USDA): | | | |
| Alaska, early or June, solids & liq. | 4 oz. | 62 | 11.1 |
| Alaska, early or June, drained solids | 4 oz. | 88 | 16.2 |
| Sweet, solids & liq. | 4 oz. | 53 | 9.5 |
| Sweet, drained solids | 4 oz. | 82 | 14.7 |
| (Blue Boy) sweet, solids & liq. | ½ cup | 80 | 15.0 |
| (Diet Delight) solids & liq. | ½ cup (4.3 oz.) | 47 | 7.4 |
| (Featherweight) sweet, solids & liq. | ½ cup | 50 | 10.0 |
| (Tillie Lewis) *Tasti Diet*, solids & liq. | ½ cup (4.4 oz.) | 40 | 7.5 |
| Frozen: | | | |
| (USDA) boiled, drained | ½ cup (3 oz.) | 57 | 9.9 |

| Food and Description | Measure or Quantity | Calories | Carbo-hydrates (grams) |
|---|---|---|---|
| (Birds Eye): | | | |
|   With cream sauce | ⅓ of 8-oz. pkg. | 134 | 13.7 |
|   With sliced mushrooms | ⅓ of 10-oz. pkg. | 65 | 10.7 |
|   Sweet, 5-minute style | ⅓ of 10-oz. pkg. | 70 | 12.0 |
|   Tender tiny, deluxe | ⅓ of 10-oz. pkg. | 55 | 8.6 |
| (Green Giant): | | | |
|   Creamed, with bread crumb topping, *Bake 'n Serve* | ⅓ of 10-oz. pkg. | 106 | 11.2 |
|   Early, small | ¼ of 16-oz. pkg. | 76 | 12.5 |
|   Sweet | ¼ of 18-oz. pkg. | 85 | 14.1 |
|   Sweet, in butter sauce | ⅓ of 10-oz. pkg. | 74 | 8.6 |
| (Le Sueur) early, in butter sauce | ⅓ of 10-oz. pkg. | 71 | 9.7 |
| (McKenzie) | ⅓ of 10-oz. pkg. | 77 | 13.1 |
| (Seabrook Farms) | ⅓ of 10-oz. pkg. | 77 | 13.1 |
| (Seabrook Farms) petite | ⅓ of 10-oz. pkg. | 62 | 10.3 |
| | | | |
| **PEA & CARROT:** | | | |
| Canned, regular pack: | | | |
|   (Del Monte): | | | |
|     Solids & liq. | ½ cup (4 oz.) | 49 | 9.4 |
|     Drained solids | ½ cup (2.8 oz.) | 44 | 8.2 |
|   (Libby's) solids & liq. | ½ cup (4.2 oz.) | 52 | 10.3 |
| Canned, dietetic or low calorie, solids & liq.: | | | |
|   (Blue Boy) | ½ cup | 60 | 11.0 |
|   (Diet Delight) | ½ cup (4.3 oz.) | 36 | 6.2 |
| Frozen: | | | |
|   (USDA) boiled, without salt, drained | ½ cup (3.1 oz.) | 46 | 8.8 |
|   (Birds Eye) | ⅓ pkg. | 50 | 9.0 |
| | | | |
| **PEA & CAULIFLOWER,** frozen (Birds Eye) with cream sauce | ½ of 10-oz. pkg. | 111 | 11.9 |

(USDA): United States Department of Agriculture
(HEW/FAO): Health, Education and Welfare/Food and Agriculture Organization
* Prepared as Package Directs

| Food and Description | Measure or Quantity | Calories | Carbo-hydrates (grams) |
|---|---|---|---|
| **PEA, MATURE SEED,** dry (USDA): | | | |
| Whole | 1 lb. | 1542 | 272.5 |
| Whole | 1 cup | 680 | 120.6 |
| Split | 1 lb. | 1579 | 284.4 |
| Split | 1 cup (7.2 oz.) | 706 | 127.3 |
| Cooked, split, drained solids | ½ cup (3.4 oz.) | 112 | 20.2 |
| **PEA & ONION,** frozen (Birds Eye) | ⅓ of 10-oz. pkg. | 67 | 11.7 |
| **PEA POD:** | | | |
| Raw (USDA) edible-podded or Chinese | 1 lb. (weighed untrimmed) | 228 | 51.7 |
| Boiled (USDA) drained solids | 4 oz. | 49 | 10.8 |
| Frozen (La Choy) | 6-oz. pkg. | 90 | 20.4 |
| **PEA & POTATO,** frozen (Birds Eye) with cream sauce | ⅓ of 8-oz. pkg. | 145 | 16.3 |
| **PEA SOUP, GREEN** (See also PEA SOUP, SPLIT): | | | |
| Canned, regular pack: | | | |
| (USDA) condensed | 8 oz. (by wt.) | 240 | 41.7 |
| *(USDA) condensed, prepared with equal volume water | 1 cup (8.6 oz.) | 130 | 22.5 |
| *(USDA) condensed, prepared with equal volume milk | 1 cup (8.6 oz.) | 208 | 28.7 |
| *(Campbell) condensed | 8-oz. serving | 144 | 23.2 |
| Canned, dietetic or low calorie: | | | |
| (Campbell) low sodium | 7½-oz. can | 150 | 24.0 |
| *(Dia-Mel) | 8-oz. serving | 110 | 18.0 |
| (Featherweight) | 8-oz. can | 180 | 32.0 |
| Mix: | | | |
| *(USDA) | 1 cup (8.5 oz.) | 121 | 20.3 |
| *(Lipton): | | | |
| Regular | 1 cup | 130 | 22.0 |

| Food and Description | Measure or Quantity | Calories | Carbo-hydrates (grams) |
|---|---|---|---|
| *Cup-A-Soup* | 6 fl. oz. | 120 | 20.0 |
| *(Nestle) *Souptime* | 6 fl. oz. | 70 | 14.0 |
| *Frozen (USDA) condensed, with ham, prepared with equal volume water | 8-oz. serving | 129 | 18.1 |
| **PEA SOUP, SPLIT, canned:** | | | |
| *(USDA) condensed, prepared with equal volume water | 1 cup (8.6 oz.) | 145 | 20.6 |
| *(Ann Page) with ham | 1 cup | 180 | 26.9 |
| *(Campbell) with ham & bacon | 8-oz. serving | 168 | 24.0 |
| (Campbell) with ham, *Chunky* | 19-oz. can | 420 | 58.0 |
| **PEACH:** | | | |
| Fresh (USDA): | | | |
| Whole, without skin | 1 lb. (weighed unpeeled) | 150 | 38.3 |
| Whole | 4-oz. peach (2″ dia.) | 38 | 9.6 |
| Diced | ½ cup (4.7 oz.) | 51 | 12.9 |
| Sliced | ½ cup (3 oz.) | 32 | 8.2 |
| Canned, regular pack, solids & liq.: | | | |
| (USDA): | | | |
| Extra heavy syrup | 4 oz. | 110 | 28.5 |
| Heavy syrup | 2 med. halves & 2 T. syrup (4.1 oz.) | 91 | 23.5 |
| Juice pack | 4 oz. | 51 | 13.2 |
| Light syrup | 4 oz. | 66 | 17.1 |
| (Del Monte): | | | |
| Chunky | ½ cup | 95 | 22.8 |
| Cling halves or slices | ½ cup | 95 | 22.8 |
| Freestone, halves or slices | ½ cup | 93 | 22.4 |
| Spiced | ½ of 7¼-oz. can | 85 | 20.6 |

(USDA): United States Department of Agriculture
(HEW/FAO): Health, Education and Welfare/Food and Agriculture Organization
* Prepared as Package Directs

| Food and Description | Measure or Quantity | Calories | Carbo-hydrates (grams) |
|---|---|---|---|
| (Libby's): | | | |
| Halves, heavy syrup | ½ cup (4.5 oz.) | 105 | 25.4 |
| Sliced, heavy syrup | ½ cup (4.5 oz.) | 102 | 24.7 |
| (Stokely-Van Camp): | | | |
| Halves | ½ cup (4.4 oz.) | 95 | 24.5 |
| Slices | ½ cup (4.5 oz.) | 90 | 24.0 |
| Canned, dietetic or low calorie, unsweetened or water pack: | | | |
| (USDA) water pack | ½ cup (4.3 oz.) | 38 | 9.9 |
| (Del Monte) Lite | ½ cup | 53 | 12.6 |
| (Diet Delight) Cling halves or slices, solids & liq. | ½ cup (4.4 oz.) | 60 | 14.3 |
| (Diet Delight) Freestone, halves or slices, solids & liq. | ½ cup (4.4 oz.) | 60 | 14.3 |
| (Featherweight) Cling halves or slices, juice pack, solids & liq. | ½ cup | 50 | 14.0 |
| (Featherweight) Cling halves or slices, water pack, solids & liq. | ½ cup | 30 | 8.0 |
| (Libby's) water pack, sliced, solids & liq. | ½ cup (4.3 oz.) | 33 | 7.5 |
| (Tillie Lewis) Cling, solids & liq. | ½ cup (4.3 oz.) | 54 | 13.4 |
| Dehydrated (USDA): | | | |
| Uncooked | 1 oz. | 96 | 24.9 |
| Cooked, with added sugar, solids & liq. | ½ cup (5.4 oz.) | 184 | 47.6 |
| Dried: | | | |
| Uncooked (USDA) | ½ cup | 231 | 60.1 |
| Uncooked (Del Monte) canned | 2-oz. serving | 153 | 35.2 |
| Cooked (USDA) unsweetened | ½ cup | 111 | 28.9 |
| Cooked (USDA) sweetened | ½ cup (5.4 oz.) | 181 | 46.8 |
| Frozen: | | | |
| (USDA) unthawed, slices, sweetened | ½ cup | 104 | 26.7 |

| Food and Description | Measure or Quantity | Calories | Carbo-hydrates (grams) |
|---|---|---|---|
| (Birds Eye) quick thaw | ½ of 10-oz. pkg. | 141 | 34.1 |
| **PEACH BUTTER** (Smucker's) | 1 T. (.7 oz.) | 45 | 16.0 |
| *PEACH CREEK* (Annie Green Springs) 8% alcohol | 3 fl. oz. | 63 | 6.8 |
| **PEACH FRUIT DRINK:** | | | |
| Canned (Hi-C) | 6 fl. oz. | 90 | 23.0 |
| *Mix (Hi-C) | 6 fl. oz. | 76 | 19.0 |
| **PEACH ICE CREAM:** | | | |
| (Breyer's) | ¼ pt. | 130 | 18.0 |
| (Sealtest) old fashioned | ¼ pt. | 130 | 19.0 |
| **PEACH LIQUEUR:** | | | |
| (Bols) 60 proof | 1 fl. oz. | 96 | 8.9 |
| (DeKuyper) 60 proof | 1 fl. oz. | 82 | 8.3 |
| (Hiram Walker) 60 proof | 1 fl. oz. | 81 | 8.0 |
| (Leroux) 60 proof | 1 fl. oz. | 85 | 8.9 |
| **PEACH NECTAR,** canned (USDA) 40% fruit juice | 1 cup (8.8 oz.) | 120 | 31.0 |
| **PEACH & PEAR,** canned, dietetic (Featherweight) sliced, solids & liq. | ½ cup | 50 | 14.0 |
| **PEACH PRESERVE or JAM:** | | | |
| Sweetened (Smucker's) | 1 T. (.7 oz.) | 53 | 13.5 |
| Low calorie: | | | |
| (Dia-Mel) | 1 T. | 2 | 0. |
| (Featherweight) | 1 T. | 16 | 4.0 |
| (Featherweight) artificially sweetened | 1 T. | 6 | 1.0 |
| (Louis Sherry) | 1 tsp. | 2 | 0. |
| (Tillie Lewis) *Tasti Diet* | 1 T. | 11 | 2.7 |

(USDA): United States Department of Agriculture
(HEW/FAO): Health, Education and Welfare/Food and Agriculture
　　　　　　Organization
* Prepared as Package Directs

| Food and Description | Measure or Quantity | Calories | Carbohydrates (grams) |
|---|---|---|---|
| **PEANUT:** | | | |
| Raw: | | | |
| In shell (USDA) | 1 lb. (weighed in shell) | 1868 | 61.6 |
| In shell (A&P) fancy | 1 oz. | 171 | 5.3 |
| With skins (USDA) | 1 oz. | 160 | 5.3 |
| Without skins (USDA) | 1 oz. | 161 | 5.0 |
| Roasted: | | | |
| (USDA): | | | |
| Whole | 1 lb. (weighed in shell) | 1769 | 62.6 |
| With skins, unsalted | 1 oz. | 165 | 5.8 |
| Chopped | ½ cup | 404 | 13.0 |
| Halves | ½ cup | 421 | 13.5 |
| (A&P): | | | |
| Dry roasted | 1 oz. | 176 | 5.7 |
| In shell | 1 oz. | 178 | 5.8 |
| Oil roasted | 1 oz. | 181 | 4.7 |
| (Excel) halves | 1 oz. | 185 | 4.8 |
| (Frito-Lay's): | | | |
| Regular | 1 oz. | 172 | 6.2 |
| Salted in the shell | 1-oz. shelled | 163 | 5.7 |
| (Planters): | | | |
| Dry roasted | 1 oz. (jar) | 170 | 5.4 |
| Oil roasted | ¾-oz. bag | 133 | 3.7 |
| Spanish, roasted: | | | |
| (Ann Page) oil roasted | 1 oz. | 180 | 5.2 |
| *Freshnut*, oil roasted | 1 oz. | 170 | 5.1 |
| (Frito-Lay's) | 1 oz. | 168 | 6.6 |
| (Planters): | | | |
| Dry roasted | 1 oz. (jar) | 175 | 3.4 |
| Oil roasted | 1 oz. (can) | 182 | 3.4 |
| **PEANUT BUTTER:** | | | |
| (Ann Page): | | | |
| Creamy smooth | 1 T. (.6 oz.) | 107 | 3.6 |
| Krunchy | 1 T. (.6 oz.) | 105 | 3.6 |
| (Jif) creamy | 1 T. | 93 | 2.7 |
| (Kitchen King) creamy or crunchy | 1 T. | 95 | 4.0 |
| (Peter Pan): | | | |
| Crunchy | 1 T. | 101 | 3.0 |
| Smooth | 1 T. (.6 oz.) | 94 | 3.1 |

| Food and Description | Measure or Quantity | Calories | Carbo- hydrates (grams) |
|---|---|---|---|
| Low sodium | 1 T. | 106 | 2.3 |
| (Planters) creamy or crunchy | 1 T. (.6 oz.) | 95 | 3.0 |
| (Skippy): | | | |
| Creamy | 1 T. (.6 oz.) | 101 | 2.7 |
| Old fashioned, creamy or super chunk | 1 T. | 101 | 2.4 |
| Super chunk | 1 T. (.6 oz.) | 109 | 2.6 |
| (Smucker's): | | | |
| Creamy or crunchy | 1 T. | 90 | 3.0 |
| Natural | 1 T. | 100 | 3.0 |
| (Sultana): | | | |
| Regular grind | 1 T. (.6 oz.) | 107 | 3.6 |
| Krunchy | 1 T. (.6 oz.) | 105 | 3.9 |
| **PEANUT BUTTER BAKING CHIPS** (Reese's) | 3 T. (1 oz.) | 151 | 12.8 |
| **PEAR:** | | | |
| Fresh (USDA): | | | |
| Whole | 1 lb. (weighed with stems & core) | 252 | 63.2 |
| Whole | 6.4-oz. pear 3" x 2½" dia.) | 101 | 25.4 |
| Quartered | 1 cup (6.8 oz.) | 117 | 29.4 |
| Slices | ½ cup (6.8 oz.) | 50 | 12.5 |
| Canned, regular pack, solids & liq.: | | | |
| (USDA): | | | |
| Extra heavy syrup | 4 oz. | 104 | 26.8 |
| Heavy syrup | ½ cup | 87 | 22.3 |
| Juice pack | 4 oz. | 52 | 13.4 |
| Light syrup | 4 oz. | 69 | 17.7 |
| (Del Monte) Bartlett halves or slices, regular or chunky | ½ cup (4 oz.) | 88 | 21.3 |
| (Libby's) halves, heavy syrup | ½ cup (4.5 oz.) | 102 | 25.1 |

(USDA): United States Department of Agriculture
(HEW/FAO): Health, Education and Welfare/Food and Agriculture Organization
* Prepared as Package Directs

| Food and Description | Measure or Quantity | Calories | Carbohydrates (grams) |
|---|---|---|---|
| (Stokely-Van Camp): | | | |
| Halves | ½ cup (4.5 oz.) | 105 | 25.0 |
| Slices | ½ cup (4.5 oz.) | 100 | 23.5 |
| Canned, unsweetened or dietetic, solids & liq.: | | | |
| (USDA) water pack | ½ cup (4.3 oz.) | 39 | 10.1 |
| (Del Monte) Lite: | | | |
| Bartlett halves | ½ cup | 58 | 13.8 |
| Bartlett slices | ½ cup | 59 | 14.1 |
| (Diet Delight): | | | |
| Syrup pack | ½ cup (4.4 oz.) | 64 | 15.5 |
| Water pack | ½ cup (4.3 oz.) | 35 | 9.0 |
| (Featherweight): | | | |
| Bartlett halves, unsweetened | ½ cup | 57 | 14.0 |
| Bartlett halves, water pack | ½ cup | 37 | 9.0 |
| (Libby's) halves, water pack | ½ cup (4.3 oz.) | 40 | 9.8 |
| (Tillie Lewis) Tasti Diet, Bartlett halves | ½ cup (4.3 oz.) | 49 | 12.2 |
| Dried (USDA): | | | |
| Uncooked | 1 lb. | 1216 | 305.3 |
| Cooked, without added sugar | 4 oz. | 143 | 36.0 |
| Cooked, with added sugar, solids & liq. | 4 oz. | 171 | 43.1 |
| **PEAR, CANDIED** (USDA) | 1 oz. | 86 | 21.5 |
| **PEAR NECTAR,** canned (Del Monte) | 6 fl. oz. | 122 | 30.3 |
| *PEBBLES,* cereal (Post): | | | |
| Cocoa | ⅞ cup (1 oz.) | 117 | 24.2 |
| Fruity | ⅞ cup (1 oz.) | 116 | 24.4 |
| **PECAN:** | | | |
| In shell (USDA) | 1 lb. (weighed in shell) | 1652 | 35.1 |
| Shelled (USDA): | | | |
| Whole | 1 lb. | 3116 | 66.2 |
| Chopped | ½ cup (1.8 oz.) | 357 | 7.6 |

| Food and Description | Measure or Quantity | Calories | Carbohydrates (grams) |
|---|---|---|---|
| Chopped | 1 T. (7 grams) | 48 | 1.0 |
| Halves | 12–14 (.5 oz.) | 96 | 2.0 |
| Halves | ½ cup (1.9 oz.) | 371 | 7.9 |
| Dry roasted: | | | |
| (Flavor House) | 1 oz. | 195 | 4.1 |
| (Planters) | 1 oz. | 206 | 3.5 |

**PECAN PIE** (See PIE, Pecan)

**PEP,** cereal (Kellogg's) | ¾ cup (1 oz.) | 100 | 24.0

**PEPPER, BLACK:**

| (French's) | 1 tsp. (2.3 grams) | 9 | 1.5 |
|---|---|---|---|
| (French's) seasoned | 1 tsp. (2.9 grams) | 8 | 1.0 |

**PEPPER, HOT CHILI:**
Green:
(USDA):

| Raw, whole | 4 oz. | 31 | 7.5 |
|---|---|---|---|
| Raw, without seeds | 4 oz. | 42 | 10.3 |
| Canned, chili sauce | 1 oz. | 6 | 1.4 |
| (Ortega) canned, diced, strips or whole | 1 oz. | 7 | 1.1 |

Red:
(USDA):

| Raw, whole | 4 oz. (weighed with seeds) | 105 | 20.5 |
|---|---|---|---|
| Raw, trimmed, pods only | 4 oz. | 54 | 13.1 |
| Canned, chili sauce | 1 oz. | 6 | 1.1 |
| (Ortega) canned, diced or whole | 1 oz. | 8 | 1.6 |

**PEPPERONI:**

| (Hormel) sliced | 1 oz. | 142 | .3 |
|---|---|---|---|
| (Swift) | 1 oz. | 152 | 1.0 |

**\*PEPPER POT SOUP,** canned

| (Campbell) condensed | 10-oz. serving | 120 | 11.0 |
|---|---|---|---|

(USDA): United States Department of Agriculture
(HEW/FAO): Health, Education and Welfare/Food and Agriculture Organization
\* Prepared as Package Directs

| Food and Description | Measure or Quantity | Calories | Carbo-hydrates (grams) |
|---|---|---|---|
| **PEPPER STEAK, frozen:** | | | |
| *(Chun King) stir fry | ⅛ of pkg. | 70 | 3.0 |
| (Stouffer's) green pepper, with rice | 10½-oz. pkg. | 354 | 34.9 |
| **PEPPER, STUFFED:** | | | |
| Home recipe (USDA) with beef & crumbs | 2¾" x 2½" pepper with 1⅛ cups stuffing (6.5 oz.) | 314 | 31.1 |
| Frozen: | | | |
| (Green Giant) with beef, in Creole sauce | 7-oz. serving | 202 | 18.1 |
| (Stouffer's) green pepper & beef in tomato sauce | ½ of 15½-oz. pkg. | 210 | 17.8 |
| (Weight Watchers) with veal stuffing | 13-oz meal | 366 | 51.0 |
| **PEPPER, SWEET (USDA):** | | | |
| Green: | | | |
| Raw: | | | |
| Whole | 1 lb. (weighed untrimmed) | 82 | 17.9 |
| Without stems & seeds | 1 med. pepper (2.6 oz.) | 13 | 2.9 |
| Chopped | ½ cup (2.6 oz.) | 16 | 3.6 |
| Slices | ½ cup (1.4 oz.) | 9 | 2.0 |
| Strips | ½ cup (1.7 oz.) | 11 | 2.4 |
| Boiled strips, drained | ½ cup (2.4 oz.) | 12 | 2.6 |
| Boiled, drained | 1 med. pepper (2.6 oz.) | 13 | 2.8 |
| Red: | | | |
| Raw, whole | 1 lb. (weighed with stems & seeds) | 112 | 25.8 |
| Raw, without stems & seeds | 1 med. pepper (2.2 oz.) | 19 | 2.4 |
| **PERCH, raw (USDA):** | | | |
| White, whole | 1 lb. (weighed whole) | 193 | 0. |
| White, meat only | 4 oz. | 134 | 0. |

| Food and Description | Measure or Quantity | Calories | Carbohydrates (grams) |
|---|---|---|---|
| Yellow, whole | 1 lb. (weighed whole) | 161 | 0. |
| Yellow, meat only | 4 oz. | 103 | 0. |
| **PERCH DINNER or LUNCHEON, frozen:** | | | |
| (Banquet) | 8¾-oz. dinner | 434 | 49.8 |
| (Mrs. Paul's) fillets, breaded & french fried | 2-oz. fillet | 127 | 8.8 |
| (Van de Kamp's) batter dipped, french fried | 2.4-oz. piece | 145 | 10.0 |
| (Weight Watchers): | | | |
| 2-compartment meal | 8½-oz. meal | 206 | 13.0 |
| 3-compartment meal | 16-oz. meal | 294 | 15.0 |
| **PERNOD** (Julius Wile) 90 proof | 1 fl. oz. | 79 | 1.1 |
| **PERSIMMON** (USDA): | | | |
| Japanese or Kaki, fresh: | | | |
| With seeds | 1 lb. (weighed with skin, calyx & seeds) | 286 | 78.3 |
| With seeds | 4.4-oz. persimmon | 79 | 20.1 |
| Seedless | 1 lb. (weighed with skin & calyx) | 293 | 75.1 |
| Seedless | 4.4-oz. persimmon (2½" dia.) | 81 | 20.7 |
| Native, fresh, whole | 1 lb. (weighed with seeds & calyx) | 472 | 124.6 |
| Native, fresh, flesh only | 4 oz. | 144 | 38.0 |
| **PHEASANT, raw** (USDA): | | | |
| Ready-to-cook | 1 lb. (weighed ready-to-cook) | 596 | 0. |
| Meat & skin | 4 oz. | 172 | 0. |
| Meat only | 4 oz. | 184 | 0. |

(USDA): United States Department of Agriculture
(HEW/FAO): Health, Education and Welfare/Food and Agriculture Organization
* Prepared as Package Directs

| Food and Description | Measure or Quantity | Calories | Carbohydrates (grams) |
|---|---|---|---|
| **PICKEREL**, chain, raw (USDA): | | | |
| Whole | 1 lb. (weighed whole) | 194 | 0. |
| Meat only | 4 oz. | 95 | 0. |
| **PICKLE:** | | | |
| Chowchow (See CHOWCHOW) | | | |
| Cucumber, fresh or bread & butter: | | | |
| (USDA) | 3 slices (¼″ x 1½″) | 15 | 3.8 |
| (Bond's) | 3 pieces | 23 | 5.0 |
| (Fanning's) | 14-fl.-oz. jar | 196 | 45.7 |
| (Featherweight) dietetic, slices or whole | 1 oz. | 12 | 2.6 |
| (Nalley's) chips | 1-oz. serving | 27 | 6.5 |
| Dill: | | | |
| (USDA) | 4.8-oz. pickle | 15 | 3.0 |
| (Bond's) | 1 pickle | 1 | .2 |
| (Bond's) fresh pack | 1 spear | 2 | .2 |
| (Featherweight) low sodium | 1-oz. serving | 5 | .9 |
| *L & S Dills* | 1 large pickle | 15 | 2.0 |
| (Nalley's) regular and Polish style | 1-oz. serving | 3 | .6 |
| (Smucker's): | | | |
| Candied stick | 4″ pickle (.8 oz.) | 45 | 11.0 |
| Hamburger | 1 slice (.13 oz.) | <1 | 0. |
| Polish, whole | 3½″ pickle (1.8 oz.) | 8 | 1.0 |
| Spears | 3½″ spear (1.4 oz.) | 6 | 1.0 |
| Hamburger (Nalley's) chips | 1-oz. serving | 3 | .6 |
| Kosher dill: | | | |
| (Bond's) | 1 pickle | 2 | .2 |
| (Claussen): | | | |
| Halves | 2-oz. serving | 7 | 1.3 |
| Whole | 2-oz. serving | 7 | 1.1 |
| (Featherweight) low sodium | 1 oz. | 5 | .9 |

| Food and Description | Measure or Quantity | Calories | Carbo-hydrates (grams) |
|---|---|---|---|
| (Nalleys') | 2-oz. serving | 12 | 1.7 |
| (Smucker's): | | | |
|   Baby | 2¾" pickle (.8 oz.) | 4 | .5 |
|   Slices | 1 slice (.1 oz.) | <1 | 0. |
|   Whole | 3½" pickle (.5 oz.) | 8 | 1.0 |
| Sour: | | | |
|   (USDA) cucumber | 1¾" x 4" (4.8 oz.) | 14 | 2.7 |
|   (Aunt Jane's) | 2-oz. pickle | 6 | 1.1 |
| Sweet: | | | |
|   (USDA): | | | |
|     Cucumber, whole | 1-oz. whole | 41 | 10.3 |
|     Cucumber, chopped | 1 T. (9 grams) | 13 | 3.3 |
|   (Aunt Jane's) | 1.5-oz. pickle | 62 | 15.5 |
|   (Nalley's): | | | |
|     Regular | 1-oz. serving | 37 | 10.5 |
|     Chips | 1-oz. serving | 34 | 9.7 |
|     Nubbins | 1-oz. serving | 28 | 7.9 |
|   (Smucker's): | | | |
|     Candied mix | 1 piece (.3 oz.) | 14 | 3.3 |
|     Gherkins | 2" long pickle (.32 oz.) | 15 | 3.5 |
|     Slices | 1 slice (.2 oz.) | 11 | 2.3 |
|     Sticks | 4" long stick | 30 | 7.0 |
|     Whole | 2½" long pickle (.4 oz.) | 18 | 4.0 |
| PIE: | | | |
|   Commercial type: | | | |
|     Apple: | | | |
|       Home recipe (USDA) 2-crust | ⅛ of 9" pie (5.6 oz.) | 404 | 60.2 |
|       (Hostess) | 4½-oz. pie | 409 | 53.7 |
|       (Tastykake) | 4-oz. pie | 348 | DNA |
|       (Tastykake) French | 4¼-oz. pie | 405 | DNA |

(USDA): United States Department of Agriculture
(HEW/FAO): Health, Education and Welfare/Food and Agriculture Organization
* Prepared as Package Directs

| Food and Description | Measure or Quantity | Calories | Carbo-hydrates (grams) |
|---|---|---|---|
| Banana, home recipe (USDA) cream or custard unenriched or enriched | 1/8 of 9" pie (5.4 oz.) | 336 | 46.7 |
| Berry (Hostess) | 4½-oz. pie | 404 | 51.1 |
| Blackberry, home recipe (USDA) 2-crust, made with vegetable shortening | 1/8 of 9" pie (5.6 oz.) | 384 | 54.4 |
| Blueberry: | | | |
| Home recipe (USDA) 2-crust, made with lard | 1/8 of 9" pie (5.6 oz.) | 382 | 55.1 |
| (Hostess) | 4½-oz. pie | 394 | 49.9 |
| (Tastykake) | 4-oz. pie | 366 | DNA |
| Boston cream, home recipe (USDA) | 1/12 of 8" pie (2.4 oz.) | 208 | 34.4 |
| Butterscotch, home recipe (USDA) | 1/8 of 9" pie (5.4 oz.) | 406 | 58.2 |
| Cherry: | | | |
| Home recipe (USDA) 2-crust | 1/8 of 9" pie (5.6 oz.) | 412 | 60.7 |
| (Hostess) | 4½-oz. pie | 435 | 58.8 |
| (Tastykake) | 4-oz. pie | 381 | DNA |
| Chocolate chiffon, home recipe (USDA) made with lard | 1/8 of 9" pie (3.8 oz.) | 354 | 47.2 |
| Chocolate meringue, home recipe (USDA) made with vegetable shortening | 1/8 of 9" pie (4.9 oz.) | 353 | 46.9 |
| Coconut custard, home recipe (USDA) | 1/8 of 9" pie (5.4 oz.) | 357 | 37.8 |

| Food and Description | Measure or Quantity | Calories | Carbo-hydrates (grams) |
|---|---|---|---|
| Custard, home recipe (USDA) enriched or unenriched | ⅛ of 9″ pie (5.4 oz.) | 331 | 35.6 |
| Lemon: | | | |
| Chiffon, home recipe (USDA) made with lard or vegetable shortening | ⅛ of 9″ pie | 338 | 47.3 |
| Meringue, home recipe, (USDA) 1-crust | ⅛ of 9″ pie (4.9 oz.) | 357 | 52.8 |
| (Hostess) | 4½-oz. pie | 415 | 52.4 |
| (Tastykake) | 4-oz. pie | 370 | DNA |
| Mince, home recipe (USDA) 2-crust, enriched or unenriched | ⅛ of 9″ pie (5.6 oz.) | 428 | 65.1 |
| Peach: | | | |
| Home recipe (USDA) 2-crust | ⅛ of 9″ pie (5.6 oz.) | 405 | 60.4 |
| (Hostess) | 4½-oz. pie | 409 | 52.4 |
| (Tastykake) | 4-oz. pie | 349 | DNA |
| Pecan: | | | |
| Home recipe (USDA) 1-crust, made with lard or vegetable shortening | ⅛ of 9″ pie | 577 | 70.8 |
| (Frito-Lay's) | 3-oz. serving | 353 | 53.5 |
| Pineapple, home recipe (USDA) 2-crust, made with lard or vegetable shortening | ⅛ of 9″ pie (5.6 oz.) | 400 | 60.2 |

(USDA): United States Department of Agriculture
(HEW/FAO): Health, Education and Welfare/Food and Agriculture Organization
* Prepared as Package Directs

| *Food and Description* | *Measure or Quantity* | *Calories* | *Carbo-hydrates (grams)* |
|---|---|---|---|
| Pineapple custard, home recipe (USDA) made with lard or vegetable shortening | ⅙ of 9″ pie (5.4 oz.) | 334 | 48.8 |
| Pumpkin, home recipe (USDA) 1-crust, made with lard or vegetable shortening | ⅙ of 9″ pie (5.4 oz.) | 321 | 37.2 |
| Raisin, home recipe (USDA) 2-crust, made with lard or vegetable shortening | ⅙ of 9″ pie (5.6 oz.) | 427 | 67.9 |
| Rhubarb, home recipe (USDA) 2-crust, made with lard or vegetable shortening | ⅙ of 9″ pie (5.6 oz.) | 400 | 60.4 |
| Strawberry, home recipe (USDA) made with lard or vegetable shortening | ⅙ of 9″ pie (5.6 oz.) | 313 | 48.8 |
| Frozen: | | | |
| Apple: | | | |
| (USDA) baked | 5-oz. serving | 361 | 56.8 |
| (Banquet) | ⅙ of 20-oz. pie | 288 | 42.6 |
| (Morton): | | | |
| Regular | ⅙ of 24-oz. pie | 295 | 40.9 |
| *Great Little Desserts* | 8-oz. pie | 598 | 88.6 |
| *Great Little Desserts*, Dutch | 7.8-oz. pie | 607 | 95.3 |
| (Pepperidge Farm) tart | 3-oz. tart | 276 | 32.8 |
| (Sara Lee): | | | |
| Regular | ⅙ of pie (5.2 oz.) | 422 | 53.4 |
| Dutch | ⅙ of pie (5 oz.) | 393 | 60.4 |
| Banana: | | | |
| (Banquet) cream | ⅙ of 14-oz. pie | 172 | 19.9 |

| Food and Description | Measure or Quantity | Calories | Carbohydrates (grams) |
|---|---|---|---|
| (Morton): | | | |
| Cream | ⅙ of 16-oz. pie | 174 | 19.7 |
| Cream, *Great Little Desserts* | 3½-oz. pie | 237 | 25.8 |
| Blueberry: | | | |
| (Banquet) | ⅙ of 20-oz. pie | 253 | 37.5 |
| (Morton): | | | |
| Regular | ⅙ of 24-oz. pie | 285 | 38.6 |
| *Great Little Desserts* | 8-oz. pie | 589 | 86.4 |
| (Pepperidge Farm) tart | 3-oz. tart | 277 | 34.5 |
| (Sara Lee) | ⅛ of pie (5.2 oz.) | 228 | 33.8 |
| Cherry: | | | |
| (Banquet) | ⅙ of 20-oz. pie | 228 | 33.8 |
| (Morton): | | | |
| Regular | ⅙ of 24-oz. pie | 300 | 42.0 |
| *Great Little Desserts* | 8-oz. pie | 589 | 86.4 |
| (Pepperidge Farm) tart | 3-oz. tart | 277 | 34.3 |
| (Sara Lee) | ⅛ of pie (5.2 oz.) | 396 | 48.0 |
| Chocolate cream: | | | |
| (Banquet) | ⅙ of 14-oz. pie | 177 | 21.8 |
| (Morton): | | | |
| Regular | ⅙ of 16-oz. pie | 199 | 22.8 |
| *Great Little Desserts* | 3½-oz. pie | 266 | 28.8 |
| Chocolate tart | | | |
| (Pepperidge Farm) | 3-oz. tart | 306 | 35.2 |
| Coconut: | | | |
| Cream: | | | |
| (Banquet) | ⅙ of 14-oz. pie | 178 | 19.1 |
| (Morton): | | | |
| Regular | ⅙ of 16-oz. pie | 197 | 22.0 |
| *Great Little Desserts* | 3½-oz. pie | 266 | 28.8 |
| (Pepperidge Farm) tart | 3-oz. tart | 310 | 29.0 |

(USDA): United States Department of Agriculture
(HEW/FAO): Health, Education and Welfare/Food and Agriculture Organization
* Prepared as Package Directs

| *Food and Description* | *Measure or Quantity* | *Calories* | *Carbo-hydrates (grams)* |
|---|---|---|---|
| Custard: | | | |
| (Banquet) | ⅙ of 20-oz. pie | 203 | 28.3 |
| (Morton) *Great Little Desserts* | 6½-oz. pie | 369 | 53.5 |
| Custard (Banquet) | ⅙ of 20-oz. pie | 247 | 38.1 |
| Lemon: | | | |
| Cream: | | | |
| (Banquet) | ⅙ of 14-oz. pie | 168 | 21.8 |
| (Morton): | | | |
| Regular | ⅙ of 16-oz. pie | 182 | 22.0 |
| *Great Little Desserts* | 3½-oz. pie | 245 | 27.8 |
| Tart (Pepperidge Farm) | 3-oz. tart | 317 | 36.4 |
| Mince: | | | |
| (Banquet) | ⅙ of 20-oz. pie | 252 | 38.5 |
| (Morton) | ⅙ of 24-oz. pie | 314 | 45.5 |
| Neapolitan (Morton) | ⅙ of 16-oz. pie | 195 | 23.0 |
| Peach: | | | |
| (Banquet) | ⅙ of 20-oz. pie | 263 | 35.8 |
| (Morton) | ⅙ of 24-oz. pie | 286 | 38.7 |
| (Sara Lee) | ⅛ of 31-oz. pie | 458 | 56.3 |
| Pumpkin: | | | |
| (Banquet) | ⅙ of 20-oz. pie | 206 | 32.3 |
| (Morton) | ⅙ of 24-oz. pie | 235 | 36.4 |
| (Sara Lee) | ⅛ of pie (5.6 oz.) | 354 | 49.4 |
| Strawberry cream: | | | |
| (Banquet) | ⅙ of 14-oz. pie | 169 | 22.5 |
| (Morton) | ⅙ of 16-oz. pie | 182 | 22.0 |
| **PIE CRUST** (See also **PASTRY SHELL**): | | | |
| Home recipe (USDA) baked | 1 9" pie crust (6.3 oz.) | 900 | 78.8 |
| Home recipe (USDA) baked | 2 9" pie crusts (12.7 oz.) | 1800 | 157.7 |
| Mix: | | | |
| (USDA) dry | 10-oz. pkg. | 1482 | 140.6 |
| (USDA) prepared with water, baked | 4 oz. | 526 | 49.9 |
| (Betty Crocker) | 1/16 pkg. | 120 | 10.0 |
| (Betty Crocker) | ⅛ stick | 120 | 10.0 |
| *(Flako) | ⅙ of 9" pie shell | 260 | 29.0 |

| Food and Description | Measure or Quantity | Calories | Carbo-hydrates (grams) |
|---|---|---|---|
| *(Pillsbury): | | | |
| Double crust | ⅛ of 2 crusts | 290 | 27.0 |
| Sticks | ⅛ of 2-crust pie | 290 | 27.0 |
| PIE FILLING (See also PUDDING or PIE FILLING): | | | |
| Apple: | | | |
| (Comstock): | | | |
| Regular | 21-oz. can | 780 | 174.0 |
| Pie-sliced | 21-oz. can | 270 | 60.0 |
| (Lucky Leaf): | | | |
| Sweetened | 8-oz. serving | 248 | 60.8 |
| Unsweetened | 8-oz. serving | 98 | 23.2 |
| (Musselman's) | 1 cup (8.7 oz.) | 283 | DNA |
| (Wilderness) | 30-oz. can | 846 | 251.7 |
| (Wilderness) French | 21-oz. can | 703 | 164.8 |
| Apricot: | | | |
| (Comstock) | 21-oz. can | 660 | 144.0 |
| (Lucky Leaf) | 8-oz. serving | 316 | 77.6 |
| (Wilderness) | 21-oz. can | 756 | 176.7 |
| Banana (Comstock) cream | 21-oz. can | 660 | 132.0 |
| Blackberry (Lucky Leaf) | 8-oz. serving | 258 | 62.4 |
| Blueberry: | | | |
| (Comstock) | 21-oz. can | 720 | 156.0 |
| (Lucky Leaf) | 8-oz. serving | 256 | 61.4 |
| (Musselman's) | 1 cup (8.8 oz.) | 321 | DNA |
| (Wilderness) | 32-oz. can | 1100 | 263.1 |
| Cherry: | | | |
| (Comstock) | 21-oz. can | 720 | 156.0 |
| (Lucky Leaf) | 8-oz. serving | 242 | 58.2 |
| (Musselman's) | 1 cup (8.7 oz.) | 400 | DNA |
| (Wilderness) | 32-oz. can | 1100 | 258.6 |
| Chocolate cream (Comstock) | 21-oz. can | 840 | 162.0 |
| Coconut cream (Comstock) | 21-oz. can | 720 | 144.0 |
| Lemon: | | | |
| (Comstock) | 21-oz. can | 960 | 198.0 |

(USDA): United States Department of Agriculture
(HEW/FAO): Health, Education and Welfare/Food and Agriculture Organization
* Prepared as Package Directs

| Food and Description | Measure or Quantity | Calories | Carbohydrates (grams) |
|---|---|---|---|
| (Lucky Leaf) | 8-oz. serving | 412 | 95.4 |
| (Wilderness) | 22-oz. can | 1104 | 230.2 |
| Mincemeat: | | | |
| (Comstock) | 21-oz. can | 1020 | 216.0 |
| (Wilderness) | 22-oz. can | 1291 | 260.4 |
| Peach: | | | |
| (Comstock) | 21-oz. can | 660 | 150.0 |
| (Lucky Leaf) | 8-oz. serving | 300 | 74.0 |
| (Musselman's) | 1 cup (8.8 oz.) | 292 | DNA |
| (Wilderness) | 21-oz. can | 679 | 148.3 |
| Pineapple: | | | |
| (Comstock) | 21-oz. can | 660 | 150.0 |
| (Lucky Leaf) | 8-oz. serving | 240 | 59.0 |
| Pumpkin (See also PUMPKIN, canned) | | | |
| (Comstock) | 4½-oz. serving | 170 | 38.0 |
| Raisin: | | | |
| (Comstock) | 21-oz. can | 840 | 180.0 |
| (Lucky Leaf) | 8-oz. serving | 292 | 67.8 |
| (Wilderness) | 22-oz. can | 773 | 180.7 |
| Strawberry: | | | |
| (Comstock) | 21-oz. can | 780 | 168.0 |
| (Lucky Leaf) | 8-oz. serving | 248 | 60.0 |
| (Wilderness) | 21-oz. can | 738 | 180.9 |
| | | | |
| *PIE MIX: | | | |
| Boston cream (Betty Crocker) | ⅛ of pie | 260 | 48.0 |
| Chocolate cream (Pillsbury) no bake | ⅛ of pie | 410 | 53.0 |
| Lemon chiffon (Pillsbury) no bake | ⅛ of pie | 330 | 50.0 |
| Vanilla (Pillsbury) marble, no bake | ⅛ of pie | 390 | 49.0 |
| | | | |
| PIESPORTER RIESLING (Julius Kayser) 10% alcohol | 3 fl. oz. | 57 | 1.7 |
| | | | |
| PIGEON (See SQUAB) | | | |
| | | | |
| PIGEONPEA (USDA) | | | |
| Raw, immature seeds in pods | 1 lb. | 207 | 37.7 |
| Dry seeds | 1 lb. | 1551 | 288.9 |

| Food and Description | Measure or Quantity | Calories | Carbo-hydrates (grams) |
|---|---|---|---|
| **PIGNOLIA** (See **PINE NUT**) | | | |
| **PIGS FEET**, pickled | | | |
| (USDA) | 4 oz. | 226 | 0. |
| **PIKE**, raw (USDA): | | | |
| Blue, whole | 1 lb. (weighed whole) | 180 | 0. |
| Blue, meat only | 4 oz. | 102 | 0. |
| Northern, whole | 1 lb. (weighed whole) | 104 | 0. |
| Northern, meat only | 4 oz. | 100 | 0. |
| Walleye, whole | 1 lb. (weighed whole) | 240 | 0. |
| Walleye, meat only | 4 oz. | 105 | 0. |
| **PILI NUT** (USDA): | | | |
| In shell | 1 lb. (weighed in shell) | 546 | 6.9 |
| Shelled | 4 oz. | 759 | 9.5 |
| **PIMIENTO**, canned: | | | |
| (USDA) solids & liq. | 4 oz. | 31 | 6.6 |
| (Dromedary) diced, sliced or whole, drained | 1-oz. serving | 10 | 2.0 |
| (Ortega) drained | ¼ cup (1.7 oz.) | 6 | 1.3 |
| **PIÑA COLADA:** | | | |
| Canned: | | | |
| (Mr. Boston) 12½% alcohol | 3 fl. oz. | 240 | 34.2 |
| (Party Tyme) 12½% alcohol | 2 fl. oz. | 63 | 5.1 |
| Mix: | | | |
| Dry (Holland House) | 1 serving (.6 oz.) | 66 | 16.0 |
| Dry (Party Tyme) | ½-oz. pkg. | 50 | 13.2 |
| Liquid (Holland House) | 1½ fl. oz. | 90 | 22.5 |

(USDA): United States Department of Agriculture
(HEW/FAO): Health, Education and Welfare/Food and Agriculture Organization
* Prepared as Package Directs

| Food and Description | Measure or Quantity | Calories | Carbohydrates (grams) |
|---|---|---|---|
| **PINEAPPLE:** | | | |
| Fresh (USDA): | | | |
| Whole | 1 lb. (weighed untrimmed) | 123 | 32.3 |
| Diced | ½ cup (2.8 oz.) | 41 | 10.7 |
| Sliced | ¾" x 3½" slice (3 oz.) | 44 | 11.5 |
| Canned, regular pack, solids & liq.: (USDA): | | | |
| Heavy syrup, crushed | ½ cup (5.6 oz.) | 97 | 25.4 |
| Heavy syrup, slices | 1 large slice & 2 T. syrup (4.3 oz.) | 90 | 23.7 |
| Heavy syrup, tidbits | ½ cup (4.6 oz.) | 95 | 25.0 |
| Juice pack | 4 oz. | 66 | 17.1 |
| Light syrup | 4 oz. | 67 | 17.5 |
| (Del Monte): | | | |
| Crushed | ½ cup (4 oz.) | 94 | 22.7 |
| Chunks | ½ cup | 91 | 22.2 |
| Slices, medium | ½ cup | 92 | 22.4 |
| Slices, large | ½ cup | 103 | 25.2 |
| Tidbits | ½ cup | 95 | 22.9 |
| (Dole): | | | |
| Heavy syrup, chunks | ½ cup | 84 | 22.0 |
| Heavy syrup, crushed or tidbits | ½ cup | 84 | 21.7 |
| Heavy syrup, slices | 2 med. slices & 2½ T. syrup (4 oz.) | 83 | 21.7 |
| Juice pack, chunks or crushed | ½ cup | 64 | 16.5 |
| Juice pack, sliced | 2 med. slices & 2½ T. syrup | 66 | 15.5 |
| Canned, unsweetened or water pack, dietetic or low calorie, solids & liq.: | | | |
| (USDA) | 4 oz. | 44 | 11.6 |
| (Del Monte): | | | |
| Chunks | ½ cup | 70 | 16.8 |
| Crushed | ½ cup | 77 | 18.5 |
| Slices | ½ cup | 81 | 19.6 |
| (Diet Delight) chunks, slices or tidbits | ½ cup | 79 | 19.1 |

| Food and Description | Measure or Quantity | Calories | Carbo-hydrates (grams) |
|---|---|---|---|
| (Featherweight) syrup pack, chunks, crushed or sliced | ½ cup | 70 | 18.0 |
| (Featherweight) water pack, sliced | ½ cup | 60 | 15.0 |
| (Tillie Lewis) *Tasti Diet*, syrup pack, chunks or slices | ½ cup | 72 | 17.9 |
| (Tillie Lewis) *Tasti Diet*, water pack, tidbits | ½ cup | 60 | 14.9 |
| **PINEAPPLE, CANDIED** | | | |
| (USDA) | 1 oz. | 90 | 22.7 |
| **PINEAPPLE & GRAPE-FRUIT JUICE DRINK,** canned: | | | |
| (USDA) 40% fruit juices | ½ cup (4.4 oz.) | 68 | 17.0 |
| (Del Monte) pink | 6 fl. oz. | 97 | 23.9 |
| (Dole) regular or pink | 6 fl. oz. | 91 | 23.0 |
| **PINEAPPLE JUICE:** Canned, unsweetened: | | | |
| (Del Monte): | | | |
| Regular | 6 fl. oz. | 98 | 23.7 |
| With vitamin C | 6 fl. oz. | 108 | 26.2 |
| (Dole) with vitamin C | 6 fl. oz. | 93 | 22.8 |
| Frozen, unsweetened: | | | |
| *(USDA) | ½ cup (4.4 oz.) | 64 | 15.9 |
| *(Minute Maid) | 6 fl. oz. | 92 | 22.7 |
| **PINEAPPLE & ORANGE JUICE DRINK:** Canned: | | | |
| (USDA) 40% fruit juices | ½ cup (4.4 oz.) | 67 | 16.7 |
| (Del Monte) | 6 fl. oz. | 97 | 24.0 |
| (Hi-C) | 8 fl. oz. | 125 | 30.7 |
| *Frozen (Minute Maid) | 6 fl. oz. | 94 | 23.0 |

(USDA): United States Department of Agriculture
(HEW/FAO): Health, Education and Welfare/Food and Agriculture Organization
* Prepared as Package Directs

| Food and Description | Measure or Quantity | Calories | Carbo-hydrates (grams) |
|---|---|---|---|
| **PINEAPPLE PRESERVE:** | | | |
| Sweetened (Smucker's) | 1 T. | 53 | 13.5 |
| Dietetic (Featherweight) | 1 T. | 16 | 4.0 |
| **PINE NUT (USDA):** | | | |
| Pignolias, shelled | 4 oz. | 626 | 13.2 |
| Piñon, whole | 4 oz. (weighed in shell) | 418 | 13.5 |
| Piñon, shelled | 4 oz. | 720 | 23.2 |
| **PINK SQUIRREL COCK-TAIL MIX, dry** (Holland House) | .6-oz. pkg. | 69 | 17.0 |
| **PINOT CHARDONNAY WINE** (Louis M. Martini) 12½% alcohol | 3 fl. oz. | 90 | .2 |
| **PINOT NOIR WINE:** | | | |
| (Inglenook) Estate, 12% alcohol | 3 fl. oz. | 58 | .3 |
| (Louis M. Martini) 12½% alcohol | 3 fl. oz. | 90 | .2 |
| **PISTACHIO NUT:** | | | |
| (USDA): | | | |
| In shell | 4 oz. (weighed in shell) | 337 | 10.8 |
| Shelled | ½ cup (2.2 oz.) | 368 | 11.8 |
| Shelled | 1 T. (8 grams) | 46 | 1.5 |
| (Flavor House) dry roasted | 1 oz. | 168 | 5.4 |
| (Frito-Lay's) | 1 oz. | 175 | 5.8 |
| (Planters) dry roasted | 1 oz. | 170 | 6.0 |
| **PITANGA, fresh** (USDA): | | | |
| Whole | 1 lb. (weighed whole) | 187 | 45.9 |
| Flesh only | 4 oz. | 58 | 14.2 |
| **PIZZA PIE** (See also **PIZZA PIE MIX**): | | | |
| Regular (Pizza Hut): | | | |
| Beef | ½ of 10" pizza (7.6 oz.) | 488 | 55.0 |

| Food and Description | Measure or Quantity | Calories | Carbo- hydrates (grams) |
|---|---|---|---|
| Cheese | ½ of 10" pie | 436 | 53.2 |
| Pepperoni | ½ of 10" pie | 459 | 54.4 |
| Pork | ½ of 10" pie | 466 | 54.6 |
| Supreme | ½ of 10" pie | 474 | 54.4 |
| Frozen: | | | |
| Cheese: | | | |
| (Celeste) | ½ of 7-oz. pie | 247 | 31.8 |
| (Celeste) | ¼ of 19-oz. pie | 320 | 36.2 |
| (Jeno's) | ½ of 13-oz. pie | 420 | 54.0 |
| (Jeno's) deluxe | ⅓ of 20-oz. pie | 490 | 57.0 |
| (La Pizzeria) | ¼ of 20-oz. pie | 330 | 42.0 |
| (La Pizzeria) | ⅓ of 18½-oz. pie | 410 | 46.0 |
| (Stouffer's) *French* Bread | ½ of 10¼-oz. pie | 327 | 42.8 |
| *Tostino's* | ½ pie | 440 | 53.0 |
| (Weight Watchers) | 6-oz. pie | 386 | 37.2 |
| (Weight Watchers) | 7-oz. pie | 450 | 43.4 |
| Cheese & mushroom (Celeste): | | | |
| Small size | ½ of 9-oz. pie | 285 | 29.0 |
| Large size | ¼ of 21-oz. pie | 298 | 30.1 |
| Cheese, Sicilian style (Celeste) | ¼ of 20-oz. pie | 329 | 42.5 |
| Combination: | | | |
| (Jeno's) deluxe | ⅓ of 23-oz. pie | 560 | 55.0 |
| (La Pizzeria) | ½ of 13½-oz. pie | 420 | 43.0 |
| (La Pizzeria) | ¼ of 24½-oz. pie | 380 | 39.0 |
| *Tostino's:* | | | |
| Classic | ⅓ of pie | 520 | 48.0 |
| Deep crust | ⅙ of pie | 310 | 33.0 |
| (Van de Kamp's) thick crust | ¼ of 23.4-oz. pie | 310 | 24.0 |
| Deluxe: | | | |
| (Celeste): | | | |
| Small pie | ½ of 9-oz. pie | 298 | 27.7 |
| Large pie | ½ of 23½-oz. pie | 367 | 33.9 |
| (Stouffer's) *French* Bread | ½ of 12⅜-oz. pkg. | 404 | 45.7 |

(USDA): United States Department of Agriculture
(HEW/FAO): Health, Education and Welfare/Food and Agriculture
        Organization
* Prepared as Package Directs

| *Food and Description* | *Measure or Quantity* | *Calories* | *Carbo-hydrates (grams)* |
|---|---|---|---|
| Hamburger: | | | |
| (Jeno's) | ½ of 13½-oz. pie | 440 | 57.0 |
| (Stouffer's) *French Bread* | ½ of 12¼-oz. pkg. | 397 | 37.8 |
| *Tostino's* | ½ of pie | 460 | 51.0 |
| Pepperoni: | | | |
| (Celeste): | | | |
| Small size | ½ of 7½-oz. pie | 264 | 25.9 |
| Large size | ¼ of 20-oz. pie | 356 | 31.7 |
| (Jeno's) | ½ of 12-oz. pie | 450 | 57.0 |
| (La Pizzeria) | ¼ of 21-oz. pie | 330 | 42.0 |
| (Stouffer's) *French Bread* | ½ of 11¼-oz. pie | 401 | 43.8 |
| *Tostino's:* | | | |
| Regular | ½ of pie | 460 | 52.0 |
| Deep crust | ⅙ of pie | 300 | 34.0 |
| (Van de Kamp's) thick crust | ¼ of 22-oz. pie | 370 | 38.0 |
| Sausage: | | | |
| (Celeste): | | | |
| Small size | ½ of 8-oz. pie | 281 | 25.8 |
| Large size | ¼ of 22-oz. pie | 375 | 33.9 |
| (Jeno's): | | | |
| Regular | ½ of 13½-oz. pie | 450 | 57.0 |
| Deluxe | ⅓ of 21-oz. pie | 500 | 53.0 |
| (La Pizzeria): | | | |
| Small size | ½ of 13-oz. pie | 430 | 41.0 |
| Large size | ¼ of 23-oz. pie | 380 | 42.0 |
| (Stouffer's) *French Bread* | ½ of 12-oz. pkg. | 417 | 43.8 |
| *Tostino's:* | | | |
| Regular | ½ of pie | 470 | 54.0 |
| Classic | ⅓ of pie | 500 | 50.0 |
| Deep crust | ⅙ of pie | 300 | 33.0 |
| (Weight Watchers): | | | |
| Small | 6-oz. pie | 330 | 30.7 |
| Large | 7-oz. pie | 385 | 35.8 |
| Sausage & mushroom: | | | |
| (Celeste): | | | |
| Small | ½ of 9-oz. pie | 285 | 29.0 |
| Large | ¼ of 24-oz. pie | 379 | 34.3 |

| Food and Description | Measure or Quantity | Calories | Carbo-hydrates (grams) |
|---|---|---|---|
| (Stouffer's) *French Bread* | ½ of 12½-oz. pkg. | 388 | 39.8 |
| **PIZZA PIE MIX:** | | | |
| Regular (Jeno's) | ½ of pkg. | 420 | 67.0 |
| Cheese: | | | |
| (Jeno's) | ½ of mix | 420 | 62.0 |
| *(Kraft) | 4 oz. | 265 | 26.1 |
| *Skillet Pizza* (General Mills) | ¼ pkg. | 210 | 30.0 |
| Pepperoni: | | | |
| (Jeno's) | ½ pkg. | 510 | 67.0 |
| *Skillet Pizza* (General Mills) | ¼ pkg. | 220 | 31.0 |
| Sausage: | | | |
| (Jeno's) | ½ of pkg. | 530 | 66.0 |
| *(Kraft) | 4 oz. | 274 | 23.9 |
| *Skillet Pizza* (General Mills) | ¼ pkg. | 230 | 29.0 |
| **PIZZA ROLL** (Jeno's) frozen, 12 to pkg.: | | | |
| Cheeseburger | ½-oz. roll | 45 | 4.5 |
| Pepperoni & cheese | ½-oz. roll | 43 | 4.2 |
| Sausage & cheese | ½-oz. roll | 43 | 4.2 |
| Shrimp & cheese | ½-oz roll | 37 | 3.8 |
| **PIZZA SAUCE, canned:** | | | |
| (Contadina) | 8 oz. | 130 | 20.0 |
| (Ragu) | 5 oz. | 120 | 15.0 |
| **PIZZA SAUCE MIX:** | | | |
| (French's) | 1-oz. pkg. | 77 | 17.2 |
| *(French's) | 2 T. | 18 | 4.1 |
| **PLANTAIN, raw** (USDA): | | | |
| Whole | 1 lb. (weighed with skin) | 389 | 101.9 |

(USDA): United States Department of Agriculture
(HEW/FAO): Health, Education and Welfare/Food and Agriculture Organization
* Prepared as Package Directs

| Food and Description | Measure or Quantity | Calories | Carbohydrates (grams) |
|---|---|---|---|
| Flesh only | 4 oz. | 135 | 35.4 |
| **PLUM:** | | | |
| Damson, fresh (USDA): | | | |
|   Whole | 1 lb. (weighed with pits) | 272 | 73.5 |
|   Flesh only | 4 oz. | 75 | 20.2 |
| Japanese & hybrid, fresh (USDA): | | | |
|   Whole | 1 lb. (weighed with pits) | 205 | 52.4 |
|   Whole | 2.1-oz. plum (2" dia.) | 27 | 6.9 |
|   Diced | ½ cup (2.9 oz.) | 39 | 10.1 |
|   Halves | ½ cup (3.1 oz.) | 42 | 10.8 |
|   Slices | ½ cup (3 oz.) | 40 | 10.3 |
| Prune type, fresh (USDA): | | | |
|   Whole | 1 lb. (weighed with pits) | 320 | 84.0 |
|   Halves | ½ cup (2.8 oz.) | 60 | 15.8 |
| Canned, purple, regular pack, solids & liq.: (USDA): | | | |
|   Extra heavy syrup | 4 oz. | 116 | 30.3 |
|   Heavy syrup, with pits | ½ cup (4.5 oz.) | 106 | 27.6 |
|   Heavy syrup, without pits | ½ cup (4.2 oz.) | 100 | 25.9 |
|   Light syrup | 4 oz. | 71 | 18.8 |
|   (Stokely-Van Camp) | ½ cup | 120 | 30.0 |
| Canned, unsweetened or low calorie, solids & liq.: | | | |
|   (Diet Delight) purple | ½ cup | 77 | 18.6 |
|   (Featherweight) purple, juice pack | ½ cup | 67 | 18.0 |
|   (Featherweight) purple, water pack | ½ cup | 39 | 9.0 |
|   (Tillie Lewis) *Tasti Diet* | ½ cup (4.3 oz.) | 73 | 18.2 |
| **PLUM HOLLOW WINE** (Annie Green Springs) | | | |
|   8% alcohol | 3 fl. oz. | 63 | 6.8 |

| Food and Description | Measure or Quantity | Calories | Carbo- hydrates (grams) |
|---|---|---|---|
| **PLUM JELLY:** | | | |
| Sweetened (Smucker's) | 1 T. (.7 oz.) | 53 | 13.5 |
| Dietetic or low calorie (Featherweight) | 1 T. | 16 | 4.0 |
| **PLUM PRESERVE** or **JAM,** sweetened (Smucker's) | 1 T. (.7 oz.) | 53 | 13.5 |
| **P.M. FRUIT DRINK** (Mott's) | 6 fl. oz. | 90 | 22.0 |
| **POLISH-STYLE SAUSAGE:** | | | |
| (USDA) | 1 oz. | 86 | .3 |
| (Frito-Lay's) smoked beef | 1 oz. | 73 | .6 |
| (Hormel) *Kolbase* | 1 oz. | 82 | .4 |
| (Vienna) beef | 3-oz. piece | 240 | 1.3 |
| (Wilson) | 1 oz. | 82 | .3 |
| **POLYNESIAN STYLE DINNER,** frozen (Swanson) | 13-oz. dinner | 490 | 65.0 |
| **POMEGRANATE, raw** (USDA): | | | |
| Whole | 1 lb. (weighed whole) | 160 | 41.7 |
| Pulp only | 4 oz. | 71 | 18.6 |
| **POMMARD WINE,** French red Burgundy: | | | |
| (Barton & Guestier) 13% alcohol | 3 fl. oz. | 67 | .4 |
| (Chanson) *St. Vincent,* 11½% alcohol | 3 fl. oz. | 60 | 6.3 |
| **POMPANO, raw** (USDA): | | | |
| Whole | 1 lb. (weighed whole) | 422 | 0. |

(USDA): United States Department of Agriculture
(HEW/FAO): Health, Education and Welfare/Food and Agriculture Organization

* Prepared as Package Directs

| Food and Description | Measure or Quantity | Calories | Carbohydrates (grams) |
|---|---|---|---|
| Meat only | 4 oz. | 188 | 0. |
| **POPCORN:** | | | |
| (USDA) unpopped | 1 oz. | 103 | 20.4 |
| (3 Minute) | ¼ cup (1 oz.) | 102 | 19.8 |
| Popped: | | | |
| (USDA): | | | |
| Plain | 1 oz. | 109 | 21.7 |
| Plain, large kernel | 1 cup (6 grams) | 23 | 4.6 |
| Butter or oil & salt added | 1 oz. | 129 | 16.8 |
| Butter or oil & salt added | 1 cup (9 grams) | 41 | 2.3 |
| Sugar-coated | 1 cup (1.2 oz.) | 134 | 29.9 |
| (Bachman): | | | |
| Plain | 1 oz. | 160 | 13.0 |
| Caramel-coated | 1 oz. | 130 | 23.0 |
| Cheese-flavored | 1 oz. | 180 | 14.0 |
| *Cracker Jack* | ¾-oz. bag | 90 | 16.7 |
| *Cracker Jack* | 3-oz. box | 350 | 65.5 |
| (Jiffy Pop): | | | |
| Plain | ½ pkg. (2½ oz.) | 244 | 29.8 |
| Buttered | ½ pkg. (2½ oz.) | 247 | 29.4 |
| (Jolly Time): | | | |
| Plain | 1 cup (.5 oz.) | 55 | 10.8 |
| Added oil & salt | 1 cup (.5 oz.) | 64 | 8.3 |
| (Old London): | | | |
| Buttered | 1 cup | 57 | 6.4 |
| Without peanuts | 1¾-oz. bag | 195 | 43.6 |
| With peanuts | 1 cup | 142 | 30.2 |
| Cheese flavored | 1 cup | 74 | 6.6 |
| Seasoned | 1¼-oz. bag | 174 | 22.4 |
| (Super Pop Brand) yellow or white | 1 cup (.2 oz.) | 22 | 4.3 |
| (Tom Huston) | 1 cup (.5 oz.) | 68 | 8.9 |
| (Wise): | | | |
| Buttered | 1 cup | 57 | 6.4 |
| Cheese-flavored | 1 cup (.5 oz.) | 74 | 6.6 |
| **POPOVER:** | | | |
| Home recipe (USDA) | 1 average popover (2 oz.) | 128 | 14.7 |
| *(Mix (Flako) | 1 popover | 170 | 25.0 |

| Food and Description | Measure or Quantity | Calories | Carbo-hydrates (grams) |
|---|---|---|---|
| **POPPY SEED** (French's) | 1 tsp. | 13 | .8 |
| **POP TARTS** (Kellogg's) | | | |
| Regular: | | | |
| Blueberry, concord grape, raspberry and strawberry | 1.8-oz. tart | 210 | 36.0 |
| Brown sugar cinnamon | 1.8-oz. tart | 210 | 34.0 |
| Cherry | 1.8-oz. tart | 210 | 35.0 |
| Frosted: | | | |
| Blueberry, concord grape, raspberry | 1.8-oz. tart | 210 | 37.0 |
| Brown sugar cinnamon | 1¾-oz. tart | 210 | 33.0 |
| Cherry, Dutch apple, strawberry | 1.8-oz. tart | 210 | 36.0 |
| Chocolate fudge, chocolate peppermint | 1.8-oz. tart | 210 | 35.0 |
| Chocolate vanilla creme | 1.8-oz. tart | 210 | 34.0 |
| **PORK**, medium-fat: | | | |
| Fresh (USDA): | | | |
| Boston butt: | | | |
| Raw | 1 lb. (weighed with bone & skin) | 1220 | 0. |
| Roasted, lean & fat | 4 oz. | 400 | 0. |
| Roasted, lean only | 4 oz. | 277 | 0. |
| Chop: | | | |
| Broiled, lean & fat | 1 chop (4 oz., weighed with bone) | 295 | 0. |
| Broiled, lean & fat | 1 chop (3 oz., weighed with bone) | 332 | 0. |
| Broiled, lean only | 1 chop (3 oz., weighed without bone) | 230 | 0. |
| Fat, separable, cooked | 1 oz. | 219 | 0. |

(USDA): United States Department of Agriculture
(HEW/FAO): Health, Education and Welfare/Food and Agriculture
　　　　　　Organization
* Prepared as Package Directs

| Food and Description | Measure or Quantity | Calories | Carbo-hydrates (grams) |
|---|---|---|---|
| Ham (See also HAM): | | | |
| Raw | 1 lb. (weighed with bone & skin) | 1188 | 0. |
| Roasted, lean & fat | 4 oz. | 424 | 0. |
| Roasted, lean only | 4 oz. | 246 | 0. |
| Loin: | | | |
| Raw | 1 lb. (weighed with bone) | 1065 | 0. |
| Roasted, lean & fat | 4 oz. | 411 | 0. |
| Roasted, lean only | 4 oz. | 288 | 0. |
| Picnic: | | | |
| Raw | 1 lb. (weighed with bone & skin) | 1083 | 0. |
| Simmered, lean & fat | 4 oz. | 424 | 0. |
| Simmered, lean only | 4 oz. | 240 | 0. |
| Spareribs: | | | |
| Raw, with bone | 1 lb. (weighed with bone) | 976 | 0. |
| Braised, lean & fat | 4 oz. | 499 | 0. |
| Cured, light commercial cure: | | | |
| Bacon (See BACON) | | | |
| Bacon butt (USDA): | | | |
| Raw | 1 lb. (weighed with bone & skin) | 1227 | 0. |
| Roasted, lean & fat | 4 oz. | 374 | 0. |
| Roasted, lean only | 4 oz. | 276 | 0. |
| Ham (See also HAM): | | | |
| Raw (USDA) | 1 lb. (weighed with bone & skin) | 1100 | 0. |
| Roasted, lean & fat (USDA) | 4 oz. | 328 | 0. |
| Roasted, lean only (USDA) | 4 oz. | 212 | 0. |
| Fully cooked, boneless: | | | |
| Parti-Style (Armour Star) | 4 oz. | 167 | .1 |
| (Wilson) rolled | 4 oz. | 222 | 0. |

| Food and Description | Measure or Quantity | Calories | Carbohydrates (grams) |
|---|---|---|---|
| Picnic: | | | |
| Raw (USDA) | 1 lb. (weighed with bone & skin) | 1060 | 0. |
| Raw (Wilson) smoked | 4 oz. | 279 | 0. |
| Roasted, lean & fat (USDA) | 4 oz. | 366 | 0. |
| Roasted, lean only (USDA) | 4 oz. | 239 | 0. |
| Cured, long-cure, country-style Virginia ham, raw: | | | |
| (USDA) | 1 lb. (weighed with bone & skin) | 1535 | 1.2 |
| (USDA) | 1 lb. (weighed without bone & skin) | 1765 | 1.4 |

**PORK & BEANS** (See **BEAN, BAKED**)

**PORK, CANNED,** chopped luncheon meat:

| | | | |
|---|---|---|---|
| (USDA) | 1 oz. | 83 | .4 |
| (USDA) chopped | 1 cup (4.8 oz.) | 400 | 1.8 |
| (USDA) diced | 1 cup | 415 | 1.8 |

**PORK DINNER,** frozen:

| | | | |
|---|---|---|---|
| (Swanson) loin of pork | 11¼-oz. dinner | 470 | 48.0 |

**PORK RINDS,** fried, *Baken-Ets*

| | | | |
|---|---|---|---|
| | 1 oz. | 150 | 1.0 |

**PORK SAUSAGE:**
Uncooked (USDA) links or bulk

| | | | |
|---|---|---|---|
| | 1 oz. | 141 | Tr. |

(USDA): United States Department of Agriculture
(HEW/FAO): Health, Education and Welfare/Food and Agriculture
Organization
* Prepared as Package Directs

| Food and Description | Measure or Quantity | Calories | Carbo-hydrates (grams) |
|---|---|---|---|
| Cooked (USDA) links or bulk | 1 oz. | 135 | Tr. |
| Cooked (Hormel): | | | |
| Little Sizzlers | 1 sausage | 65 | Tr. |
| Smoked | 1 oz. | 98 | .2 |
| Cooked (Oscar Mayer) | | | |
| Little Friers | .6-oz. link | 64 | .4 |
| Canned (USDA): | | | |
| Solids & liq. | 1 oz. | 118 | .7 |
| Drained | 1 oz. | 108 | .5 |
| **PORK, SWEET & SOUR,** | | | |
| frozen (La Choy) | ½ of 15-oz. entree | 229 | 45.2 |
| **PORT WINE:** | | | |
| (Gallo) 16% alcohol | 3 fl. oz. | 94 | 7.8 |
| (Gallo) ruby, 20% alcohol | 3 fl. oz. | 112 | 8.7 |
| (Gallo) tawny, Old Decanter, 20% alcohol | 3 fl. oz. | 112 | 8.4 |
| (Gallo) white, 20% alcohol | 3 fl. oz. | 111 | 8.4 |
| (Gold Seal) 19% alcohol | 3 fl. oz. | 158 | 9.4 |
| (Great Western) Solera, 18% alcohol | 3 fl. oz. | 138 | 11.5 |
| (Great Western) Solera, tawny, 18% alcohol | 3 fl. oz. | 136 | 11.4 |
| (Italian Swiss Colony-Gold Medal) 19.7% alcohol | 3 fl. oz. | 130 | 8.7 |
| (Louis M. Martini) 19½% alcohol | 3 fl. oz. | 165 | 2.0 |
| (Louis M. Martini) tawny, 19½% alcohol | 3 fl. oz. | 165 | 2.0 |
| (Robertson's) ruby, 20% alcohol | 3 fl. oz. | 138 | 9.9 |
| (Robertson's) tawny, Dry Humour, 21% alcohol | 3 fl. oz. | 145 | 9.9 |
| (Robertson's) tawny, Game Bird, 21% alcohol | 3 fl. oz. | 145 | 9.9 |
| (Robertson's) Rebello Valente, 20½% alcohol | 3 fl. oz. | 141 | 9.9 |
| (Taylor) 18.5% alcohol | 3 fl. oz. | 144 | 13.2 |
| (Taylor) tawny, 18.5% alcohol | 3 fl. oz. | 138 | 12.0 |

| Food and Description | Measure or Quantity | Calories | Carbo-hydrates (grams) |
|---|---|---|---|
| *POSTUM, cereal beverage (General Foods): | | | |
| Ground, brewed | 6 fl. oz. | 8 | 2.1 |
| Instant, regular | 6 fl. oz. | 11 | 2.5 |
| Instant, coffee flavored | 6 fl. oz. | 11 | 2.5 |
| POTATO (See also POTATO CHIP, POTATO MIX, POTATO SALAD, POTATO STICK, and others): | | | |
| Raw (USDA): | | | |
| Whole | 1 lb. (weighed unpared) | 279 | 62.8 |
| Pared, chopped | 1 cup (5.2 oz.) | 112 | 25.1 |
| Pared, diced | 1 cup (5.5 oz.) | 119 | 26.8 |
| Pared, sliced | 1 cup (5.2 oz.) | 113 | 25.5 |
| Cooked (USDA): | | | |
| Au gratin or scalloped, with cheese | ½ cup (4.3 oz.) | 127 | 17.9 |
| Au gratin or scalloped, without cheese | ½ cup (4.3 oz.) | 177 | 16.6 |
| Baked, peeled after baking | 2½" dia. potato (3 raw to 1 lb.) | 92 | 20.9 |
| Boiled, peeled after boiling | 1 med. (3 raw to 1 lb.) | 103 | 23.3 |
| Boiled, peeled before boiling: | | | |
| Whole | 1 med. (3 raw to 1 lb.) | 79 | 17.7 |
| Diced | ½ cup (2.8 oz.) | 51 | 11.3 |
| Mashed | ½ cup (3.7 oz.) | 68 | 15.1 |
| Riced | ½ cup (4 oz.) | 74 | 16.5 |
| Sliced | ½ cup (2.8 oz.) | 52 | 11.6 |
| French fried in deep fat | 10 pieces (2" x ½" x ½", 2 oz.) | 156 | 20.5 |

(USDA): United States Department of Agriculture
(HEW/FAO): Health, Education and Welfare/Food and Agriculture Organization
* Prepared as Package Directs

| Food and Description | Measure or Quantity | Calories | Carbohydrates (grams) |
|---|---|---|---|
| Hash browned, after holding overnight | ½ cup (3.4 oz.) | 223 | 28.4 |
| Mashed, milk added | ½ cup (3.5 oz.) | 64 | 12.7 |
| Mashed, milk & butter added | ½ cup (3.4 oz.) | 92 | 12.1 |
| Pan fried from raw | ½ cup (3 oz.) | 228 | 27.7 |
| Scalloped (See Au Gratin) | | | |
| Canned: | | | |
| (USDA) solids & liq. | 1 cup (8.8 oz.) | 110 | 24.5 |
| (Butter Kernel) white | 3-4 small potatoes (4.1 oz.) | 96 | 22.0 |
| (Del Monte): | | | |
| White, solids & liq. | 1 cup | 84 | 19.8 |
| White, drained solids | 1 cup | 265 | 28.4 |
| (Stokely-Van Camp) whole, solids & liq. | ½ cup (4.4 oz.) | 50 | 11.0 |
| Dehydrated, mashed (See also POTATO MIX): | | | |
| (USDA) flakes, without milk, dry | ½ cup (.8 oz.) | 84 | 19.3 |
| *(USDA) flakes, prepared with water, milk & fat | ½ cup (3.8 oz.) | 100 | 15.5 |
| (USDA) granules, without milk, dry | ½ cup | 352 | 80.4 |
| *(USDA) granules, prepared with water, milk & butter | ½ cup (3.7 oz.) | 101 | 15.1 |
| Frozen: | | | |
| (USDA): | | | |
| French-fried, heated | 10 pieces (2" x ½") (2 oz.) | 125 | 19.2 |
| Mashed, heated | 4 oz. | 105 | 17.8 |
| (Birds Eye): | | | |
| Cottage fries | ⅛ of 14-oz. pkg. | 120 | 17.0 |
| Crinkle cuts | ⅓ of 9-oz. pkg. | 115 | 18.4 |
| French fries | 3-oz. serving | 113 | 16.8 |
| French fries, Tasti Fries | 2.5-oz. serving | 140 | 17.0 |
| Hash browns | 4-oz. serving | 75 | 16.6 |
| Hash browns O'Brien | 4-oz. serving | 60 | 14.0 |
| Hash browns, shredded | 3-oz. serving | 60 | 13.0 |

| Food and Description | Measure or Quantity | Calories | Carbo-hydrates (grams) |
|---|---|---|---|
| Shoestring | 3.3-oz. serving | 140 | 20.0 |
| Steak fries | 3-oz. serving | 110 | 18.0 |
| *Tasti Puffs* | 2.5-oz. serving | 190 | 19.0 |
| *Tiny Taters* | 3.2-oz. serving | 200 | 22.0 |
| Whole, peeled | ⅒ of 32-oz. pkg. | 60 | 13.0 |
| (Green Giant): | | | |
| Au gratin, *Bake'n Serve* | ⅓ of 10-oz. pkg. | 141 | 12.1 |
| & sweet peas in bacon cream sauce | ⅓ of 10-oz. pkg. | 88 | 12.6 |
| Shoestring, in butter sauce | ⅓ of 10-oz. pkg. | 123 | 14.7 |
| Slices in butter sauce | ⅓ of 10-oz. pkg. | 76 | 10.9 |
| Stuffed with cheese-flavored topping | 5-oz. serving | 237 | 30.0 |
| Stuffed with sour cream & chives | 5-oz. serving | 232 | 30.0 |
| Vermicelli, with mushrooms & cheese sauce, *Bake'n Serve* | ⅓ of 10-oz. pkg. | 135 | 14.3 |
| (McKenzie) white, whole | 3½-oz. serving | 69 | 14.9 |
| (Ore-Ida): | | | |
| Cottage fries | ⅒ of 32-oz. pkg. | 149 | 23.5 |
| *Country Style Dinner Fries* | ⅛ of 24-oz. pkg. | 120 | 18.0 |
| *Crispers* | ⅒ of 32-oz. pkg. | 245 | 27.7 |
| *Golden Fries* | ⅕ of 16-oz. pkg. | 138 | 23.4 |
| *Golden Crinkles* | ⅕ of 16-oz. pkg. | 130 | 21.0 |
| Hash browns, shredded | ½ of 12-oz. pkg. | 120 | 24.0 |
| Hash browns, Southern style | ⅒ of 32-oz. pkg. | 75 | 17.1 |
| Hash browns, Southern style, with butter sauce | ⅛ of 24-oz. pkg. | 120 | 15.0 |
| Hash browns, Southern style, with butter sauce & onions | ⅛ of 24-oz. pkg. | 130 | 17.0 |
| O'Brien style | ⅛ of 24-oz. pkg. | 60 | 14.0 |

(USDA): United States Department of Agriculture
(HEW/FAO): Health, Education and Welfare/Food and Agriculture Organization
* Prepared as Package Directs

| *Food and Description* | *Measure or Quantity* | *Calories* | *Carbo-hydrates (grams)* |
|---|---|---|---|
| *Pixie Crinkles* | 1/6 of 1¼-lb. pkg. | 187 | 27.5 |
| Shoestrings | 1/6 of 1¼-lb. pkg. | 171 | 21.3 |
| *Tater Tots,* plain | ⅕ of 16-oz. pkg. | 171 | 21.3 |
| *Tater Tots,* bacon flavored | ⅕ of 16-oz. pkg. | 170 | 22.4 |
| *Tater Tots,* with onion | ⅕ of 16-oz. pkg. | 170 | 22.4 |
| Whole, small, peeled | 1/10 of 32-oz. pkg. | 74 | 17.1 |
| (Seabrook Farms) white, whole, boiled | 3½-oz. serving | 69 | 14.9 |
| (Stouffer's): | | | |
| Au gratin | ⅓ of 11½-oz. pkg. | 135 | 12.9 |
| Scalloped | ⅓ of 12-oz. pkg. | 130 | 13.9 |
| **POTATO CHIP:** | | | |
| (USDA) | 1 oz. | 161 | 14.2 |
| (Bachman) | 1 oz. | 150 | 14.0 |
| (Frito-Lay's) natural style | 1 oz. | 157 | 15.1 |
| *Lay's* | 1 oz. | 150 | 14.0 |
| *Lay's,* Bar-B-Q-flavored | 1 oz. | 160 | 14.0 |
| *Lay's,* sour cream & onion flavor | 1 oz. | 160 | 15.0 |
| (Nalley's) | 1 oz. | 165 | 14.2 |
| (Nalley's) barbecue flavor | 1 oz. | 166 | 14.2 |
| (Planters) stackable | 1 oz. | 150 | 17.0 |
| *Pringle's,* country style | 1 oz. | 157 | 14.5 |
| *Pringle's,* original | 1 oz. | 153 | 14.4 |
| *Pringle's,* rippled | 1 oz. | 156 | 15.1 |
| *Ruffles* | 1 oz. | 150 | 15.0 |
| **POTATO MIX:** | | | |
| Au gratin: | | | |
| *(Betty Crocker) | 1/6 pkg. | 150 | 20.0 |
| *(French's) | ½ cup | 190 | 28.6 |
| *(Buds) Betty Crocker | ⅓ cup | 130 | 15.0 |
| *Creamed (Betty Crocker) made in saucepan | 1/6 pkg. | 160 | 20.0 |
| Hash brown: | | | |
| *(Betty Crocker) with onion | 1/6 pkg. | 150 | 22.0 |
| *(French's) *Big Tate,* with seasonings | ½ cup | 165 | 22.0 |
| *Julienne (Betty Crocker) | 1/6 pkg. | 130 | 17.0 |

| Food and Description | Measure or Quantity | Calories | Carbo- hydrates (grams) |
|---|---|---|---|
| Mashed: | | | |
| *(French's) *Big Tate* | ½ cup | 140 | 16.0 |
| *(French's) Idaho | ½ cup | 120 | 16.0 |
| *(Pillsbury) *Hungry Jack* | ½ cup | 140 | 16.0 |
| *Potatoes'n Cream (Betty Crocker) | ¼ pkg. | 140 | 16.0 |
| Scalloped: | | | |
| *(Betty Crocker) | ⅙ pkg. | 150 | 20.0 |
| *(French's) | ½ cup | 190 | 30.0 |
| *Sour cream & chives (Betty Crocker) | ⅛ pkg. | 140 | 18.0 |
| **POTATO PANCAKE MIX** (French's) *Big Tate* | 3″ pancake | 43 | 5.7 |
| **POTATO SALAD:** | | | |
| Home recipe (USDA) with cooked salad dressing & seasonings | 4 oz. | 112 | 18.5 |
| Home recipe (USDA) with mayonnaise & French dressing, hard-cooked eggs, seasonings | 4 oz. | 164 | 15.2 |
| Canned (Nalley's): | | | |
| Regular | 4-oz. serving | 139 | 17.0 |
| German style | 4-oz. serving | 143 | 18.2 |
| **POTATO SOUP**, canned (Campbell) cream of, condensed | 10-oz. serving | 90 | 14.0 |
| **POTATO STICK, O & C:** | | | |
| Regular | 1½-oz. can | 231 | 22.0 |
| *Snackin' Crisp* | 4-oz. can | 620 | 60.0 |
| **POUILLY-FUISSÉ WINE,** French white Burgundy: | | | |
| (Barton & Guestier) 12½% alcohol | 3 fl. oz. | 64 | .3 |

(USDA): United States Department of Agriculture
(HEW/FAO): Health, Education and Welfare/Food and Agriculture Organization
* Prepared as Package Directs

| Food and Description | Measure or Quantity | Calories | Carbo-hydrates (grams) |
|---|---|---|---|
| (Chanson) *St. Vincent*, 12% alcohol | 3 fl. oz. | 84 | 6.3 |
| **POUILLY-FUMÉ**, French white Loire Valley (Barton & Guestier) 12% alcohol | 3 fl. oz. | 60 | .1 |
| **POUND CAKE** (See **CAKE**, Pound) | | | |
| **PRESERVE** (See also individual listings by flavor): Sweetened: | | | |
| (Ann Page) all flavors | 2 tsps. (.5 oz.) | 38 | 9.6 |
| (Crosse & Blackwell) all flavors | 1 T. | 60 | 14.8 |
| **PRETZEL:** | | | |
| (Bachman): | | | |
| *Nutzel* | 1 oz. | 110 | 21.0 |
| *Thins* | 1 oz. | 110 | 21.0 |
| (Nabisco): | | | |
| *Mister Salty* | 1 piece | 20 | 4.0 |
| *Mister Salty*, Dutch | 1 piece | 55 | 11.0 |
| *Mister Salty*, Little Shaper | 1 piece | 6 | 1.2 |
| *Mister Salty Veri Thin*, sticks | 1 piece (.3 grams) | 1 | .2 |
| (Old London): | | | |
| Nuggets | 1 oz. | 112 | 22.5 |
| Rings | 1 oz. | 104 | 21.9 |
| (Planters) sticks and twists | 1 oz. | 110 | 22.0 |
| (Wise): | | | |
| Nuggets | 1 oz. | 112 | 22.5 |
| Old fashioned | 1 oz. | 103 | 21.3 |
| Rods | 1 oz. | 102 | 22.2 |
| Sticks | 1 oz. | 108 | 22.7 |
| Thins | 1 oz. | 106 | 22.2 |
| **PRICKLY PEAR**, fresh (USDA): | | | |
| Whole | 1 lb. (weighed with rind & seeds) | 84 | 21.8 |
| Flesh only | 4 oz. | 48 | 12.4 |

| Food and Description | Measure or Quantity | Calories | Carbohydrates (grams) |
|---|---|---|---|
| **PRODUCT 19**, cereal (Kellogg's) | ¾ cup (1 oz.) | 110 | 24.0 |
| **PRUNE:** | | | |
| Canned: | | | |
| (Del Monte) stewed, with pits, solids & liq. | 1 cup (8 oz.) | 262 | 62.5 |
| (Del Monte) *Moist Pak,* with pits | 2 oz. | 142 | 33.5 |
| (Sunsweet) cooked, pitted, solids & liq. | 5-6 prunes (1.8 oz.) | 138 | 32.9 |
| Dietetic (Featherweight) water pack, stewed, solids & liq. | ½ cup | 130 | 35.0 |
| Dried: | | | |
| (USDA) dried, cooked, with sugar | 1 cup (16-18 prunes & ⅔ cup liq.) | 504 | 132.1 |
| (Del Monte): | | | |
| Breakfast, with pits | 2 oz. | 152 | 35.4 |
| Medium, with pits | 2 oz. | 152 | 35.6 |
| Large, with pits | 2 oz. | 153 | 36.2 |
| Extra large, with pits | 2 oz. | 150 | 35.3 |
| Jumbo, with pits | 2 oz. | 157 | 37.0 |
| Pitted | 2 oz. | 151 | 35.4 |
| (Sun-Maid): | | | |
| With pits | 2 oz. | 120 | 32.0 |
| Pitted | 2 oz. | 140 | 36.0 |
| **PRUNE JUICE**, canned: | | | |
| (USDA) | ½ cup (4.5 oz.) | 99 | 24.3 |
| (Ann Page) | ½ cup (4.5 oz.) | 92 | 22.4 |
| (Del Monte) | 6 fl. oz. | 137 | 33.2 |
| (Mott's): | | | |
| Regular | 6 fl. oz. | 140 | 34.0 |
| With prune pulp | 6 fl. oz. | 120 | 30.0 |

(USDA): United States Department of Agriculture
(HEW/FAO): Health, Education and Welfare/Food and Agriculture Organization
\* Prepared as Package Directs

| Food and Description | Measure or Quantity | Calories | Carbo-hydrates (grams) |
|---|---|---|---|
| (Sunsweet) | 6 fl. oz. | 136 | 32.9 |
| **PRUNE NECTAR,** canned | | | |
| (Mott's) | 6 fl. oz. | 100 | 25.0 |
| **PRUNE WHIP,** home recipe | | | |
| (USDA) | 1 cup (4.8 oz.) | 211 | 49.8 |
| **PUDDING or PIE FILLING:** | | | |
| Home recipe (USDA): | | | |
| Rice, made with raisins | ½ cup (4.7 oz.) | 193 | 35.2 |
| Tapioca: | | | |
| Apple | ½ cup (4.4 oz.) | 146 | 36.8 |
| Cream | ½ cup (2.9 oz.) | 110 | 14.0 |
| Canned, regular pack: | | | |
| Banana: | | | |
| (Del Monte) | 5-oz. container | 183 | 30.1 |
| (Hunt's) *Snack Pack* | 5-oz. container | 180 | 24.0 |
| Butterscotch: | | | |
| (Del Monte) | 5-oz. container | 186 | 30.8 |
| (Hunt's) *Snack Pack* | 5-oz. container | 170 | 27.0 |
| (Thank You) | ½ cup (4.5 oz.) | 169 | 29.2 |
| Chocolate: | | | |
| (Betty Crocker) | 5-oz. serving | 180 | 30.0 |
| (Betty Crocker) fudge | 5-oz. serving | 180 | 30.0 |
| (Del Monte) | 5-oz. container | 173 | 33.0 |
| (Del Monte) fudge | 5-oz. container | 193 | 31.0 |
| (Hunt's) *Snack Pack:* | | | |
| Regular | 5-oz. container | 180 | 28.0 |
| Fudge | 5-oz. container | 180 | 26.0 |
| German | 5-oz. container | 170 | 25.0 |
| Marshmallow | 5-oz. container | 170 | 25.0 |
| (Thank You) | ½ cup (4.5 oz.) | 175 | 29.2 |
| Lemon: | | | |
| (Hunt's) *Snack Pack* | 5-oz. container | 150 | 32.0 |
| (Thank You) | ½ cup (4.5 oz.) | 183 | 36.2 |
| Rice: | | | |
| (Betty Crocker) | ½ cup (4.3 oz.) | 150 | 25.0 |
| (Comstock) | ¼ of 15-oz. can | 120 | 23.0 |
| (Hunt's) *Snack Pack* | 5-oz. container | 190 | 27.0 |
| (Menner's) | ½ cup (3.9 oz.) | 119 | 24.5 |
| Tapioca: | | | |
| (Betty Crocker) | ½ cup (4.3 oz.) | 150 | 22.0 |

| Food and Description | Measure or Quantity | Calories | Carbo-hydrates (grams) |
|---|---|---|---|
| (Del Monte) | 5-oz. container | 174 | 30.1 |
| (Hunt's) *Snack Pack* | 5-oz. container | 140 | 23.0 |
| Vanilla: | | | |
| (Betty Crocker) | ½ cup (5 oz.) | 190 | 29.0 |
| (Del Monte) | 5-oz. container | 189 | 32.1 |
| (Hunt's) *Snack Pack* | 5-oz. container | 180 | 29.0 |
| (Thank You) | ½ cup (4.5 oz.) | 169 | 29.2 |
| Canned, dietetic or low calorie (Sego): | | | |
| Banana | 8-oz. container | 250 | 39.0 |
| Butterscotch | 8-oz. container | 250 | 39.0 |
| Vanilla | 8-oz. container | 250 | 39.0 |
| Chilled, *Swiss Miss:* | | | |
| Butterscotch | 4½-oz. container | 174 | 25.1 |
| Chocolate | 4½-oz. container | 180 | 25.1 |
| Chocolate, dark | 4½-oz. container | 190 | 28.0 |
| Tapioca | 4½-oz. container | 176 | 29.3 |
| Vanilla | 4½-oz. container | 192 | 29.5 |
| Frozen (Rich's): | | | |
| Banana | 3-oz. container | 142 | 19.3 |
| Butterscotch | 4½-oz. container | 199 | 27.4 |
| Chocolate | 4½-oz. container | 214 | 27.1 |
| Vanilla | 4½-oz. container | 199 | 27.5 |
| Mix, regular pack: | | | |
| Banana: | | | |
| (Ann Page) regular | ¼ of 2⅛-oz. pkg. | 84 | 21.0 |
| *(Jell-O) cream: | | | |
| Regular | ⅛ of 8″ pie, excluding crust | 110 | 18.0 |
| Instant | ½ cup | 180 | 30.0 |
| *(My-T-Fine) cream, regular | ½ cup | 175 | 32.6 |
| *(Royal): | | | |
| Regular | ½ cup | 160 | 27.0 |
| Instant | ½ cup | 180 | 29.0 |
| *Butter pecan (Jell-O) instant | ½ cup | 180 | 29.0 |

(USDA): United States Department of Agriculture
(HEW/FAO): Health, Education and Welfare/Food and Agriculture
        Organization
* Prepared as Package Directs

| Food and Description | Measure or Quantity | Calories | Carbohydrates (grams) |
|---|---|---|---|
| Butterscotch: | | | |
| (Ann Page): | | | |
| Regular | ¼ of 3⅝-oz. pkg. | 96 | 24.1 |
| Instant | ¼ of 3¼-oz. pkg. | 85 | 21.3 |
| *(Jell-O): | | | |
| Regular | ½ cup | 180 | 30.0 |
| Instant | ½ cup | 180 | 30.0 |
| *(My-T-Fine) regular | ½ cup | 143 | 28.0 |
| *(Royal): | | | |
| Regular | ½ cup | 160 | 27.0 |
| Instant | ½ cup | 180 | 29.0 |
| Chocolate: | | | |
| (Ann Page): | | | |
| Regular | ¼ of 3⅝-oz. pkg. | 102 | 23.7 |
| Instant | ¼ of 4-oz. pkg. | 110 | 25.6 |
| *(Jell-O): | | | |
| Regular: | | | |
| Plain | ½ cup | 170 | 29.0 |
| Fudge | ½ cup | 170 | 28.0 |
| Milk | ½ cup | 170 | 29.0 |
| Instant: | | | |
| Plain | ½ cup | 190 | 34.0 |
| Fudge | ½ cup | 190 | 33.0 |
| *(My-T-Fine) regular: | | | |
| Plain | ½ cup | 133 | 28.0 |
| Almond | ½ cup | 169 | 27.0 |
| Fudge | ½ cup | 151 | 27.0 |
| *(Royal): | | | |
| Regular: | | | |
| Plain | ½ cup | 180 | 33.0 |
| Dark N' Sweet | ½ cup | 180 | 33.0 |
| Instant: | | | |
| Plain | ½ cup | 190 | 35.0 |
| Dark N' Sweet | ½ cup | 190 | 35.0 |
| Coconut: | | | |
| (Ann Page) cream | ¼ of 3½-oz. pkg. | 100 | 18.1 |
| (Ann Page) instant, toasted | ¼ of 3¼-oz. pkg. | 96 | 19.9 |
| *(Jell-O) cream: | | | |
| Regular | ⅙ of 8" pie, excluding crust | 110 | 17.0 |
| Instant | ½ cup | 190 | 28.0 |
| *(Royal) instant | ½ cup | 170 | 30.0 |

| *Food and Description* | *Measure or Quantity* | *Calories* | *Carbo-hydrates (grams)* |
|---|---|---|---|
| *Coffee (Royal) instant | ½ cup | 180 | 29.0 |
| Custard: | | | |
| (Ann Page) egg | ¼ of 2¾-oz. pkg. | 73 | 15.4 |
| **Jell-O Americana,* | | | |
| golden egg | ½ cup | 170 | 24.0 |
| *(Royal) regular | ½ cup | 150 | 22.0 |
| *Flan (Royal) regular | ½ cup | 150 | 22.0 |
| Lemon: | | | |
| (Ann Page): | | | |
| Regular | ¼ of 2-oz. pkg. | 80 | 20.0 |
| Instant | ¼ of 3¾-oz. pkg. | 100 | 25.0 |
| *(Jell-O): | | | |
| Regular | ⅙ of 9″ pie, excluding crust | 180 | 38.0 |
| Instant | ½ cup | 180 | 31.0 |
| *(My-T-Fine) regular | ½ cup | 164 | 30.0 |
| *(Royal): | | | |
| Regular | ½ cup | 160 | 30.0 |
| Instant | ½ cup | 180 | 29.0 |
| *Lime (Royal) regular, Key Lime | ½ cup | 160 | 30.0 |
| *Pineapple (Jell-O) instant, cream | ½ cup | 180 | 31.0 |
| Pistachio: | | | |
| (Ann Page) instant | ¼ of 3½-oz. pkg. | 97 | 22.7 |
| *(Jell-O) instant | ½ cup | 190 | 30.0 |
| *(Royal) instant | ½ cup | 170 | 30.0 |
| *Rice, *Jell-O Americana* | ½ cup | 180 | 30.0 |
| Tapioca: | | | |
| (Ann Page): | | | |
| Chocolate | ¼ of 3½-oz. pkg. | 97 | 22.6 |
| Vanilla | ¼ of 3¼-oz. pkg. | 89 | 22.3 |
| **Jell-O Americana:* | | | |
| Chocolate | ½ cup | 160 | 27.0 |
| Vanilla | ½ cup | 160 | 27.0 |
| *(My-T-Fine) vanilla | ½ cup | 130 | 28.0 |
| *(Royal): | | | |
| Chocolate | ½ cup | 180 | 33.0 |

(USDA): United States Department of Agriculture
(HEW/FAO): Health, Education and Welfare/Food and Agriculture Organization
* Prepared as Package Directs

| Food and Description | Measure or Quantity | Calories | Carbohydrates (grams) |
|---|---|---|---|
| Vanilla | ½ cup | 160 | 27.0 |
| Vanilla: | | | |
| (Ann Page): | | | |
| Regular | ¼ of 3⅛-oz. pkg. | 84 | 21.0 |
| Regular, cherry | ¼ of 3¼-oz. pkg. | 86 | 21.4 |
| *(Jell-O): | | | |
| Regular: | | | |
| Plain | ½ cup | 160 | 27.0 |
| French | ½ cup | 180 | 30.0 |
| Instant: | | | |
| Plain | ½ cup | 180 | 31.0 |
| French | ½ cup | 180 | 30.0 |
| *(My-T-Fine) regular | ½ cup | 133 | 28.0 |
| *(Royal): | | | |
| Regular | ½ cup | 160 | 27.0 |
| Instant | ½ cup | 180 | 29.0 |
| *Mix, dietetic pack: | | | |
| Butterscotch: | | | |
| (D-Zerta) | ½ cup | 70 | 13.0 |
| (Featherweight): | | | |
| Regular | 4-oz. serving | 12 | 10.0 |
| Artificially sweetened | 4-oz. serving | 12 | 3.0 |
| Chocolate: | | | |
| (Dia-Mel) | 4-oz. serving | 60 | 8.2 |
| (D-Zerta) | 4-oz. serving | 70 | 12.0 |
| (Estee) | 4-oz. serving | 85 | 16.0 |
| (Featherweight) | 4-oz. serving | 40 | 9.0 |
| (Featherweight) artificially sweetened | 4-oz. serving | 14 | 2.0 |
| Custard (Featherweight) | 4-oz. serving | 40 | 9.0 |
| Lemon (Dia-Mel) | 4-oz. serving | 53 | 8.2 |
| Vanilla: | | | |
| (Dia-Mel) | 4-oz. serving | 53 | DNA |
| (D-Zerta) | ½ cup | 70 | 13.0 |
| (Estee) | ½ cup | 85 | 16.0 |
| (Featherweight) | 4-oz. serving | 40 | 10.0 |
| (Featherweight) artificially sweetened | 4-oz. serving | 12 | 3.0 |
| PUFFED CORN, cereal (USDA) added nutrients | 1 oz. | 113 | 22.9 |

| Food and Description | Measure or Quantity | Calories | Carbo-hydrates (grams) |
|---|---|---|---|
| **PUFFED OAT,** cereal (USDA): | | | |
| Plain, added nutrients | 1 oz. | 113 | 21.3 |
| Sugar coated, added nutrients | 1 oz. | 112 | 24.3 |
| **PUFFED RICE,** cereal: | | | |
| (Malt-O-Meal) | 1 cup (½ oz.) | 52 | 11.9 |
| (Quaker) | 1 cup (½ oz.) | 55 | 12.7 |
| **PUFFED WHEAT,** cereal: | | | |
| (Malt-O-Meal) | 1 cup (½ oz.) | 48 | 9.9 |
| (Quaker) | 1 cup (½ oz.) | 54 | 10.8 |
| **PUFFS,** frozen (Rich's) vanilla | 1.8-oz. puff | 167 | 23.4 |
| **PUMPKIN:** | | | |
| Fresh (USDA): | | | |
| Whole | 1 lb. (weighed with rind & seeds) | 83 | 20.6 |
| Flesh only | 4 oz. | 29 | 7.4 |
| Canned: | | | |
| (Del Monte) | ½ cup (4.3 oz.) | 45 | 9.5 |
| (Libby's) solid pack | ¼ of 16-oz. can | 47 | 9.9 |
| (Stokely-Van Camp) | ½ cup (4.3 oz.) | 45 | 9.5 |
| **PUMPKIN PIE** (See **PIE,** Pumpkin) | | | |
| **PUMPKIN SEED,** dry (USDA): | | | |
| Whole | 4 oz. (weighed in hull | 464 | 12.6 |
| Hulled | 4 oz. | 627 | 17.0 |

(USDA): United States Department of Agriculture
(HEW/FAO): Health, Education and Welfare/Food and Agriculture Organization
* Prepared as Package Directs

| Food and Description | Measure or Quantity | Calories | Carbo-hydrates (grams) |
|---|---|---|---|

# Q

**QUAIL,** raw (USDA):
| | | | |
|---|---|---|---|
| Ready-to-cook | 1 lb. (weighed with bones) | 686 | 0. |
| Meat & skin only | 4 oz. | 195 | 0. |

**QUIK** (Nestlé):
| | | | |
|---|---|---|---|
| Chocolate | 3 heaping tsps. (.7 oz.) | 70 | 19.0 |
| Strawberry | 3 heaping tsps. (.7 oz.) | 80 | 21.0 |

**QUINCE,** fresh (USDA):
| | | | |
|---|---|---|---|
| Untrimmed | 1 lb. (weighed with skin & seeds) | 158 | 42.3 |
| Flesh only | 4 oz. | 65 | 17.4 |

**QUINCE JAM,** sweetened (Smucker's)
| | | | |
|---|---|---|---|
| | 1 T. | 53 | 13.5 |

**QUISP,** cereal (Quaker)
| | | | |
|---|---|---|---|
| | 1⅛ cups (1 oz.) | 121 | 23.1 |

# R

**RABBIT** (USDA):
Domesticated:
| | | | |
|---|---|---|---|
| Raw, ready-to-cook | 1 lb. (weighed with bones) | 581 | 0. |
| Stewed, flesh only | 4 oz. | 245 | 0. |
| Wild, ready-to-cook | 1 lb. (weighed with bones) | 490 | 0. |

**RACCOON,** roasted, meat only (USDA)
| | | | |
|---|---|---|---|
| | 4 oz. | 289 | 0. |

**RADISH** (USDA):
Common, raw:
| | | | |
|---|---|---|---|
| Without tops | ½ lb. (weighed untrimmed) | 34 | 7.4 |
| Trimmed, whole | 4 small radishes (1.4 oz.) | 7 | 1.4 |

| Food and Description | Measure or Quantity | Calories | Carbohydrates (grams) |
|---|---|---|---|
| Trimmed, sliced | ½ cup (2 oz.) | 10 | 2.1 |
| Oriental, raw, without tops | ½ lb. (weighed unpared) | 34 | 7.4 |
| Oriental, raw, trimmed & pared | 4 oz. | 22 | 4.8 |
| **RAISIN:** | | | |
| Dried: | | | |
| (USDA): | | | |
| Whole, pressed down | ½ cup (2.9 oz.) | 237 | 63.5 |
| Chopped | ½ cup (2.9 oz.) | 234 | 62.7 |
| Ground | ½ cup (4.7 oz.) | 387 | 103.7 |
| (Del Monte): | | | |
| Golden seedless | 3 oz. | 287 | 67.8 |
| Thompson seedless | 3 oz. | 283 | 66.5 |
| (Sun-Maid) seedless, natural Thompson | ½ cup (3 oz.) | 276 | 65.5 |
| Cooked (USDA) added sugar, solids & liq. | ½ cup (4.3 oz.) | 260 | 68.8 |
| ***RALSTON***, cereal, instant and regular | ¼ cup (1 oz.) | 110 | 20.0 |
| **RASPBERRY:** | | | |
| Black (USDA): | | | |
| Fresh: | | | |
| Whole | 1 lb. (weighed with caps & stems) | 160 | 34.6 |
| Without caps & stems | ½ cup (2.4 oz.) | 49 | 10.5 |
| Canned, water pack, unsweetened, solids & liq. | 4 oz. | 58 | 12.1 |
| Red (USDA): | | | |
| Fresh: | | | |
| Whole | 1 lb. (weighed with caps & stems) | 126 | 29.9 |

(USDA): United States Department of Agriculture
(HEW/FAO): Health, Education and Welfare/Food and Agriculture
        Organization
* Prepared as Package Directs

| Food and Description | Measure or Quantity | Calories | Carbohydrates (grams) |
|---|---|---|---|
| Without caps & stems | ½ cup (2.5 oz.) | 41 | 9.8 |
| Canned, water pack, unsweetened or low calorie, solids & liq. | 4 oz. | 40 | 10.0 |
| Frozen (Birds Eye) quick thaw | ½ of 10-oz. pkg. | 145 | 34.8 |
| **RASPBERRY JELLY,** sweetened (Smucker's) black or red | 1 T. | 53 | 13.5 |
| **RASPBERRY LIQUEUR** (Leroux) 50 proof | 1 fl. oz. | 74 | 8.3 |
| **RASPBERRY PRESERVE or JAM:** | | | |
| Sweetened (Smucker's) Black or red | 1 T. | 53 | 13.5 |
| Dietetic or low calorie: | | | |
| (Dia-Mel) black | 1 T. | 6 | 0. |
| (Featherweight) | 1 T. | 16 | 4.0 |
| (Louis Sherry) black or red | 1 tsp. | 2 | 0. |
| **RASPBERRY SPREAD,** low sugar (Smucker's) | 1 T. | 24 | 6.0 |
| **RASPBERRY SYRUP:** | | | |
| Sweetened (Smucker's) red | 1 T. | 43 | 11.1 |
| Dietetic (Featherweight) | 1 T. | 14 | 3.0 |
| **RAVIOLI:** | | | |
| Canned, regular pack: | | | |
| (Franco-American): | | | |
| Beef: | | | |
| In meat sauce | ½ of 15-oz. can | 220 | 36.0 |
| In meat sauce, *Raviolios* | ½ of 15-oz. can | 220 | 32.0 |
| Cheese, in tomato sauce, *Raviolios* | ½ of 15-oz. can | 260 | 39.0 |
| (Nalley's): | | | |
| Beef | 8-oz. serving | 214 | 34.1 |
| Chicken | 8-oz. serving | 225 | 34.1 |

| Food and Description | Measure or Quantity | Calories | Carbo-hydrates (grams) |
|---|---|---|---|
| Canned, dietetic or low calorie: | | | |
| (Dia-Mel) beef, in sauce | 8-oz. can | 230 | 35.0 |
| (Featherweight) beef, low sodium | 8-oz. can | 230 | 35.0 |
| **REDFISH** (See **DRUM, RED & OCEAN PERCH,** Atlantic) | | | |
| **RED & GRAY SNAPPER,** raw (USDA): | | | |
| Whole | 1 lb. (weighed whole) | 219 | 0. |
| Meat only | 4 oz. | 105 | 0. |
| **RELISH:** | | | |
| Regular pack: | | | |
| Hamburger (Nalley's) | 1 T. (.6 oz.) | 17 | 4.1 |
| Hot dog (Nalley's) | 1 T. (.7 oz.) | 24 | 4.8 |
| Sour (USDA) | 1 T. (.5 oz.) | 3 | .4 |
| Sweet: | | | |
| (USDA) finely chopped | 1 T. (.5 oz.) | 21 | 5.1 |
| (Aunt Jane's) | 1 rounded tsp. (.4 oz.) | 14 | 3.4 |
| (Lutz & Schramm) | 1 T. | 14 | 4.0 |
| (Nalley's) | 1 T. (.5 oz.) | 17 | 3.9 |
| (Smucker's) | 1 T. (.6 oz.) | 23 | 4.8 |
| Dietetic or low calorie, cucumber (Featherweight) | 1-oz. serving | 11 | 2.3 |
| **RHINESKELLER WINE** (Italian Swiss Colony) 12% alcohol | 3 fl. oz. | 66 | 3.0 |
| **RHINE WINE:** (Deinhard) Rheinritter, 11% alcohol | 3 fl. oz. | 60 | 3.6 |

(USDA): United States Department of Agriculture
(HEW/FAO): Health, Education and Welfare/Food and Agriculture Organization

* Prepared as Package Directs

| Food and Description | Measure or Quantity | Calories | Carbohydrates (grams) |
|---|---|---|---|
| (Gallo) 12% alcohol | 3 fl. oz. | 50 | .8 |
| (Gallo) Rhine Garten, 12% alcohol | 3 fl. oz. | 59 | 3.0 |
| (Gold Seal) 12% alcohol | 3 fl. oz. | 82 | .4 |
| (Great Western) 12% alcohol | 3 fl. oz. | 73 | 2.9 |
| (Great Western) Dutchess, 12% alcohol | 3 fl. oz. | 72 | 2.9 |
| (Inglenook): | | | |
| Navalle, 12% alcohol | 3 fl. oz. | 76 | 4.3 |
| Vintage, 12% alcohol | 3 fl. oz. | 63 | 1.7 |
| (Italian Swiss Colony) 11% alcohol | 3 fl. oz. | 59 | .6 |
| (Louis M. Martini) 12.5% alcohol | 3 fl. oz. | 90 | .2 |
| (Taylor) 12.5% alcohol | 3 fl. oz. | 75 | 3.0 |
| **RHUBARB:** | | | |
| Fresh: | | | |
| Partly trimmed (USDA) | 1 lb. (weighed with part leaves, ends & trimmings) | 54 | 12.6 |
| Trimmed (USDA) | 4 oz. | 18 | 4.2 |
| Diced (USDA) | ½ cup (2.2 oz.) | 10 | 2.3 |
| Cooked, sweetened, solids & liq. (USDA) | ½ cup (4.2 oz.) | 169 | 43.2 |
| Frozen, sweetened, cooked, added sugar (USDA) | ½ cup (4.4 oz.) | 177 | 44.9 |
| **RICE:** | | | |
| Brown: | | | |
| Raw (USDA) | ½ cup (3.7 oz.) | 374 | 80.5 |
| Parboiled (Uncle Ben's) dry, long-grain | 1 oz. | 107 | 21.2 |
| Cooked (Uncle Ben's) parboiled, no added butter or salt | ⅔ cup | 133 | 26.4 |
| Cooked (Uncle Ben's) parboiled, with butter & salt | ⅔ cup (4.2 oz.) | 152 | 26.4 |

| Food and Description | Measure or Quantity | Calories | Carbo- hydrates (grams) |
|---|---|---|---|
| **White:** | | | |
| Instant or precooked: | | | |
| Dry: | | | |
| (USDA) long-grain | 1 oz. | 106 | 23.4 |
| (Uncle Ben's) long-grain | 1 oz. | 101 | 22.5 |
| Cooked: | | | |
| (Minute Rice) no added butter or salt | ⅔ cup | 120 | 27.0 |
| (Uncle Ben's Quick) long-grain, no added butter or salt | ⅔ cup (4.2 oz.) | 119 | 27.4 |
| (Uncle Ben's Quick) long-grain, with butter & salt | ⅔ cup (4.3 oz.) | 143 | 27.4 |
| (Uncle Ben's Converted) long-grain, no butter or salt | ⅔ cup (4.6 oz.) | 129 | 28.9 |
| Regular: | | | |
| Dry (USDA) | ½ cup (3.3 oz.) | 336 | 74.4 |
| Cooked (USDA) | ⅔ cup (4.8 oz.) | 149 | 33.2 |
| Cooked (Carolina) long-grain | ½ cup | 100 | 22.0 |
| Cooked (Mahatma) long-grain | ½ cup | 100 | 22.0 |
| Cooked (Success Rice) long-grain | ½ cup (½ bag) | 110 | 23.0 |
| **RICE BRAN** (USDA) | 1 oz. | 78 | 14.4 |
| **RICE CHEX**, cereal (Ralston Purina) | 1⅛ cups (1 oz.) | 110 | 25.0 |
| **RICE, FRIED:** | | | |
| Canned: | | | |
| *(La Choy): Chicken | ½ cup (4 oz.) | 209 | 40.1 |

(USDA): United States Department of Agriculture
(HEW/FAO): Health, Education and Welfare/Food and Agriculture
   Organization
* Prepared as Package Directs

| *Food and Description* | *Measure or Quantity* | *Calories* | *Carbo-hydrates (grams)* |
|---|---|---|---|
| Chinese style | ½ cup (4 oz.) | 207 | 42.8 |
| (Chun King) with pork | ½ of 10-oz. pkg. | 180 | 24.0 |
| *Seasoning mix (Durkee) | 1 cup | 215 | 46.5 |
| **RICE, FRIED, & PORK ENTREE,** frozen (La Choy) | ½ of 12-oz. entree | 245 | 38.8 |
| ***RICE KRINKLES,*** cereal (Post) | ⅞ cup (1 oz.) | 113 | 26.3 |
| ***RICE KRISPIES,*** cereal (Kellogg's) | 1 cup (1 oz.) | 110 | 25.0 |
| **RICE MIX:** | | | |
| Beef: | | | |
| (Ann Page) *Rice'n Easy* | 1.3-oz. dry | 131 | 26.2 |
| *(Carolina) *Bake-it-Easy* | ⅙ of 6-oz. pkg. | 110 | 23.0 |
| *Rice-A-Roni* | 1.6 of 8-oz. pkg. | 130 | 27.0 |
| *Brown & wild (Uncle Ben's): | | | |
| Without butter | ½ cup | 126 | 24.7 |
| With butter | ½ cup | 150 | 24.7 |
| Chicken: | | | |
| *(Ann Page) *Rice'n Easy* | 1.3-oz. serving | 137 | 27.4 |
| *(Carolina) *Bake-it-Easy* | ⅙ of 6-oz. pkg. | 110 | 23.0 |
| *Rice-A-Roni* | ⅕ of 8-oz. pkg. | 160 | 33.2 |
| *Drumstick (Minute Rice) | ½ cup | 150 | 25.0 |
| *Fried (Minute Rice) | ½ cup | 160 | 25.0 |
| *Oriental (Carolina) *Bake-it-Easy* | ⅙ of 6-oz. pkg. | 120 | 25.0 |
| *Rib roast (Minute Rice) | ½ cup | 150 | 25.0 |
| Spanish: | | | |
| *(Carolina) *Bake-it-Easy* | ⅙ of 6-oz. pkg. | 110 | 24.0 |
| *(Minute Rice) | ½ cup | 150 | 25.0 |
| *Rice-A-Roni* | ⅙ of 7½-oz. pkg. | 120 | 25.9 |

**RICE PUDDING** (See **PUDDING or PIE FILLING**)

| Food and Description | Measure or Quantity | Calories | Carbo-hydrates (grams) |
|---|---|---|---|
| **RICE, SPANISH:** | | | |
| Home recipe (USDA) | 4 oz. | 99 | 18.8 |
| Canned, regular pack: | | | |
| (Comstock) | 7½-oz. serving | 140 | 27.0 |
| (Libby's) | ½ of 15-oz. can | 135 | 27.5 |
| (Van Camp) | ½ cup | 95 | 15.5 |
| Canned, dietetic or low calorie (Featherweight) | ½ of 7¼-oz. can | 70 | 14.0 |
| **RICE & VEGETABLES,** frozen: | | | |
| (Birds Eye) rice, peas & mushrooms | ⅓ of 7-oz. pkg. | 106 | 22.4 |
| (Green Giant): | | | |
| & broccoli in cheese sauce | ½ of 11-oz. pkg. | 149 | 22.7 |
| Continental, with green beans and almonds | ½ of 11-oz. pkg. | 138 | 21.4 |
| *Medley,* with sweet peas & mushrooms | ½ of 11-oz. pkg. | 134 | 23.7 |
| Pilaf, with mushrooms & onions | ½ of 11-oz. pkg. | 141 | 28.7 |
| *Verdi,* with bell peppers & parsley | ½ of 11-oz. pkg. | 175 | 32.0 |
| White & wild, medley, with peas, celery, mushrooms & almonds | ½ of 11½-oz. pkg. | 195 | 27.9 |
| White & wild, oriental, with bean sprouts, pea pods & water chestnuts | ⅓ of 12-oz. pkg. | 94 | 16.5 |
| **RICE WINE (HEW/FAO):** | | | |
| Chinese, 20.7% alcohol | 3 fl. oz. | 114 | 3.3 |
| Japanese, 10.6% alcohol | 3 fl. oz. | 215 | 39.4 |
| **ROAST BEEF SPREAD,** canned (Underwood) | 1 oz. | 58 | .3 |

(USDA): United States Department of Agriculture
(HEW/FAO): Health, Education and Welfare/Food and Agriculture Organization
* Prepared as Package Directs

| Food and Description | Measure or Quantity | Calories | Carbo-hydrates (grams) |
|---|---|---|---|
| **ROCK & RYE** (Mr. Boston) | 1 fl. oz. | 74 | 7.2 |
| **ROE** (USDA): | | | |
| Raw: | | | |
| Carp, cod, haddock, herring, pike or shad | 4 oz. | 147 | 1.7 |
| Salmon, sturgeon or turbot | 4 oz. | 235 | 1.6 |
| Baked or broiled, cod & shad | 4 oz. | 143 | 2.2 |
| Canned, cod, haddock or herring, solids & liq. | 4 oz. | 134 | .3 |
| **ROLAIDS** (Warner-Lambert) | 1 piece | 4 | 1.4 |
| **ROLL or BUN** (See also ROLL DOUGH and ROLL MIX): | | | |
| Commercial type: | | | |
| Biscuit (Wonder) | 2.5-oz. roll | 214 | 34.1 |
| *Brown'n Serve* (Wonder): | | | |
| With buttermilk | 1-oz. roll | 87 | 13.1 |
| French style | 1-oz. roll | 86 | 13.6 |
| Gem style | 1-oz. roll | 86 | 13.6 |
| Half & Half | 1-oz. roll | 88 | 13.6 |
| Home bake | 1-oz. roll | 88 | 13.6 |
| Butter crescent (Pepperidge Farm) | 1 roll | 120 | 13.0 |
| Club (Pepperidge Farm) | 1 roll | 100 | 20.0 |
| Deli twist (Arnold) | 1.3-oz. roll | 110 | 17.0 |
| Dinner: | | | |
| *Home Pride* | 1-oz. roll | 93 | 13.6 |
| (Pepperidge Farm) | 1 roll | 60 | 10.0 |
| (Wonder) | 2.5-oz. roll | 214 | 34.1 |
| *Dinner Party Rounds* (Arnold) | .7-oz. roll | 55 | 10.0 |
| Finger: | | | |
| (Arnold) *Dinner Party* | .7-oz. roll | 55 | 10.0 |
| (Pepperidge Farm) poppyseed or white | 1 roll | 53 | 8.0 |
| (Pepperidge Farm) sesame | 1 roll | 57 | 8.7 |

| Food and Description | Measure or Quantity | Calories | Carbo-hydrates (grams) |
| --- | --- | --- | --- |
| Frankfurter: | | | |
| (Arnold) hot dog | 1.3-oz. bun | 110 | 20.0 |
| (Wonder) | 2-oz. bun | 162 | 28.9 |
| French: | | | |
| (Arnold) *Francisco,* enriched | 2-oz. roll | 160 | 31.0 |
| (Arnold) *Francisco,* sourdough | 1.1-oz. roll | 90 | 16.0 |
| (Pepperidge Farm): | | | |
| Large | 1 roll | 380 | 76.0 |
| Small | 1 roll | 240 | 48.0 |
| Golden twist (Pepperidge Farm) | 1 roll | 110 | 14.0 |
| Hamburger: | | | |
| (Arnold) | 1.4-oz. bun | 110 | 21.0 |
| (Pepperidge Farm) | 1 bun | 120 | 19.0 |
| (Wonder) | 2-oz. bun | 162 | 29.1 |
| *Hearth* (Pepperidge Farm) | 1 roll | 55 | 10.0 |
| Honey (Hostess) | 4¾-oz. piece | 579 | 63.4 |
| Kaiser-Hogie (Wonder) | 6-oz. roll | 465 | 81.8 |
| Old-fashioned (Pepperidge Farm) | 1 roll | 53 | 7.7 |
| Pan (Wonder) | 2.5-oz. roll | 214 | 34.1 |
| Parkerhouse: | | | |
| (Arnold) *Dinner Party* | .7-oz. roll | 55 | 10.0 |
| (Pepperidge Farm) | 1 roll | 57 | 9.0 |
| Party pan (Pepperidge Farm) | 1 roll | 33 | 5.3 |
| Sandwich: | | | |
| (Arnold): | | | |
| *Dutch Egg* | 1.6-oz. bun | 130 | 22.0 |
| *Francisco* | 2-oz. roll | 160 | 30.0 |
| Soft, plain or poppy seeds | 1.3-oz. roll | 110 | 18.0 |
| Soft, sesame seeds | 1.3-oz. roll | 110 | 19.0 |
| Sesame crisp (Pepperidge Farm) | 1 roll | 63 | 11.0 |

(USDA): United States Department of Agriculture
(HEW/FAO): Health, Education and Welfare/Food and Agriculture Organization
* Prepared as Package Directs

| Food and Description | Measure or Quantity | Calories | Carbo- hydrates (grams) |
|---|---|---|---|
| Frozen: | | | |
| Apple crunch (Sara Lee) | 1 oz. roll | 102 | 13.5 |
| Caramel pecan (Sara Lee) | 1.3-oz. roll | 145 | 14.6 |
| Caramel sticky (Sara Lee) | 1-oz. bun | 118 | 15.0 |
| Cinnamon (Sara Lee) | .9-oz. roll | 100 | 13.9 |
| Croissant (Sara Lee) | .9-oz. roll | 109 | 11.2 |
| Honey: | | | |
| (Morton): | | | |
| Regular | 2½-oz. piece | 231 | 30.7 |
| Mini | 1.3-oz. piece | 133 | 17.7 |
| (Sara Lee) | 1-oz. roll | 112 | 14.6 |
| Parkerhouse (Sara Lee) | .8-oz. roll | 73 | 10.3 |
| Party (Sara Lee) | .6-oz. roll | 55 | 7.7 |
| Sesame seeds (Sara Lee) | .6-oz. roll | 55 | 7.7 |
| **ROLL DOUGH:** | | | |
| Frozen (Rich's) onion | 2½-oz. roll | 196 | 36.7 |
| Refrigerated (Pillsbury): | | | |
| Caramel bun | 1 bun | 120 | 19.0 |
| Cinnamon, *Ballard,* with icing | 1 bun | 10 | 17.0 |
| Cinnamon, *Hungry Jack,* with icing, *Butter Tastin'* | 1 roll | 145 | 19.5 |
| Danish, caramel, with nuts | 1 roll | 150 | 19.5 |
| Danish, cinnamon & raisins | 1 roll | 135 | 21.0 |
| Danish, orange | 1 roll | 130 | 21.0 |
| Dinner, butterflake | 1 roll | 100 | 17.0 |
| Dinner, crescent, | 1 roll | 95 | 12.5 |
| Dinner, *Oven Lovin'* | 1 roll | 55 | 9.5 |
| **\*ROLL MIX** (Pillsbury) hot roll | 1 roll | 95 | 15.5 |
| **ROSEMARY LEAVES** (French's) | 1 tsp. | 5 | .8 |
| **ROSÉ WINE:** | | | |
| (Antinori) 12% alcohol | 3 fl. oz. | 84 | 6.3 |

| Food and Description | Measure or Quantity | Calories | Carbo-hydrates (grams) |
|---|---|---|---|
| *Chateau Ste. Roseline,* 11–14% alcohol | 3 fl. oz. | 84 | 6.3 |
| (Chanson) *Rosé des Anges,* 12% alcohol | 3 fl. oz. | 84 | 6.3 |
| (Cruse) 12% alcohol | 3 fl. oz. | 72 | |
| (Gallo) 13% alcohol | 3 fl. oz. | 55 | 1.8 |
| (Gallo) *Gypsy,* 20% alcohol | 3 fl. oz. | 112 | 12.0 |
| (Great Western) 12% alcohol | 3 fl. oz. | 80 | 2.4 |
| (Great Western) Isabella, 12% alcohol | 3 fl. oz. | 77 | 4.0 |
| (Inglenook) Gamay, Estate, 12% alcohol | 3 fl. oz. (2.9 oz.) | 60 | .5 |
| (Inglenook) Navalle, 12% alcohol | 3 fl. oz. (2.9 oz.) | 62 | 1.3 |
| (Inglenook) Vintage, 12% alcohol | 3 fl. oz. (2.9 oz.) | 61 | .9 |
| (Italian Swiss Colony-Gold Medal) Grenache, 12.4% alcohol | 3 fl. oz. | 69 | 2.2 |
| (Italian Swiss Colony) Grenache, 12% alcohol | 3 fl. oz. | 61 | .5 |
| (Louis M. Martini) Gamay, 12.5% alcohol | 3 fl. oz. | 90 | .2 |
| (Mogen David) 12% alcohol | 3 fl. oz. | 75 | 8.9 |
| *Nectarosé, vin rosé d' Anjou,* 12% alcohol | 3 fl. oz. | 70 | 2.6 |
| (Taylor) 12.5% alcohol | 3 fl. oz. | 72 | 3.0 |
| **ROSÉ WINE, SPARKLING** (Chanson) | 3 fl. oz. | 72 | 3.6 |
| **ROTINI,** canned (Franco-American): | | | |
| In tomato sauce | ½ of 15-oz. can | 200 | 36.0 |
| & meatballs in tomato sauce | ½ of 14¾-oz. can | 235 | 27.6 |

(USDA): United States Department of Agriculture
(HEW/FAO): Health, Education and Welfare/Food and Agriculture
         Organization
* Prepared as Package Directs

| Food and Description | Measure or Quantity | Calories | Carbo-hydrates (grams) |
|---|---|---|---|
| **RUM** (See **DISTILLED LIQUOR**) | | | |
| **RUM & COLA**, canned (Party Tyme) 10% alcohol | 2 fl. oz. | 55 | 5.2 |
| **RUTABAGA:** | | | |
| Raw, without tops (USDA) | 1 lb. (weighed with skin) | 177 | 42.4 |
| Raw, diced (USDA) | ½ cup (2.5 oz.) | 32 | 7.7 |
| Boiled, drained, diced (USDA) | ½ cup (3 oz.) | 30 | 7.1 |
| Boiled, drained, mashed (USDA) | ½ cup (4.3 oz.) | 43 | 10.0 |
| **RYE**, whole grain (USDA) | 1 oz. | 95 | 20.8 |
| **RYE FLOUR** (See **FLOUR**) | | | |
| **RYE WHISKEY** (See **DISTILLED LIQUOR**) | | | |

# S

| Food and Description | Measure or Quantity | Calories | Carbo-hydrates (grams) |
|---|---|---|---|
| **SABLEFISH**, raw (USDA): | | | |
| Whole | 1 lb. (weighed whole) | 362 | 0. |
| Meat only | 4 oz. | 215 | 0. |
| **SAFFLOWER SEED KERNELS**, dry (USDA) | 1 oz. | 174 | 3.5 |
| **SAGE** (French's) | 1 tsp. (.9 grams) | 4 | .6 |
| **SAINT-EMILION WINE,** French Bordeaux (Barton & Guestier) 12% alcohol | 3 fl. oz. | 63 | .7 |
| **SAINT JOHN'S BREAD FLOUR** (See **FLOUR**, Carob) | | | |

| Food and Description | Measure or Quantity | Calories | Carbo- hydrates (grams) |
|---|---|---|---|
| **SAKE WINE**, 19.8% alcohol (HEW/FAO) | 3 fl. oz. | 116 | 4.3 |
| **SALAD DRESSING** (See also **SALAD DRESSING MIX**): | | | |
| Regular: | | | |
| Avocado Goddess (Marie's) | 1 T. (.5 oz.) | 95 | 1.0 |
| Bacon: | | | |
| (Marie's) | 1 T. (.5 oz.) | 95 | 1.0 |
| (Seven Seas) creamy | 1 T. | 60 | 1.0 |
| Bell pepper (Seven Seas) *Viva* | 1 T. | 45 | 1.0 |
| Bleu or blue cheese: | | | |
| (Bernstein's) Danish | 1 T. (.5 oz.) | 60 | .6 |
| (Marie's) | 1 T. (.5 oz.) | 100 | 1.0 |
| (Seven Seas) creamy | 1 T. | 70 | 1.0 |
| (Wish-Bone) chunky | 1 T. (.5 oz.) | 80 | 1.0 |
| Boiled, home recipe (USDA) | 1 T. (.6 oz.) | 26 | 2.4 |
| Caesar: | | | |
| (Pfeiffer) | ½ oz. | 70 | .5 |
| (Seven Seas) *Viva* | 1 T. | 60 | 1.0 |
| (Wish-Bone) | 1 T. | 80 | 1.0 |
| Capri (Seven Seas) | 1 T. | 70 | 3.0 |
| Coleslaw (Kraft) | 1 T. (.5 oz.) | 66 | 3.6 |
| French: | | | |
| (Bernstein's) creamy | 1 T. (.5 oz.) | 56 | 2.1 |
| (Bernstein's) chutney | 1 T. (.5 oz.) | 62 | 3.6 |
| (Kraft) | 1 T. (.5 oz.) | 59 | 2.1 |
| (Kraft) *Catalina* | 1 T. (.5 oz.) | 64 | 3.7 |
| (Nalley's) | 1 T. (.5 oz.) | 56 | 2.1 |
| (Nalley's) chutney | 1 T. (.5 oz.) | 62 | 3.6 |
| (Nalley's) original | 1 T. (.5 oz.) | 60 | 3.1 |
| (Pfeiffer) homo | ½ oz. | 55 | 3.5 |
| (Seven Seas) creamy | 1 T. (.5 oz.) | 60 | 2.0 |
| (Seven Seas) family style | 1 T. (.5 oz.) | 60 | 3.0 |

(USDA): United States Department of Agriculture
(HEW/FAO): Health, Education and Welfare/Food and Agriculture Organization
\* Prepared as Package Directs

| Food and Description | Measure or Quantity | Calories | Carbohydrates (grams) |
|---|---|---|---|
| (Wish-Bone) deluxe | 1 T. | 50 | 2.0 |
| (Wish-Bone) garlic | 1 T. (.5 oz.) | 70 | 3.0 |
| (Wish-Bone) *Sweet'n Spicy* | 1 T. | 70 | 3.0 |
| Garlic (Wish-Bone) creamy | 1 T. | 80 | 1.0 |
| German style (Marzetti) | 1 T. (.5 oz.) | 55 | 2.4 |
| Green Goddess: | | | |
| (Kraft) | 1 T. (.5 oz.) | 79 | .8 |
| (Nalley's) | 1 T. (.5 oz.) | 68 | 1.2 |
| (Seven Seas) | 1 T. | 60 | 0. |
| Green onion (Kraft) | 1 T. (.5 oz.) | 75 | 1.1 |
| Herb & spice (Seven Seas) | 1 T. | 60 | 1.0 |
| Italian: | | | |
| (Bernstein's) | 1 T. (.5 oz.) | 50 | .8 |
| (Bernstein's) with cheese | 1 T. (.5 oz.) | 56 | .8 |
| (Kraft) | 1 T. (.5 oz.) | 75 | 1.1 |
| (Marie's) with garlic | 1 T. (.5 oz.) | 100 | 1.1 |
| (Pfeiffer) chef | ½ oz. | 60 | .5 |
| (Seven Seas) | 1 T. | 70 | 1.0 |
| (Seven Seas) creamy | 1 T. | 70 | 1.0 |
| (Seven Seas) family style | 1 T. | 70 | 0. |
| (Seven Seas) *Viva Italian* | 1 T. | 70 | 1.0 |
| (Wish-Bone) | 1 T. | 80 | 1.0 |
| Louis dressing (Nalley's) | 1 T. | 69 | 1.8 |
| Mayonnaise-type (USDA) | 1 T. (.5 oz.) | 65 | 2.2 |
| Oil & vinegar (Kraft) | 1 T. (.5 oz.) | 68 | .6 |
| Onion: | | | |
| (Marie's) creamy | 1 T. | 90 | 1.4 |
| (Wish-Bone) *California* | 1 T. | 80 | 1.0 |
| Onion & chive (Seven Seas) creamy | 1 T. | 60 | 1.0 |
| Potato salad (Marzetti) | 1 T. (.5 oz.) | 62 | 2.9 |
| Ranch (Marie's) | 1 T. | 105 | 1.3 |
| Red wine vinegar & oil (Seven Seas) | 1 T. (.6 oz.) | 60 | 1.0 |
| *Rich'n Tangy* (Dutch Pantry) | 1 T. (.6 oz.) | 68 | 4.4 |

| Food and Description | Measure or Quantity | Calories | Carbo-hydrates (grams) |
|---|---|---|---|
| Roquefort: | | | |
| (Bernstein's) | 1 T. (.5 oz.) | 65 | .8 |
| (Marie's) | 1 T. (.5 oz.) | 105 | 1.1 |
| Russian: | | | |
| (Kraft) | 1 T. (.5 oz.) | 55 | 4.3 |
| (Pfeiffer) | ½ oz. | 65 | 2.0 |
| (Seven Seas) creamy | 1 T. | 80 | 1.0 |
| (Wish-Bone) | 1 T. | 60 | 7.0 |
| (Saffola) | 1 T. (.5 oz.) | 51 | 2.2 |
| Sesame (Sahadi) creamy | 1 T. (.5 oz.) | 60 | 2.0 |
| Sesame (Sahadi) spice | 1 T. (.5 oz.) | 80 | 1.0 |
| *Spin Blend* (Hellmann's) | 1 T. (.6 oz.) | 56 | 2.7 |
| Sweet'n Sour (Dutch Pantry) | 1 T. (.6 oz.) | 80 | 3.9 |
| Sweet'n Sour (Dutch Pantry) creamy | 1 T. | 77 | 4.0 |
| Sweet'n Sour (Nalley's) | 1 T. (.5 oz.) | 59 | 2.3 |
| Thousand Island: | | | |
| (Bernstein's) | 1 T. (.5 oz.) | 63 | 1.7 |
| (Kraft) | 1 T. (.5 oz.) | 59 | 2.5 |
| (Marie's) | 1 T. (.5 oz.) | 85 | 1.6 |
| (Marzetti) | 1 T. (.5 oz.) | 70 | 2.3 |
| (Nalley's) | 1 T. (.5 oz.) | 59 | 2.3 |
| (Pfeiffer) | ½ oz. | 65 | 2.0 |
| (Seven Seas) | 1 T. | 50 | 2.0 |
| (Wish-Bone) | 1 T. | 70 | 2.0 |
| *Tomato'n Spice* (Dutch Pantry) | 1 T. (.6 oz.) | 66 | 3.6 |
| Vinaigrette (Bernstein's) French | 1 T. (.5 oz.) | 49 | .2 |
| Dietetic or low calorie: | | | |
| Bleu or blue cheese: | | | |
| (Ann Page) | 1 T. | 13 | .5 |
| (Dia-Mel) | 1 T. (.5 oz.) | 15 | 0. |
| (Featherweight) imitation | 1 T. | 16 | 1.0 |
| (Marie's) | 1 T. (.5 oz.) | 30 | 3.3 |

(USDA): United States Department of Agriculture
(HEW/FAO): Health, Education and Welfare/Food and Agriculture Organization

* Prepared as Package Directs

| Food and Description | Measure or Quantity | Calories | Carbohydrates (grams) |
|---|---|---|---|
| (Tillie Lewis) *Tasti Diet* | 1 T. (.5 oz.) | 11 | .5 |
| Caesar: | | | |
| (Dia-Mel) | 1 T. (.5 oz.) | 50 | .5 |
| (Pfeiffer) | 1 oz. | 20 | 2.0 |
| Chef style (Ann Page) | 1 T. (.5 oz.) | 20 | 3.2 |
| Cucumber & onion (Featherweight) creamy | 1 T. | 16 | 0. |
| French: | | | |
| (Ann Page) | 1 T. | 24 | 2.0 |
| (Dia-Mel) | 1 T. (.5 oz.) | 30 | 1.0 |
| (Featherweight) imitation | 1 T. | 14 | 1.0 |
| (Kraft) | 1 T. (.5 oz.) | 21 | 2.0 |
| (Pfeiffer) | ½ oz. | 17 | 2.5 |
| (Tillie Lewis) *Tasti Diet* | 1 T. (.5 oz.) | 12 | 2.5 |
| (Wish-Bone) | 1 T. | 25 | 4.0 |
| Imitation (Featherweight) | 1 T. | 16 | 1.0 |
| Italian: | | | |
| (Ann Page) | 1 T. | 12 | .7 |
| (Dia-Mel) | 1 T. | 2 | .5 |
| (Featherweight) creamy | 1 T. | 18 | 0. |
| (Kraft) | 1 T. (.5 oz.) | 7 | .6 |
| (Pfeiffer) | ½ oz. | 10 | 1.5 |
| (Tillie Lewis) *Tasti Diet* | 1 T. (.5 oz.) | 6 | Tr. |
| (Weight Watchers) | 1 T. (.5 oz.) | 50 | 2.0 |
| (Wish-Bone) | 1 T. | 20 | 1.0 |
| Red wine (Pfeiffer) | ½ oz. | 10 | 1.0 |
| Russian: | | | |
| (Dia-Mel) | 1 T. (.5 oz.) | 9 | .5 |
| (Featherweight) creamy | 1 T. | 14 | 1.0 |
| (Kraft) | 1 T. (.5 oz.) | 30 | 4.3 |
| (Pfeiffer) | ½ oz. | 15 | 2.0 |
| (Tillie Lewis) *Tasti Diet* | 1 T. | 12 | 2.4 |
| (Weight Watchers) | 1 T. (.5 oz.) | 50 | 2.0 |
| (Wish-Bone) | 1 T. | 25 | 5.0 |

| Food and Description | Measure or Quantity | Calories | Carbohydrates (grams) |
|---|---|---|---|
| Thousand Island: | | | |
| (Ann Page) | 1 T. (.6 oz.) | 22 | 2.1 |
| (Dia-Mel) | 1 T. (.5 oz.) | 30 | 1.0 |
| (Featherweight) | 1 T. | 16 | 1.0 |
| (Kraft) | 1 T. (.5 oz.) | 28 | 2.2 |
| (Pfeiffer) | ½ oz. | 15 | 2.0 |
| (Tillie Lewis) *Tasti Diet* | 1 T. (.5 oz.) | 15 | 2.3 |
| (Weight Watchers) | 1 T. (.5 oz.) | 50 | 2.0 |
| (Wish-Bone) | 1 T. | 25 | 3.0 |
| 2-calorie Low Sodium | | | |
| (Featherweight) | 1 T. | 2 | 0. |
| Whipped: | | | |
| (Dia-Mel) | 1 T. | 22 | 2.1 |
| (Tillie Lewis) *Tasti Diet* | 1 T. (.5 oz.) | 20 | 1.0 |
| **SALAD DRESSING MIX:** | | | |
| *Regular (Good Seasons): | | | |
| Bleu or blue cheese: | | | |
| Regular | 1 T. | 90 | .5 |
| *Thick'n Creamy* | 1 T. | 80 | .5 |
| Buttermilk, farm style | 1 T. | 60 | 1.0 |
| French: | | | |
| Regular | 1 T. | 80 | 3.0 |
| Old-fashioned | 1 T. | 80 | 1.0 |
| *Riviera* | 1 T. | 90 | 3.0 |
| *Thick'n Creamy* | 1 T. | 75 | 2.0 |
| Garlic | 1 T. | 80 | 1.0 |
| Garlic, with cheese | 1 T. | 90 | 1.0 |
| Italian: | | | |
| Regular | 1 T. | 80 | 1.0 |
| Cheese | 1 T. | 90 | 1.0 |
| Mild | 1 T. | 90 | 1.0 |
| *Thick'n Creamy* | 1 T. | 85 | 1.0 |
| Onion | 1 T. | 80 | 1.0 |
| Thousand Island, *Thick'n Creamy* | 1 T. (.6 oz.) | 75 | 2.0 |

(USDA): United States Department of Agriculture
(HEW/FAO): Health, Education and Welfare/Food and Agriculture Organization

* Prepared as Package Directs

| Food and Description | Measure or Quantity | Calories | Carbo-hydrates (grams) |
|---|---|---|---|
| Dietetic or low calorie: | | | |
| *Blue cheese (Weight Watchers) | 1 T. | 10 | 1.0 |
| French: | | | |
| (Dia-Mel) | ½-oz. packet | 18 | 0. |
| (Louis Sherry) | ½-oz. packet | 18 | 0. |
| *(Weight Watchers) | 1 T. | 4 | 1.0 |
| Garlic (Dia-Mel) creamy | ½-oz. packet | 21 | 1.0 |
| Italian: | | | |
| (Dia-Mel) | ½-oz. packet | 2 | 0. |
| *(Good Seasons) | 1 T. | 8 | 2.0 |
| (Louis Sherry) | ½-oz. packet | 2 | 0. |
| *(Weight Watchers) | 1 T. | 2 | 0. |
| *(Weight Watchers) creamy | 1 T. | 4 | 1.0 |
| Russian: | | | |
| (Louis Sherry) | ½-oz. packet | 20 | 0. |
| *(Weight Watchers) | 1 T. | 4 | 1.0 |
| Thousand Island: | | | |
| (Dia-Mel) | ½-oz. packet | 20 | 0. |
| *(Weight Watchers) | 1 T. | 12 | 1.0 |
| **SALAD FIXIN'S** (Arnold): | | | |
| Danish style bleu cheese | ½ oz. | 66 | 8.8 |
| French onion | ½ oz. | 67 | 8.7 |
| Spicy Italian | ½ oz. | 67 | 9.3 |
| **SALAD SEASONING** (Durkee): | | | |
| Regular | 1 tsp. | 4 | .7 |
| With cheese | 1 tsp. | 10 | .4 |
| **SALAMI:** | | | |
| Dry (USDA) | 1 oz. | 128 | .3 |
| Cooked (USDA) | 1 oz. | 88 | .4 |
| (Hormel): | | | |
| Genoa, *DiLusso* | 1 oz. | 101 | Tr. |
| Genoa, sliced | 1 oz. | 127 | .6 |
| Hard | 1 oz. | 117 | .2 |
| Hard, sliced | 1 oz. | 118 | .5 |
| Party, sliced | 1 oz. | 94 | .1 |
| (Oscar Mayer): | | | |
| For beer | .8-oz. slice | 54 | .3 |

| Food and Description | Measure or Quantity | Calories | Carbohydrates (grams) |
|---|---|---|---|
| Cotto | .8-oz. slice | 53 | .6 |
| Cotto, beef | .8-oz. slice | 50 | .5 |
| Hard, all meat | .3-oz. slice | 33 | .1 |
| (Swift): | | | |
| Genoa | 1 oz. | 114 | .3 |
| Hard | 1 oz. | 115 | .9 |
| (Vienna) beef | 1 oz. | 79 | .8 |
| **SALISBURY STEAK:** | | | |
| Canned (Morton House) | ⅓ of 12½-oz. can | 160 | 7.0 |
| Frozen: | | | |
| (Banquet): | | | |
| Cooking bag | 5-oz. bag | 246 | 7.8 |
| Dinner | 11-oz. dinner | 390 | 24.0 |
| *Man-Pleaser* | 19-oz. dinner | 873 | 71.7 |
| (Green Giant): | | | |
| With gravy, oven bake | 7-oz. entree | 290 | 14.0 |
| With tomato sauce, boil-in-bag | 9-oz. entree | 390 | 22.0 |
| (Morton): | | | |
| Regular | 11-oz. dinner | 287 | 25.1 |
| *Country Table* | 15-oz. dinner | 515 | 37.9 |
| *Country Table* | 10¼-oz. entree | 494 | 60.0 |
| King Size | 19-oz. dinner | 772 | 64.8 |
| (Stouffer's) with onion gravy | 12-oz. pkg. | 470 | 9.8 |
| (Swanson): | | | |
| Regular | 11½-oz. dinner | 500 | 40.0 |
| With crinkle cut potatoes | 5½-oz. entree | 370 | 28.0 |
| With gravy | 10-oz. entree | 440 | 16.0 |
| *Hungry Man*, dinner | 17-oz. dinner | 870 | 65.0 |
| *Hungry Man*, entree | 12½-oz. entree | 640 | 39.0 |
| 3-course | 16-oz. dinner | 490 | 48.0 |
| **SALMON:** | | | |
| Atlantic (USDA): | | | |
| Raw, whole | 1 lb. (weighed whole) | 640 | 0. |

(USDA): United States Department of Agriculture
(HEW/FAO): Health, Education and Welfare/Food and Agriculture Organization
* Prepared as Package Directs

| Food and Description | Measure or Quantity | Calories | Carbo- hydrates (grams) |
|---|---|---|---|
| Meat only | 4 oz. | 246 | 0. |
| Canned, solids & liq., including bones | 4 oz. | 230 | 0. |
| Chinook or King (USDA): | | | |
| Raw steak | 1 lb. (weighed whole) | 886 | 0. |
| Raw, meat only | 4 oz. | 252 | 0. |
| Canned, solids & liq., including bones | 4 oz. | 238 | 0. |
| Chum, canned (USDA), solids & liq., including bones | 4 oz. | 158 | 0. |
| Coho, canned (USDA), solids & liq., including bones | 4 oz. | 174 | 0. |
| Pink or Humpback: | | | |
| Raw, steak (USDA) | 1 lb. (weighed whole) | 475 | 0. |
| Raw, meat only (USDA) | 4 oz. | 135 | 0. |
| Canned: | | | |
| (USDA) solids & liq., including bones | 4 oz. | 160 | 0. |
| (Del Monte) solids & liq. | 7¾-oz. can | 277 | 0. |
| (Icy Point) solids & liq. | 7¾-oz. can | 310 | 0. |
| (Pink Beauty) solids & liq. | 7¾-oz. can | 310 | 0. |
| Sockeye or Red or Blueback, canned, solids & liq.: | | | |
| (USDA) | 4 oz. | 194 | 0. |
| (Bumble Bee) | 3¾-oz. can | 179 | 0. |
| (Bumble Bee) | 7¾-oz. can | 370 | 0. |
| Unspecified kind of salmon (USDA) baked or broiled | 4.2-oz. steak (approx. 4" x 3" x ½") | 218 | 0. |
| **SALMON, SMOKED:** | | | |
| (USDA) | 4 oz. | 200 | 0. |
| (Vita): | | | |
| Lox, drained | 4-oz. jar | 136 | .2 |
| Nova, drained | 4-oz. can | 221 | 1.0 |

| Food and Description | Measure or Quantity | Calories | Carbo-hydrates (grams) |
|---|---|---|---|
| **SALT:** | | | |
| Regular: | | | |
| Butter-flavored (French's) imitation | 1 tsp. (3.6 grams) | 8 | 0. |
| Garlic (Lawry's) | 1 tsp. (4 grams) | 5 | 1.0 |
| Hickory smoke (French's) | 1 tsp. (4 grams) | 2 | <.5 |
| *Lite Salt* (Morton) iodized | 1 tsp. (6 grams) | 0 | 0. |
| Onion (Lawry's) | 1 tsp. | 4 | .9 |
| Seasoned (Lawry's) | 1 tsp. | 1 | .1 |
| Table: | | | |
| (USDA) | 1 tsp. (6 grams) | 0 | 0. |
| (Morton) iodized | 1 tsp. (7 grams) | 0 | 0. |
| Substitute: | | | |
| (Adolph's) | 1 tsp. (6 grams) | 1 | Tr. |
| (Adolph's) | 1 packet (8 grams) | <1 | Tr. |
| (Adolph's) seasoned | 1 tsp. | 6 | 1.1 |
| (Dia-Mel) *Salt-It* | ⅛ tsp. | 0 | 0. |
| (Morton) | 1 tsp. (6 grams) | Tr. | Tr. |
| (Morton) seasoned | 1 tsp. (6 grams) | 3 | .5 |
| **SALT PORK, raw (USDA):** | | | |
| With skin | 1 lb. (weighed with skin) | 3410 | 0. |
| Without skin | 1 oz. | 222 | 0. |
| **SANDWICH SPREAD:** | | | |
| Regular: | | | |
| (USDA) | 1 T. (.5 oz.) | 57 | 2.4 |
| (Bennett's) | 1 T. (.5 oz.) | 44 | 3.7 |
| (Best Foods) | 1 T. (.5 oz.) | 62 | 2.2 |
| (Hellmann's) | 1 T. (.5 oz.) | 62 | 2.2 |
| (Kraft) | 1 oz. | 105 | 5.6 |
| (Kraft) pimiento | 1 oz. | 117 | .8 |
| (Nalley's) | 1 T. (.5 oz.) | 38 | 3.0 |
| Dietetic or low calorie | | | |
| (USDA) | 1 T. (.5 oz.) | 17 | 1.2 |

(USDA): United States Department of Agriculture
(HEW/FAO): Health, Education and Welfare/Food and Agriculture Organization
* Prepared as Package Directs

| Food and Description | Measure or Quantity | Calories | Carbo- hydrates (grams) |
|---|---|---|---|
| **SANGRIA:** | | | |
| (Taylor) 11.6% alcohol | 3 fl. oz. | 99 | 10.8 |
| Mix (Party Tyme) | ½-oz. pkg. | 53 | 13.7 |
| **SARDINE:** | | | |
| Raw, whole (HEW/FAO) | 1 lb. (weighed whole) | 321 | 0. |
| Raw, meat only (HEW/FAO) | 4 oz. | 146 | 0. |
| Canned: | | | |
| Atlantic: | | | |
| (USDA) in oil, solids & liq. | 3¾-oz. can | 330 | .6 |
| (USDA) in oil, drained solids, with skin & bones | 3¾-oz. can | 187 | DNA |
| (Del Monte) in tomato sauce, solids & liq. | 7½-oz. can | 330 | 4.0 |
| Norwegian: | | | |
| (Snow) | 1 oz. | 66 | DNA |
| (Underwood) in mustard sauce | 3¾-oz. can | 195 | 2.3 |
| (Underwood) in soya bean oil | 3¾-oz. can | 233 | .4 |
| (Underwood) in tomato sauce | 3¾-oz. can | 169 | 4.5 |
| Pacific (USDA) in brine or mustard, solids & liq. | 4 oz. | 222 | 1.9 |
| **SAUCE (See also SAUCE MIX):** | | | |
| *A1* | 1 T. (.6 oz.) | 12 | 2.8 |
| Barbecue: | | | |
| *Chris & Pitt's* | 1 T. | 15 | 4.0 |
| (French's) regular & smoky | 1 T. | 14 | 3.0 |
| *Open Pit* | 1 T. (.6 oz.) | 15 | 3.6 |
| *Open Pit*, hickory smoked flavor | 1 T. | 16 | 4.0 |
| *Open Pit*, with minced onions | 1 T. | 18 | 4.0 |
| Cocktail: | | | |
| (Nalley's) | 2-oz. serving | 66 | 14.2 |

| Food and Description | Measure or Quantity | Calories | Carbo-hydrates (grams) |
|---|---|---|---|
| (Pfeiffer) | 2-oz. serving | 100 | 12.0 |
| *Escoffier Sauce Diable* | 1 T. (.6 oz.) | 20 | 4.2 |
| *Escoffier Sauce Robert* | 1 T. | 19 | 4.5 |
| *Famous* (Durkee) | 1 T. | 69 | 2.2 |
| Hot, *Frank's* | 1 tsp. | 14 | 2.0 |
| *H.P. Steak Sauce* (Lea & Perrins) | 1 T. (1 oz.) | 20 | 4.8 |
| Italian: | | | |
| (Carnation) | 2 fl. oz. | 43 | 7.0 |
| (Ragu) red cooking | 3½ fl. oz. | 45 | 6.0 |
| Marinara (Ragu) | 5 oz. | 120 | 15.0 |
| Mushroom (Nalley's) | 1-oz. serving | 17 | 2.0 |
| Seafood (Bernstein's) | 1 T. (.5 oz.) | 16 | 3.6 |
| Seafood cocktail (Del Monte) | 1 T. (.6 oz.) | 22 | 4.9 |
| Soy: | | | |
| (Kikkoman) | 1 T. (.7 oz.) | 11 | 1.1 |
| (La Choy) | 1 T. (.5 oz.) | 8 | .9 |
| Steak (Dawn Fresh) with mushrooms | 2-oz. serving | 18 | 3.5 |
| *Steak Supreme* | 1 T. | 20 | 4.8 |
| Sweet & Sour: | | | |
| (Carnation) | 2 fl. oz. | 20 | 4.5 |
| (La Choy) | 1-oz. serving | 51 | 12.6 |
| Swiss steak (Carnation) | 2 fl. oz. | 20 | 4.5 |
| Taco (Ortega) | 1 T. | 21 | 4.8 |
| Tartar: | | | |
| (Best Foods) | 1 T. (.5 oz.) | 74 | .2 |
| (Hellmann's) | 1 T. (.5 oz.) | 74 | .2 |
| (Nalley's) | 1 T. (.5 oz.) | 89 | .3 |
| Teriyaki (Kikkoman) | 1 T. (.7 oz.) | 16 | 3.0 |
| "*V-8*" | 1-oz. serving | 25 | 6.0 |
| White (USDA) medium | 1 cup (9 oz.) | 413 | 22.4 |
| Worcestershire: | | | |
| (French's) regular or smoke | 1 T. | 10 | 2.0 |
| (Lea & Perrins) | 1 T. (.6 oz.) | 12 | 3.0 |

(USDA): United States Department of Agriculture
(HEW/FAO): Health, Education and Welfare/Food and Agriculture Organization
* Prepared as Package Directs

| Food and Description | Measure or Quantity | Calories | Carbo- hydrates (grams) |
|---|---|---|---|
| **SAUCE MIX:** | | | |
| Regular: | | | |
| A la King (Durkee) | 1.1-oz. pkg. | 133 | 14.0 |
| Cheese: | | | |
| (Durkee) | 1.1-oz. pkg. | 175 | 7.0 |
| *(Durkee) | 1 cup | 337 | 19.0 |
| (French's) | 1.2-oz. pkg. | 163 | 14.0 |
| Enchilada: | | | |
| (Durkee) | 1.1-oz. pkg. | 89 | 18.0 |
| *(Durkee) | 1 cup | 57 | 12.5 |
| Hollandaise: | | | |
| (Durkee) | 1-oz. pkg. | 173 | 11.0 |
| (French's) | 1.1-oz. pkg. | 188 | 7.4 |
| Sour cream: | | | |
| (Durkee) | 1-oz. pkg. | 135 | 9.0 |
| *(Durkee) | ⅔ cup | 214 | 15.0 |
| (French's) | 1.2-oz. pkg. | 166 | 16.0 |
| Stroganoff: | | | |
| (Durkee) | 1.2-oz. pkg. | 90 | 18.0 |
| *(Durkee) | 1 cup | 820 | 6.5 |
| (French's) | 1¾-oz. pkg. | 213 | 26.0 |
| Sweet & sour: | | | |
| (Durkee) | 2-oz. pkg. | 230 | 45.0 |
| (French's) | 2-oz. pkg. | 223 | 55.0 |
| Tartar (Lawry's) | .6-oz. pkg. | 64 | 9.8 |
| Teriyaki (French's) | 1.6-oz. pkg. | 136 | 27.0 |
| *White (Durkee) | 1 cup | 218 | 41.0 |
| *Dietetic, lemon butter (Weight Watchers) | 1 T. | 8 | 1.0 |
| **SAUERKRAUT, canned:** | | | |
| (USDA): | | | |
| Solids & liq. | 1 cup (8.3 oz.) | 42 | 9.4 |
| Drained solids | 1 cup (5 oz.) | 31 | 6.2 |
| (Blue Boy) solids & liq. | 1 cup (8.7 oz.) | 60 | 16.0 |
| (Claussen) drained | ¼ of 32-oz. jar | 49 | 8.9 |
| (Del Monte) solids & liq. | 1 cup (8 oz.) | 55 | 10.7 |
| (Libby's) solids & liq. | ⅛ of 32-oz. jar | 21 | 4.0 |
| (Silver Floss) solids & liq.: | | | |
| Regular | ½ cup (can) | 30 | 5.0 |
| Regular | ½ cup (jar) | 25 | 5.0 |
| Bavarian Kraut | ½ cup | 35 | 8.0 |
| *Krispy Kraut* | ½ cup | 25 | 5.0 |

| Food and Description | Measure or Quantity | Calories | Carbo-hydrates (grams) |
|---|---|---|---|
| Polybag (Stokely-Van Camp): | ½ cup | 20 | 4.0 |
| Bavarian style, solids & liq. | ½ cup (4.2 oz.) | 35 | 7.0 |
| Chopped or shredded, solids & liq. | ½ cup (4.2 oz.) | 25 | 4.5 |
| **SAUERKRAUT JUICE,** canned (USDA) | ½ cup (4.3 oz.) | 12 | 2.8 |
| **SAUSAGE** (See also individual kinds): (USDA): | | | |
| Brown & serve, before browning | 1 oz. | 111 | .8 |
| Brown & serve, after browning | 1 oz. | 120 | .8 |
| (Hormel) brown & serve | .8-oz. piece | 74 | Tr. |
| (Oscar Mayer): | | | |
| Patties | 1.5-oz. pattie | 183 | 0. |
| Smoked, breakfast | .7-oz. sausage | 65 | .3 |
| Smokie links | 1.5-oz. link | 136 | .6 |
| (Swift) Brown & serve, after browning: | | | |
| Bacon & sausage flavor | .7-oz. link | 72 | .4 |
| Beef flavor | .7-oz. link | 86 | .5 |
| Kountry Kured | .7-oz. link | 86 | .3 |
| Original | .7-oz. link | 77 | .5 |
| **SAUTERNES:** | | | |
| (Barton & Guestier) French white Bordeaux, 13% alcohol | 3 fl. oz. | 95 | 7.6 |
| (Barton & Guestier) haut, French white Bordeaux, 13% alcohol | 3 fl. oz. | 99 | 8.7 |
| (Gallo) 12% alcohol | 3 fl. oz. | 50 | .9 |
| (Gallo) haut, 12% alcohol | 3 fl. oz. | 67 | 2.1 |

(USDA): United States Department of Agriculture
(HEW/FAO): Health, Education and Welfare/Food and Agriculture Organization
* Prepared as Package Directs

| Food and Description | Measure or Quantity | Calories | Carbohydrates (grams) |
|---|---|---|---|
| (Gold Seal) dry, 12% alcohol | 3 fl. oz. | 82 | .4 |
| (Gold Seal) semi-soft, 12% alcohol | 3 fl. oz. | 87 | 2.6 |
| (Great Western) Aurora, 12% alcohol | 3 fl. oz. | 79 | 4.5 |
| (Italian Swiss Colony) 12% alcohol | 3 fl. oz. (2.9 oz.) | 59 | 1.2 |
| (Louis M. Martini) dry, 12.5% alcohol | 3 fl. oz. | 90 | .2 |
| (Mogen David) cream, 12% alcohol | 3 fl. oz. | 45 | 6.2 |
| (Mogen David) dry, American, 12% alcohol | 3 fl. oz. | 30 | 1.8 |
| (Taylor) 12.5% alcohol | 3 fl. oz. | 81 | 4.8 |

**SCALLION (See ONION, GREEN)**

**SCALLOP:**

| | | | |
|---|---|---|---|
| Raw (USDA) muscle only | 4 oz. | 92 | 3.7 |
| Steamed (USDA) | 4 oz. | 127 | DNA |
| Frozen: | | | |
| (USDA) breaded, fried, reheated | 4 oz. | 220 | 11.9 |
| (Mrs. Paul's): | | | |
| Batter fried | ½ of 7-oz. pkg. | 204 | 20.9 |
| Breaded & fried | ⅓ of 12-oz. pkg. | 230 | 27.5 |
| With butter & cheese | 7-oz. pkg. | 260 | 11.0 |
| (Van de Kamp's) country seasoned | ½ of 7-oz. pkg. | 270 | 19.0 |

**SCHNAPPS, PEPPERMINT:**

| | | | |
|---|---|---|---|
| (DeKuyper) | 1 fl. oz. | 79 | 7.5 |
| (Garnier) | 1 fl. oz. | 83 | 8.4 |
| (Hiram Walker) | 1 fl. oz. | 78 | 7.2 |
| (Leroux) | 1 fl. oz. | 87 | 9.2 |
| (Mr. Boston) | 1 fl. oz. | 77 | 8.0 |

**\*SCOTCH BROTH,** canned (Campbell) condensed | 10-oz. serving | 140 | 17.0 |

**SCOTCH SOUR COCKTAIL,** canned (National Distillers)
*Duet,* 12½% alcohol | 8-fl.-oz. can | 272 | 25.6 |

| Food and Description | Measure or Quantity | Calories | Carbohydrates (grams) |
|---|---|---|---|
| SCRAPPLE (USDA) | 4 oz. | 244 | 16.6 |
| **SCREWDRIVER COCKTAIL:** | | | |
| Canned: | | | |
| (Mr. Boston) 12% alcohol | 3 fl. oz. | 111 | 12.0 |
| (National Distillers) | | | |
| *Duet*, 12½% alcohol | 8-fl.-oz. can | 288 | 25.6 |
| (Party Tyme) 12½% alcohol | 2 fl. oz. | 69 | 6.4 |
| Mix: | | | |
| (Bar-Tender's) | ⅝-oz. serving | 70 | 17.4 |
| (Holland House) | .6-oz. pkg. | 69 | 17.0 |
| **SCUP** (See **PORGY**) | | | |
| **SEA BASS, WHITE,** raw (USDA) meat only | 4 oz. | 109 | 0. |
| **SEAFOOD PLATTER,** frozen (Mrs. Paul's) combination, with potato puffs | 9-oz. pkg. | 507 | 57.1 |
| ***SEGO* DIET FOOD:** | | | |
| Bars, all flavors | 1-oz. bar | 138 | 12.0 |
| Canned: | | | |
| Chocolate & milk chocolate | 10-fl.-oz. can | 225 | 39.0 |
| Very butterscotch, very banana, very strawberry, very vanilla | 10-fl.-oz. can | 225 | 35.0 |
| Vanilla | 10-fl.-oz. can | 225 | 33.0 |
| Very chocolate malt | 10-fl.-oz. can | 225 | 40.0 |
| ***SERUTAN* (J.B. Williams):** | | | |
| Toasted granules | 1 tsp. | 6 | 1.3 |
| Concentrated powder | 1 tsp. | 5 | 1.3 |
| Fruit flavored powder | 1 tsp. | 6 | 1.5 |
| **SESAME NUT MIX,** canned (Planters) oil roasted | 1 oz. | 160 | 8.0 |

(USDA): United States Department of Agriculture
(HEW/FAO): Health, Education and Welfare/Food and Agriculture
           Organization
* Prepared as Package Directs

| Food and Description | Measure or Quantity | Calories | Carbo-hydrates (grams) |
|---|---|---|---|
| **SESAME SEEDS,** dry (USDA): | | | |
| Whole | 1 oz. | 160 | 6.1 |
| Hulled | 1 oz. | 165 | 5.0 |
| **SHAD** (USDA): | | | |
| Raw, whole | 1 lb. (weighed whole) | 370 | 0. |
| Raw, meat only | 4 oz. | 193 | 0. |
| Cooked, home recipe: | | | |
| Baked with butter or margarine & bacon slices | 4 oz. | 228 | 0. |
| Creole | 4 oz. | 172 | 1.8 |
| Canned, solids & liq. | 4 oz. | 172 | 0. |
| **SHAD, GIZZARD,** raw (USDA): | | | |
| Whole | 1 lb. (weighed whole) | 299 | 0. |
| Meat only | 4 oz. | 227 | 0. |
| *SHAKE 'N BAKE:* | | | |
| Regular: | | | |
| Chicken | 2.4-oz. pkg. | 291 | 43.0 |
| Chicken, barbecue style | 3¾-oz. pkg. | 377 | 83.2 |
| Chicken, crispy country mild | 2.4-oz. pkg. | 321 | 50.1 |
| Chicken, Italian flavor | 2.4-oz. pkg. | 294 | 41.4 |
| Fish | 2-oz. pkg. | 234 | 33.9 |
| Hamburger | 2-oz. pkg. | 169 | 33.2 |
| Pork | 2.4-oz. pkg. | 255 | 47.1 |
| Pork & ribs, barbecue style | 2.9-oz. pkg. | 305 | 61.2 |
| & homestyle gravy mix: | | | |
| Beef | 3.1-oz. pkg. | 304 | 51.4 |
| Pork | 3.7-oz. pkg. | 327 | 67.4 |
| **SHALLOT,** raw (USDA): | | | |
| With skin | 1 oz. | 18 | 4.2 |
| With skin removed | 1 oz. | 20 | 4.8 |
| **SHERBET** (See also individual kinds): | | | |
| (Dean) 1.7% fat | ¼ pt. | 137 | 30.6 |

| Food and Description | Measure or Quantity | Calories | Carbo-hydrates (grams) |
|---|---|---|---|
| (Meadow Gold) orange | ¼ pt. | 120 | 26.0 |
| (Sealtest): | | | |
| Lemon, *Light 'n Lively* | ¼ pt. | 130 | 29.0 |
| Lime, *Light 'n Lively* | ¼ pt. | 130 | 29.0 |
| Orange | ¼ pt. | 120 | 26.5 |
| Orange, *Light 'n Lively* | ¼ pt. | 130 | 30.0 |
| Pineapple, *Light 'n Lively* | ¼ pt. | 130 | 29.0 |
| Rainbow, *Light 'n Lively* | ¼ pt. | 130 | 29.0 |
| Red raspberry, *Light 'n Lively* | ¼ pt. | 130 | 28.0 |
| Strawberry, *Light 'n Lively* | ¼ pt. | 130 | 30.0 |
| **SHERRY:** | | | |
| (Gallo) 20% alcohol | 3 fl. oz. | 88 | 2.7 |
| (Gallo) 16% alcohol | 3 fl. oz. | 76 | 3.3 |
| (Gold Seal) 19% alcohol | 3 fl. oz. | 139 | 4.6 |
| (Great Western) Solera, 18% alcohol | 3 fl. oz. | 120 | 8.5 |
| Cocktail (Gold Seal) 19% alcohol | 3 fl. oz. | 122 | 1.6 |
| Cocktail (Petri) | 3 fl. oz. | 102 | |
| Cream: | | | |
| (Gallo) 20% alcohol | 3 fl. oz. | 111 | 8.4 |
| (Gallo) Old Decanter, Livingston, 20% alcohol | 3 fl. oz. | 117 | 12.8 |
| (Gold Seal) 19% alcohol | 3 fl. oz. | 158 | 9.4 |
| (Great Western) Solera, 18% alcohol | 3 fl. oz. | 141 | 12.2 |
| (Louis M. Martini) 19.5% alcohol | 3 fl. oz. | 138 | 1.2 |
| (Taylor) 17.5% alcohol | 3 fl. oz. | 138 | 13.2 |
| (Williams & Humbert) Canasta, 20½% alcohol | 3 fl. oz. | 150 | 5.4 |
| Dry: | | | |
| (Gallo) 20% alcohol | 3 fl. oz. | 84 | 1.8 |
| (Gallo) Old Decanter, very dry, 20% alcohol | 3 fl. oz. | 87 | 2.1 |

(USDA): United States Department of Agriculture
(HEW/FAO): Health, Education and Welfare/Food and Agriculture Organization
* Prepared as Package Directs

| Food and Description | Measure or Quantity | Calories | Carbohydrates (grams) |
|---|---|---|---|
| Meat only | 4 oz. | 103 | 1.7 |
| Canned: | | | |
| (USDA): | | | |
| Wet pack, solids & liq. | 4 oz. | 91 | .9 |
| Dry pack or drained | 4 oz. | 132 | .8 |
| (Bumble Bee) baby, solids & liq. | 4½-oz. can | 90 | .9 |
| (Icy Point) cocktail, tiny, drained | 4½-oz. can | 148 | .8 |
| (Pillar Rock) cocktail, drained | 4½-oz. can | 148 | .8 |
| Cooked, french-fried (USDA) | 4 oz. | 255 | 11.3 |
| Frozen (Mrs. Paul's) breaded & fried | ½ of 6-oz. pkg. | 198 | 16.8 |
| SHRIMP CAKE, frozen (Mrs. Paul's): | | | |
| Breaded & fried | 3-oz. cake | 156 | 17.2 |
| Breaded & fried thins | 2-oz. cake | 95 | 14.0 |
| SHRIMP DINNER, frozen (Van de Kamp's) | 10-oz. dinner | 370 | 40.0 |
| SHRIMP PASTE, canned (USDA) | 1 oz. | 51 | .4 |
| SHRIMP PUFF, frozen (Durkee) | 1 piece | 44 | 3.0 |
| SHRIMP SOUP: | | | |
| Canned: | | | |
| *(Campbell) cream of, condensed | 10-oz. serving | 110 | 10.0 |
| *(Campbell) cream of, condensed, made with equal part milk | 10-oz. serving | 210 | 17.0 |
| (Crosse & Blackwell) | ½ of 13-oz. can | 90 | 7.0 |

(USDA): United States Department of Agriculture
(HEW/FAO): Health, Education and Welfare/Food and Agriculture Organization
* Prepared as Package Directs

| Food and Description | Measure or Quantity | Calories | Carbo-hydrates (grams) |
|---|---|---|---|
| **SHRIMP STICKS,** frozen (Mrs. Paul's) breaded & french fried | .8-oz. piece | 48 | 5.5 |
| **SIDE CAR COCKTAIL MIX** (Holland House) canned | 1½ fl. oz. | 66 | 16.5 |
| **SIP 'N SLIM COCKTAIL MIX** (Holland House) canned | 2 fl. oz. | 19 | 5.1 |
| **SKATE,** raw, meat only (USDA) | 4 oz. | 111 | 0. |
| **SLENDER** (Carnation): | | | |
| Bars: | | | |
| Chocolate | 1 bar | 138 | 11.5 |
| Cinnamon & vanilla | 1 bar | 138 | 12.0 |
| Dry: | | | |
| Chocolate | 1-oz. pkg. | 110 | 20.0 |
| Chocolate malt | 1-oz. pkg. | 110 | 20.0 |
| Coffee | 1-oz. pkg. | 110 | 21.0 |
| Dutch chocolate | 1-oz. pkg. | 110 | 20.0 |
| French vanilla | 1-oz. pkg. | 110 | 21.0 |
| Wild strawberry | 1-oz. pkg. | 110 | 21.0 |
| Liquid, all flavors | 10-fl.-oz. can | 225 | 34.0 |
| **SLOE GIN** (See **GIN, SLOE**) | | | |
| **SLOPPY JOE:** | | | |
| Canned: | | | |
| (Hormel) *Short Orders* | 7½-oz. can | 340 | 15.0 |
| (Libby's): | | | |
| Beef | ⅔ cup (2½ oz.) | 119 | 6.0 |
| Pork | ⅔ cup (2½ oz.) | 103 | 5.7 |
| (Morton House) barbecue sauce with beef | ⅓ of 15-oz. can | 240 | 19.0 |
| (Nalley's) | 8-oz. serving | 348 | 24.0 |
| Frozen: | | | |
| (Banquet) | 5-oz. bag | 199 | 11.2 |
| (Green Giant) with tomato sauce & beef, *Toast Topper* | 5-oz. serving | 154 | 14.3 |

| Food and Description | Measure or Quantity | Calories | Carbo-hydrates (grams) |
|---|---|---|---|
| **SLOPPY JOE SEASONING MIX:** | | | |
| (Ann Page) | 1½-oz. pkg. | 127 | 28.8 |
| *(Durkee) | 1¼ cups | 727 | 30.0 |
| *(Durkee) pizza flavor | 1¼ cups | 746 | 26.0 |
| (French's) | 1½-oz. pkg. | 128 | 32.0 |
| **SMELT, Atlantic, jack & bay (USDA):** | | | |
| Raw, whole | 1 lb. (weighed whole) | 244 | 0. |
| Raw, meat only | 4 oz. | 111 | 0. |
| Canned, solids & liq. | 4 oz. | 227 | 0. |
| **SMOKIE SAUSAGE:** | | | |
| (Eckrich): | | | |
| Beef, Smok-Y-Links | .8-oz. link | 75 | 1.0 |
| Maple flavor, Smok-Y-Links | .8-oz. link | 75 | 1.0 |
| Meat | 1-oz. portion | 105 | .5 |
| Skinless | 1.2-oz. link | 115 | 1.0 |
| Skinless, Smok-Y-Link | 8-oz. link | 85 | 1.0 |
| (Vienna) | 2½-oz. serving | 196 | .9 |
| **SNACK (See CRACKER, POPCORN, POTATO CHIP, etc.)** | | | |
| **SNAIL, raw (USDA):** | | | |
| Unspecified kind | 4 oz. | 102 | 2.3 |
| Giant African | 4 oz. | 83 | 5.0 |
| **SNAPPER (See RED SNAPPER)** | | | |
| *SNO BALLS* (Hostess) | 1½-oz. cake | 140 | 25.1 |
| **SOAVE WINE,** Italian white (Antinori) 12% alcohol | 3 fl. oz. | 84 | 6.3 |

(USDA): United States Department of Agriculture
(HEW/FAO): Health, Education and Welfare/Food and Agriculture Organization
* Prepared as Package Directs

| Food and Description | Measure or Quantity | Calories | Carbo-hydrates (grams) |
|---|---|---|---|
| **SOFT DRINK:** | | | |
| Sweetened: | | | |
| *Aspen* | 6 fl. oz. | 81 | 18.6 |
| Birch beer: | | | |
| (Pennsylvania Dutch) | 6 fl. oz. | 84 | 19.7 |
| (Yukon Club) | 6 fl. oz. | 89 | 22.3 |
| Bitter lemon: | | | |
| (Canada Dry) | 6 fl. oz. | 77 | 19.2 |
| (Schweppes) | 6 fl. oz. | 84 | 20.3 |
| *Bubble Up* | 6 fl. oz. | 73 | 18.4 |
| Cherry: | | | |
| (Canada Dry) wild | 6 fl. oz. | 96 | 24.0 |
| (Cott) | 6 fl. oz. | 94 | 23.0 |
| (Mission) | 6 fl. oz. | 94 | 23.0 |
| (Shasta) black | 6 fl. oz. | 86 | 21.7 |
| Chocolate: | | | |
| (Cott) cream | 6 fl. oz. | 92 | 22.0 |
| (Mission) cream | 6 fl. oz. | 92 | 22.0 |
| (Yoo-Hoo) high protein | 6 fl. oz. | 108 | 24.1 |
| Club soda (all brands) | 6 fl. oz. | 0 | 0. |
| Coconut (Yoo-Hoo) | 6 fl. oz. | 89 | 18.0 |
| Coffee (Hoffman) | 6 fl. oz. | 70 | 17.5 |
| Cola: | | | |
| (Canada Dry) *Jamaica* | 6 fl. oz. | 79 | 19.8 |
| *Coca-Cola* | 6 fl. oz. | 72 | 18.0 |
| *Pepsi-Cola* | 6 fl. oz. | 79 | 19.8 |
| (Royal Crown) | 6 fl. oz. | 78 | 19.4 |
| (Shasta) | 6 fl. oz. | 77 | 19.4 |
| (Shasta) cherry | 6 fl. oz. | 74 | 18.4 |
| Cream: | | | |
| (Canada Dry) vanilla | 6 fl. oz. | 96 | 24.0 |
| (Schweppes) red | 6 fl. oz. | 86 | 21.3 |
| (Shasta) | 6 fl. oz. | 81 | 20.3 |
| Dr. Brown's Cel-Ray Tonic | 6 fl. oz. | 66 | 16.5 |
| *Dr. Nehi* (Royal Crown) | 6 fl. oz. | 73 | 18.3 |
| *Dr. Pepper* | 6 fl. oz. | 72 | 18.6 |
| Fruit punch (Shasta) | 6 fl. oz. | 84 | 23.0 |
| Ginger ale: | | | |
| (Canada Dry) | 6 fl. oz. | 65 | 15.6 |
| (Fanta) | 6 fl. oz. | 63 | 15.8 |
| (Royal Crown) | 6 fl. oz. | 66 | 16.4 |
| (Schweppes) | 6 fl. oz. | 66 | 16.3 |

| Food and Description | Measure or Quantity | Calories | Carbo-hydrates (grams) |
|---|---|---|---|
| (Shasta) | 6 fl. oz. | 59 | 16.0 |
| Ginger beer (Schweppes) | 6 fl. oz. | 72 | 16.8 |
| Grape: | | | |
| (Canada Dry) concord | 6 fl. oz. | 96 | 24.0 |
| (Fanta) | 6 fl. oz. | 86 | 21.8 |
| (Nehi) | 6 fl. oz. | 80 | 19.9 |
| (Patio) | 6 fl. oz. | 96 | 24.0 |
| (Schweppes) | 6 fl. oz. | 97 | 15.7 |
| (Shasta) | 6 fl. oz. | 86 | 23.5 |
| Grapefruit (Shasta) | 6 fl. oz. | 87 | 21.5 |
| *Hi Spot* (Canada Dry) | 6 fl. oz. | 74 | 18.6 |
| Lemonade: | | | |
| (Hi-C) | 6 fl. oz. | 80 | 20.0 |
| (Shasta) | 6 fl. oz. | 71 | 19.0 |
| Lemon-lime (Shasta) | 6 fl. oz. | 70 | 19.0 |
| *Mello Yello* | 6 fl. oz. | 87 | 22.5 |
| *Mountain Dew* | 6 fl. oz. | 89 | 22.2 |
| *Mr. PiBB* | 6 fl. oz. | 70 | 18.8 |
| Orange: | | | |
| (Canada Dry) *Sunripe* | 6 fl. oz. | 90 | 14.1 |
| (Fanta) | 6 fl. oz. | 88 | 22.5 |
| (Hi-C) | 6 fl. oz. | 92 | 23.0 |
| (Nedick's) | 6 fl. oz. | 91 | 22.6 |
| (Nehi) | 6 fl. oz. | 94 | 23.4 |
| (Patio) | 6 fl. oz. | 96 | 24.0 |
| (Schweppes) Sparkling | 6 fl. oz. | 89 | 22.0 |
| (Shasta) | 6 fl. oz. | 86 | 23.5 |
| (Sunkist) | 6 fl. oz. | 96 | 7.6 |
| Quinine or Tonic Water | | | |
| (Canada Dry) | 6 fl. oz. | 70 | 16.1 |
| *Rondo* (Schweppes) | 6 fl. oz. | 77 | 19.6 |
| Root beer: | | | |
| *Barrelhead* (Canada Dry) | 6 fl. oz. | 79 | 19.8 |
| (Dad's) | 6 fl. oz. | 79 | 19.6 |
| (Fanta) | 6 fl. oz. | 77 | 20.3 |
| *On Tap* | 6 fl. oz. | 81 | 20.4 |
| (Patio) | 6 fl. oz. | 83 | 21.0 |

(USDA): United States Department of Agriculture
(HEW/FAO): Health, Education and Welfare/Food and Agriculture Organization
\* Prepared as Package Directs

| Food and Description | Measure or Quantity | Calories | Carbo- hydrates (grams) |
|---|---|---|---|
| *Rooti* (Canada Dry) | 6 fl. oz. | 79 | 19.8 |
| (Royal Crown) | 6 fl. oz. | 87 | 21.7 |
| (Schweppes) | 6 fl. oz. | 79 | 19.3 |
| (Shasta) draft | 6 fl. oz. | 75 | 20.5 |
| *Seven-Up* | 6 fl. oz. | 72 | 18.1 |
| *Sprite* | 6 fl. oz. | 71 | 18.0 |
| Strawberry: | | | |
| (Canada Dry) California | 6 fl. oz. | 89 | 22.3 |
| (Shasta) | 6 fl. oz. | 72 | 19.5 |
| (Yoo-Hoo) | 6 fl. oz. | 95 | 20.9 |
| *Tahitian Treat* (Canada Dry) | 6 fl. oz. | 96 | 24.1 |
| *Teem* | 6 fl. oz. | 61 | 18.6 |
| Tom Collins or Collins mix (Canada Dry) | 6 fl. oz. | 60 | 15.0 |
| *Upper 10* (Royal Crown) | 6 fl. oz. | 76 | 19.0 |
| Vanilla (Yoo-Hoo) | 6 fl. oz. | 93 | 20.4 |
| Vanilla cream (Canada Dry) | 6 fl. oz. | 88 | 22.0 |
| *Wink* (Canada Dry) | 6 fl. oz. | 91 | 22.7 |
| Dietetic or low calorie: | | | |
| *Bubble Up* | 6 fl. oz. | 1 | .2 |
| Cherry: | | | |
| (Shasta) black | 6 fl. oz. | 0 | 0. |
| (Tab) black | 6 fl. oz. | 2 | Tr. |
| Chocolate mint (No-Cal) | 6 fl. oz. | 2 | <.1 |
| Citrus, *Flair* | 6 fl. oz. | 1 | .2 |
| Cola: | | | |
| (Canada Dry) | 6 fl. oz. | <1 | .6 |
| *Diet Rite* | 6 fl. oz. | <1 | Tr. |
| (No-Cal) | 6 fl. oz. | 0 | <.1 |
| *Pepsi,* diet | 6 fl. oz. | <1 | <.1 |
| *Pepsi Light* | 6 fl. oz. | <1 | <.1 |
| (Shasta) | 6 fl. oz. | 0 | 0. |
| (Shasta) cherry | 6 fl. oz. | 0 | 0. |
| *Tab* | 6 fl. oz. | <1 | <.1 |
| Cream: | | | |
| (No-Cal) | 6 fl. oz. | 0 | <.1 |
| (Shasta) | 6 fl. oz. | 0 | 0. |
| Dr. Brown's Cel-Ray Tonic | 6 fl. oz. | 1 | .2 |
| Dr. Pepper | 6 fl. oz. | 2 | .4 |

| Food and Description | Measure or Quantity | Calories | Carbo-hydrates (grams) |
|---|---|---|---|
| *Fresca* | 6 fl. oz. | 1 | 0. |
| Ginger ale: | | | |
| (Canada Dry) | 6 fl. oz. | <1 | 0. |
| (No-Cal) | 6 fl. oz. | 0 | Tr. |
| (Shasta) | 6 fl. oz. | 0 | 0. |
| *Tab* | 6 fl. oz. | 2 | Tr. |
| Grape: | | | |
| (Shasta) | 6 fl. oz. | 0 | 0. |
| *Tab* | 6 fl. oz. | 2 | 0. |
| Grapefruit (Shasta) | 6 fl. oz. | <1 | .2 |
| Lemon-lime: | | | |
| (Shasta) | 6 fl. oz. | 0 | 0. |
| *Tab* | 6 fl. oz. | 2 | 0. |
| *Mr. PiBB* | 6 fl. oz. | <1 | 0. |
| Orange: | | | |
| (No-Cal) | 6 fl. oz. | 0 | 0. |
| (Shasta) | 6 fl. oz. | 0 | 0. |
| *Tab* | 6 fl. oz. | <1 | 0. |
| *Red Pop* (No-Cal) | 6 fl. oz. | 0 | 0. |
| *Rondo* (Schweppes) | 6 fl. oz. | <1 | Tr. |
| Root beer: | | | |
| *Barrelhead* (Canada Dry) | 6 fl. oz. | <1 | .8 |
| (Dad's) | 6 fl. oz. | <1 | .2 |
| (No-Cal) | 6 fl. oz. | 0 | Tr. |
| (Shasta) draft | 6 fl. oz. | 0 | 0. |
| *Tab* | 6 fl. oz. | 1 | .2 |
| *Seven-Up* | 6 fl. oz. | 2 | 0. |
| *Shape-Up* (No-Cal) | 6 fl. oz. | 0 | 0. |
| *Sprite* | 6 fl. oz. | 2 | 0. |
| Strawberry: | | | |
| (Shasta) | 6 fl. oz. | 0 | 0. |
| *Tab* | 6 fl. oz. | <2 | 0. |
| *Tab* | 6 fl. oz. | <1 | .1 |
| Tea (No-Cal) | 6 fl. oz. | 0 | 0. |
| *TNT* (No-Cal) | 6 fl. oz. | 0 | 0. |

(USDA): United States Department of Agriculture
(HEW/FAO): Health, Education and Welfare/Food and Agriculture Organization
* Prepared as Package Directs

| Food and Description | Measure or Quantity | Calories | Carbo-hydrates (grams) |
|---|---|---|---|
| **SOLE:** | | | |
| Raw (USDA): | | | |
| Whole | 1 lb. (weighed whole) | 118 | 0. |
| Meat only | 4 oz. | 90 | 0. |
| Frozen: | | | |
| (Mrs. Paul's): | | | |
| Fillets, breaded & fried | ½ of 8-oz. pkg. | 225 | 21.8 |
| Fillets, with lemon butter | ½ of 8½-oz. pkg. | 155 | 9.7 |
| (Van de Kamp's) batter dipped, french fried | 2.4-oz. piece | 140 | 12.0 |
| (Weight Watchers): | | | |
| 2-compartment meal | 9½-oz. meal | 208 | 14.0 |
| 3-compartment meal | 16-oz. meal | 245 | 14.1 |
| **SORGHUM** (USDA): | | | |
| Grain | 1 oz. | 94 | 20.7 |
| Syrup | 1 T. (.7 oz.) | 54 | 12.2 |
| **SORREL** (See DOCK) | | | |
| **SOUFFLÉ,** frozen (Stouffer's): | | | |
| Cheese | ⅓ of 12-oz. pkg. | 241 | 9.3 |
| Corn | ⅓ of 12-oz. pkg. | 154 | 18.9 |
| **SOUP** (See individual listings by kind) | | | |
| **SOUP GREENS** (Durkee) | 2½-oz. jar | 216 | 43.0 |
| **SOURSOP,** raw (USDA): | | | |
| Whole | 1 lb. (weighed with skin & seeds) | 200 | 50.3 |
| Flesh only | 4 oz. | 74 | 18.5 |
| **SOUSE** (USDA) | 1 oz. | 51 | .3 |
| **SOUTHERN COMFORT:** | | | |
| 80 proof | 1 fl. oz. | 79 | 3.4 |
| 90 proof | 1 fl. oz. | 87 | 3.5 |
| 100 proof | 1 fl. oz. | 96 | 3.5 |

| Food and Description | Measure or Quantity | Calories | Carbo-hydrates (grams) |
|---|---|---|---|
| **SOYBEAN:** | | | |
| (USDA): | | | |
| Young seeds: | | | |
| Raw | 1 lb. (weighed in pod) | 322 | 31.7 |
| Boiled, drained | 4 oz. | 134 | 11.5 |
| Canned, solids & liq. | 4 oz. | 85 | 7.1 |
| Canned, drained solids | 4 oz. | 117 | 8.4 |
| Mature seeds, dry: | | | |
| Raw | 1 lb. | 1828 | 152.0 |
| Raw | 1 cup (7.4 oz.) | 846 | 70.4 |
| Cooked | 4 oz. | 147 | 12.2 |
| Oil roasted: | | | |
| (Soy Ahoy) | 1 oz. | 152 | 4.8 |
| (Soy Ahoy) barbecue or garlic | 1 oz. | 152 | 4.8 |
| (Soytown) | 1 oz. | 152 | 4.8 |
| **SOYBEAN CURD or TOFU** | | | |
| (USDA): | | | |
| Regular | 4 oz. | 82 | 2.7 |
| Cake | 4.2-oz. cake | 86 | 2.9 |
| **SOYBEAN FLOUR (See FLOUR)** | | | |
| **SOYBEAN GRITS, high fat** (USDA) | 1 cup (4.9 oz.) | 524 | 46.0 |
| **SOYBEAN MILK (USDA):** | | | |
| Fluid | 4 oz. | 37 | 1.5 |
| Powder | 1 oz. | 122 | 7.9 |
| **SOYBEAN PROTEIN** (USDA) | 1 oz. | 91 | 4.3 |
| **SOYBEAN PROTEINATE** (USDA) | 1 oz. | 88 | 2.2 |

(USDA): United States Department of Agriculture
(HEW/FAO): Health, Education and Welfare/Food and Agriculture
Organization
* Prepared as Package Directs

| Food and Description | Measure or Quantity | Calories | Carbo-hydrates (grams) |
|---|---|---|---|
| **SOYBEAN SPROUT** (See BEAN SPROUT) | | | |
| **SOY SAUCE** (See SAUCE) | | | |
| **SPAGHETTI.** Plain spaghetti products are essentially the same in caloric value and carbohydrate content on the same weight basis. The longer the cooking, the more water is absorbed and this affects the nutritive value (USDA): | | | |
| Dry | 1 oz. | 105 | 21.3 |
| Dry, broken | 1 cup (2.5 oz.) | 262 | 53.4 |
| Cooked: | | | |
| 8-10 minutes, "al dente" | 1 cup (5.1 oz.) | 216 | 43.9 |
| 8-10 minutes, "al dente" | 4 oz. | 168 | 34.1 |
| 14-20 minutes, tender | 1 cup (4.9 oz.) | 155 | 32.2 |
| 14-20 minutes, tender | 4 oz. | 126 | 26.1 |
| **SPAGHETTI MEAL:** | | | |
| Canned (Franco-American): | | | |
| With meat sauce | 7¾-oz. serving | 220 | 26.0 |
| With tomato sauce & cheese | ½ of 14¾-oz. can | 170 | 33.0 |
| *Mix (Ann Page) Italian style | ¼ of 8-oz. pkg. | 205 | 37.4 |
| **SPAGHETTI & FRANKFURTERS,** canned (Franco-American) in tomato sauce, *Spaghetti-Os* | ½ of 14¾-oz. can | 210 | 26.0 |
| **SPAGHETTI & MEATBALLS IN TOMATO SAUCE:** | | | |
| Home recipe (USDA) | 1 cup (8.7 oz.) | 332 | 38.7 |
| Canned, regular pack: | | | |
| (USDA) | 1 cup (8.8 oz.) | 258 | 28.5 |
| (Franco-American): | | | |
| Regular | 7¼-oz. can | 210 | 23.0 |
| *Spaghetti-Os* | ½ of 14¾-oz. can | 210 | 24.0 |
| (Hormel) *Short Orders* | 7½-oz. can | 210 | 24.0 |

| Food and Description | Measure or Quantity | Calories | Carbo-hydrates (grams) |
|---|---|---|---|
| (Libby's) | ½ of 15-oz. can | 189 | 27.5 |
| (Nalley's) | 8-oz. can | 245 | 31.8 |
| Canned, dietetic or low calorie: | | | |
| (Dia-Mel) | 8-oz. can | 200 | 24.0 |
| (Featherweight) | 8-oz. can | 220 | 28.0 |
| Frozen: | | | |
| (Banquet): | | | |
| Buffet | 2-lb. pkg. | 1127 | 129.1 |
| Dinner | 11½-oz. dinner | 450 | 62.9 |
| (Green Giant) | 9-oz. entree | 269 | 29.1 |
| (Morton) | 11-oz. dinner | 344 | 59.4 |
| (Swanson) | 12½-oz. dinner | 410 | 57.0 |
| (Swanson) *Hungry Man* | 18½-oz. dinner | 660 | 83.0 |
| **SPAGHETTI WITH MEAT SAUCE**, frozen: | | | |
| (Banquet) | 8-oz. entree | 311 | 31.3 |
| (Stouffer's) | 14-oz. pkg. | 442 | 61.6 |
| **SPAGHETTI SAUCE** (See also **SPAGHETTI SAUCE MIX** and **SAUCE**, Italian): | | | |
| Clam (Ragu) chopped | 5-oz. serving | 110 | 14.0 |
| Marinara: | | | |
| (Ann Page) | ¼ of 15½-oz. jar | 70 | 12.3 |
| (Prince) | 4-oz. serving | 80 | 12.4 |
| (Ragu) | 5-oz. serving | 120 | 15.0 |
| Meat-flavored: | | | |
| (Ann Page) | ¼ of 15½-oz. jar | 81 | 12.3 |
| (Ragu) | 5-oz. serving | 115 | 14.0 |
| Meat: | | | |
| (Prince) | ½ cup (4.9 oz.) | 101 | 11.1 |
| (Ragu) extra thick & zesty | 5-oz. serving | 130 | 14.0 |
| (Ronzoni) | 4-oz. serving | 87 | 11.0 |
| Meatless or plain: | | | |
| (Ann Page) with mushroom | ¼ of 15½-oz. jar | 75 | 12.5 |

(USDA): United States Department of Agriculture
(HEW/FAO): Health, Education and Welfare/Food and Agriculture Organization
* Prepared as Package Directs

| Food and Description | Measure or Quantity | Calories | Carbohydrates (grams) |
|---|---|---|---|
| (Ann Page) plain | ¼ of 15½-oz. jar | 76 | 12.9 |
| (Prince) | ½ cup (4.6 oz.) | 90 | 11.4 |
| (Ragu) | 5-oz. serving | 105 | 14.0 |
| (Ragu) extra thick & zesty | 5-oz. serving | 120 | 13.0 |
| (Ronzoni) | 4-oz. serving | 78 | 13.0 |
| Mushroom: | | | |
| (Prince) | 4-oz. serving | 77 | 11.3 |
| (Ragu) | 5-oz. serving | 105 | 13.0 |
| (Ragu) extra thick & zesty | 5-oz. serving | 110 | 14.0 |
| Pepperoni (Ragu) | 5-oz. serving | 120 | 14.0 |
| Dietetic (Featherweight) low sodium | 5-oz. serving | 80 | 10.0 |
| **SPAGHETTI SAUCE MIX:** | | | |
| (Ann Page): | | | |
| With mushrooms | 1½-oz. pkg. | 125 | 26.7 |
| Without mushrooms | 1½-oz. pkg. | 128 | 27.0 |
| *(Durkee) | 2½ cups | 224 | 52.0 |
| *(Durkee) mushroom | 2⅔ cups | 208 | 48.0 |
| (French's) Italian style | 1½-oz. pkg. | 121 | 26.8 |
| (French's) with mushroom | 1¾-oz. pkg. | 125 | 19.0 |
| *(Spatini) | 2-oz. serving | 80 | 4.0 |
| *SPAM* (Hormel): | | | |
| Regular | 3-oz. serving | 264 | 3.2 |
| & cheese, chunk | 3-oz. serving | 261 | 2.1 |
| Deviled | 1 T. (.5 oz.) | 38 | 0. |
| Smoke flavored | 3-oz. serving | 263 | .8 |
| **SPANISH MACKEREL, raw (USDA):** | | | |
| Whole | 1 lb. (weighed whole) | 490 | 0. |
| Meat only | 4 oz. | 201 | 0. |
| *SPECIAL K,* cereal (Kellogg's) | 1¼ cups (1 oz.) | 110 | 21.0 |
| **SPINACH:** | | | |
| Raw (USDA): | | | |
| Untrimmed | 1 lb. (weighed with large stems & roots) | 85 | 14.0 |
| Trimmed or packaged | 1 lb. | 118 | 19.5 |

| Food and Description | Measure or Quantity | Calories | Carbohydrates (grams) |
|---|---|---|---|
| Trimmed, whole leaves | 1 cup (1.2 oz.) | 9 | 1.4 |
| Trimmed, chopped | 1 cup (1.8 oz.) | 14 | 2.2 |
| Boiled, whole leaves | | | |
| (USDA drained | 1 cup (5.5 oz.) | 36 | 5.6 |
| Canned, regular pack: | | | |
| (USDA): | | | |
| Solids & liq. | ½ cup (4.1 oz.) | 22 | 3.5 |
| Drained solids | ½ cup | 27 | 4.0 |
| (Del Monte) solids & liq. | ½ cup (4.1 oz.) | 28 | 3.4 |
| (Libby's) solids & liq. | ½ cup (4.2 oz.) | 27 | 3.6 |
| Canned, dietetic or low calorie: | | | |
| (USDA) low sodium: | | | |
| Solids & liq. | 4 oz. | 24 | 3.9 |
| Drained solids | 4 oz. | 29 | 4.5 |
| (Blue Boy) solids & liq. | 4-oz. serving | 22 | 2.4 |
| (Featherweight) low sodium | ½ cup | 30 | 4.0 |
| Frozen: | | | |
| (USDA) chopped, boiled drained | 4 oz. | 26 | 4.2 |
| (Birds Eye): | | | |
| Chopped or leaf | ⅓ of 10-oz. pkg. | 23 | 2.7 |
| Creamed | ⅓ of 9-oz. pkg. | 57 | 4.0 |
| (Green Giant): | | | |
| In butter sauce | ⅓ of 10-oz. pkg. | 43 | 2.3 |
| Creamed | ⅓ of 10-oz. pkg. | 69 | 7.8 |
| Souffle, *Bake 'n Serve* | ⅓ of 10-oz. pkg. | 109 | 8.2 |
| (McKenzie) | ⅓ of 10-oz. pkg. | 27 | 3.3 |
| (Seabrook Farms) chopped or whole | ⅓ of 10-oz. pkg. | 27 | 3.3 |
| (Stouffer's) souffle | ⅓ of 12-oz. pkg. | 130 | 11.9 |
| **SPINY LOBSTER** (See **CRAYFISH**) | | | |
| **SPLEEN**, raw (USDA): | | | |
| Beef & calf | 4 oz. | 118 | 0. |

(USDA): United States Department of Agriculture
(HEW/FAO): Health, Education and Welfare/Food and Agriculture Organization
* Prepared as Package Directs

| Food and Description | Measure or Quantity | Calories | Carbohydrates (grams) |
|---|---|---|---|
| Hog | 4 oz. | 121 | 0. |
| Lamb | 4 oz. | 130 | 0. |
| **SQUAB**, pigeon, raw (USDA): | | | |
| Dressed | 1 lb. (weighed with feet, inedible viscera & bones) | 569 | 0. |
| Meat & skin | 4 oz. | 333 | 0. |
| Meat only | 4 oz. | 161 | 0. |
| Light meat only, without skin | 4 oz. | 142 | 0. |
| Giblets | 1 oz. | 44 | .3 |
| **SQUASH SEEDS**, dry (USDA): | | | |
| In hull | 4 oz. | 464 | 12.6 |
| Hulled | 1 oz. | 157 | 4.3 |
| **SQUASH, SUMMER:** | | | |
| Fresh (USDA): | | | |
| Crookneck & straightneck, yellow: | | | |
| Whole | 1 lb. (weighed untrimmed) | 89 | 19.1 |
| Boiled, drained, diced | ½ cup (3.6 oz.) | 15 | 3.2 |
| Boiled, drained, slices | ½ cup (3.1 oz.) | 13 | 2.7 |
| Scallop, white & pale green: | | | |
| Whole | 1 lb. (weighed untrimmed) | 93 | 22.7 |
| Boiled, drained, mashed | ½ cup (4.2 oz.) | 19 | 4.5 |
| Zucchini & cocazelle, green: | | | |
| Whole | 1 lb. (weighed untrimmed) | 73 | 15.5 |
| Boiled, drained slices | ½ cup (2.7 oz.) | 9 | 1.9 |
| Canned (Del Monte) zucchini, in tomato sauce | ½ cup (4.1 oz.) | 37 | 7.9 |
| Frozen: (USDA): | | | |
| Unthawed | 4 oz. | 24 | 5.3 |
| Boiled, drained | 4 oz. | 24 | 5.3 |

| Food and Description | Measure or Quantity | Calories | Carbohydrates (grams) |
|---|---|---|---|
| (Birds Eye): | | | |
| Sliced | ⅓ of 10-oz. pkg. | 18 | 4.0 |
| Zucchini | ⅓ of 10-oz. pkg. | 16 | 3.0 |
| (Green Giant) in cheese sauce. Southern recipe | ⅓ of 10-oz. pkg. | 41 | 5.1 |
| (McKenzie): | | | |
| Crookneck, yellow | 3.3-oz. serving | 22 | 3.8 |
| Zucchini | 3½-oz. serving | 20 | 3.6 |
| (Mrs. Paul's): | | | |
| Zucchini parmesan | ½ of 12-oz. pkg. | 493 | 93.2 |
| Zucchini sticks, batter fried | ½ of 9-oz. pkg. | 186 | 23.1 |
| (Seabrook Farms): | | | |
| Crookneck, yellow | ⅓ of 10-oz. pkg. | 22 | 3.8 |
| Zucchini | 3½-oz. serving | 20 | 3.6 |
| **SQUASH, WINTER:** | | | |
| Fresh (USDA): | | | |
| Acorn: | | | |
| Whole | 1 lb. (weighed with skin & seeds) | 152 | 38.6 |
| Baked, flesh only, mashed | ½ cup (3.6 oz.) | 56 | 14.3 |
| Boiled, mashed | ½ cup (4.1 oz.) | 39 | 9.7 |
| Butternut: | | | |
| Whole | 1 lb. (weighed with skin & seeds) | 171 | 44.4 |
| Baked, flesh only | 4 oz. | 77 | 19.8 |
| Boiled, flesh only | 4 oz. | 46 | 11.8 |
| Hubbard: | | | |
| Whole | 1 lb. (weighed with skin & seeds) | 117 | 28.1 |
| Baked, flesh only | 4 oz. | 57 | 13.3 |
| Boiled, flesh only, diced | ½ cup (4.2 oz.) | 35 | 8.1 |
| Boiled. flesh only, mashed | ½ cup (4.3 oz.) | 37 | 8.4 |
| Frozen: | | | |
| (USDA) heated | ½ cup (4.2 oz.) | 46 | 11.0 |
| (Birds Eye) | ⅓ pkg. | 50 | 11.0 |

(USDA): United States Department of Agriculture
(HEW/FAO): Health, Education and Welfare/Food and Agriculture
Organization
* Prepared as Package Directs

| Food and Description | Measure or Quantity | Calories | Carbohydrates (grams) |
|---|---|---|---|
| **SQUID**, raw, meat only (USDA) | 4 oz. | 95 | 1.7 |
| ***SQUOZE** (Pillsbury) all flavors | 8 fl. oz. | 40 | 10.0 |
| **STARCH** (See **CORNSTARCH**) | | | |
| ***START**, instant breakfast drink | ½ cup | 51 | 12.7 |
| **STEAK & GREEN PEPPERS**, frozen (Swanson) in oriental-style sauce | 8½-oz. entree | 200 | 11.0 |
| ***STOCKPOT SOUP** (Campbell) condensed, vegetable & beef | 10-oz. serving | 120 | 12.0 |
| **STOMACH, PORK**, scalded (USDA) | 4 oz. | 172 | 0. |
| **STRAINED FOOD** (See **BABY FOOD**) | | | |
| **STRAWBERRY:** | | | |
| Fresh (USDA): | | | |
| Whole | 1 lb. (weighed with caps & stems) | 161 | 36.6 |
| Whole, capped | 1 cup (5.1 oz.) | 53 | 12.1 |
| Canned (USDA) unsweetened or low calorie, water pack, solids & liq. | 4 oz. | 25 | 6.4 |
| Frozen (Birds Eye): | | | |
| Halves | ⅓ of 16-oz. pkg. | 196 | 48.2 |
| Whole | ¼ of 16-oz. pkg. | 97 | 23.2 |
| Whole, quick thaw | ½ of 10-oz. pkg. | 123 | 29.7 |
| **STRAWBERRY DRINK** (Hi-C): | | | |
| Canned | 6 fl. oz. | 89 | 22.0 |
| *Mix | 6 fl. oz. | 76 | 19.0 |

| Food and Description | Measure or Quantity | Calories | Carbo-hydrates (grams) |
|---|---|---|---|
| **STRAWBERRY ICE CREAM:** | | | |
| (Breyer's) | ¼ pt. | 130 | 17.0 |
| (Breyer's) twin | ¼ pt. | 140 | 20.0 |
| (Dean) 10.5% fat | 1 cup (5.6 oz.) | 336 | 40.0 |
| (Meadow Gold) | ¼ pt. | 140 | 19.0 |
| (Sealtest) | ¼ pt. | 130 | 18.0 |
| (Swift's) sweet cream | ½ cup | 124 | 15.3 |
| **STRAWBERRY JELLY:** | | | |
| Sweetened (Smucker's) | 1 T. | 53 | 13.5 |
| Dietetic or low calorie (Featherweight) | 1 T. | 16 | 4.0 |
| **STRAWBERRY PRESERVES** **or JAM:** | | | |
| Sweetened (Smucker's) | 1 T. | 53 | 13.5 |
| Dietetic or low calorie: | | | |
| (Dia-Mel) | 1 tsp. (6 grams) | 2 | 0. |
| (Diet Delight) | 1 T. | 13 | 3.2 |
| (Featherweight) | 1 T. | 16 | 4.0 |
| (Featherweight) artificially sweetened | 1 T. | 4 | 1.0 |
| (Louis Sherry) wild | 1 tsp. | 2 | 0. |
| (Slenderella) imitation | 1 T. | 24 | 6.0 |
| (Tillie Lewis) *Tasti Diet* | 1 T. | 11 | 2.8 |
| **STRAWBERRY SPREAD,** low sugar (Smucker's) | 1 T. | 24 | 6.0 |
| **STRAWBERRY SYRUP:** | | | |
| Sweetened (Smucker's) | 1 T. | 50 | 13.0 |
| Dietetic or low calorie (Featherweight) | 1 T. | 14 | 3.0 |
| **STUFFING MIX:** | | | |
| *Chicken, *Stove Top* | ½ cup | 170 | 21.0 |
| Cornbread: (Pepperidge Farm) | 8-oz. pkg. | 880 | 168.0 |

(USDA): United States Department of Agriculture
(HEW/FAO): Health, Education and Welfare/Food and Agriculture
Organization
* Prepared as Package Directs

| Food and Description | Measure or Quantity | Calories | Carbo-hydrates (grams) |
|---|---|---|---|
| *Stove Top | ½ cup | 170 | 20.0 |
| Herb seasoned (Pepperidge Farm) | 8-oz. pkg. | 880 | 168.0 |
| *Pork, Stove Top | ½ cup | 170 | 20.0 |
| *With rice, Stove Top | ½ cup | 180 | 23.0 |
| White bread, Mrs. Cubbison's | 1 oz. | 101 | 20.5 |
| **STURGEON** (USDA): | | | |
| Raw: | | | |
| Section | 1 lb. (weighed with skin & bones) | 362 | 0. |
| Meat only | 4 oz. | 107 | 0. |
| Smoked | 4 oz. | 169 | 0. |
| Steamed | 4 oz. | 181 | 0. |
| **SUCCOTASH:** | | | |
| Canned: | | | |
| (Libby's): | | | |
| Cream style | ½ cup (4.6 oz.) | 111 | 22.8 |
| Whole kernel | ¼ of 16-oz. can | 82 | 16.0 |
| (Stokely-Van Camp) solids & liq. | ½ cup (4.5 oz.) | 85 | 17.5 |
| Frozen: | | | |
| (USDA) boiled, drained | ½ cup (3.4 oz.) | 89 | 19.7 |
| (Birds Eye) | ⅓ of 10-oz. pkg. | 80 | 17.0 |
| **SUCKER, CARP,** raw (USDA): | | | |
| Whole | 1 lb. (weighed whole) | 196 | 0. |
| Meat only | 4 oz. | 126 | 0. |
| **SUCKER,** including **WHITE MULLET,** raw (USDA): | | | |
| Whole | 1 lb. (weighed whole) | 203 | 0. |
| Meat only | 4 oz. | 118 | 0. |
| **SUET,** raw (USDA) | 1 oz. | 242 | 0. |

| Food and Description | Measure or Quantity | Calories | Carbo-hydrates (grams) |
|---|---|---|---|
| **SUGAR,** beet or cane (there are no differences in calories and carbohydrates among brands) (USDA): | | | |
| Brown: | | | |
| Regular | 1 lb. | 1692 | 437.3 |
| Brownulated | 1 cup (5.4 oz.) | 567 | 146.5 |
| Firm-packed | 1 cup (7.5 oz.) | 791 | 204.4 |
| Firm-packed | 1 T. (.5 oz.) | 48 | 12.5 |
| Confectioners': | | | |
| Unsifted | 1 cup (4.3 oz.) | 474 | 122.4 |
| Unsifted | 1 T. (8 grams) | 30 | 7.7 |
| Sifted | 1 cup (3.4 oz.) | 366 | 94.5 |
| Sifted | 1 T. (6 grams) | 23 | 5.9 |
| Stirred | 1 cup (4.2 oz.) | 462 | 119.4 |
| Stirred | 1 T. (8 grams) | 29 | 7.5 |
| Granulated | 1 lb. | 1746 | 451.3 |
| Granulated | 1 cup (6.9 oz.) | 751 | 194.0 |
| Granulated | 1 T. (.4 oz.) | 46 | 11.9 |
| Granulated | 1 lump (1⅛" x ¾" x ⅝", 6 grams) | 23 | 6.0 |
| Maple | 1 lb. | 1579 | 408.0 |
| Maple | 1¾" x 1¼" x ½" piece (1.2 oz.) | 104 | 27.0 |
| **SUGAR APPLE,** raw (USDA): | | | |
| Whole | 1 lb. (weighed with skin & seeds) | 192 | 48.4 |
| Flesh only | 4 oz. | 107 | 26.9 |
| ***SUGAR CRISP,*** cereal (Post) | ⅞ cup (1 oz.) | 113 | 25.5 |
| **SUGAR FROSTED FLAKES,** cereal: | | | |
| (Kellogg's) | ⅔ cup (1 oz.) | 110 | 26.0 |
| (Ralston Purina) | ¾ cup (1 oz.) | 110 | 26.0 |

(USDA): United States Department of Agriculture
(HEW/FAO): Health, Education and Welfare/Food and Agriculture
              Organization
* Prepared as Package Directs

| Food and Description | Measure or Quantity | Calories | Carbohydrates (grams) |
|---|---|---|---|
| **SUGAR POPS**, cereal (Kellogg's) | 1 cup (1 oz.) | 110 | 26.0 |
| **SUGAR SMACKS**, cereal (Kellogg's) | ¾ cup (1 oz.) | 110 | 25.0 |
| **SUGAR SUBSTITUTE:** | | | |
| *Sprinkle Sweet* (Pillsbury) | 1 tsp. | 2 | .5 |
| *Sugar-Like* (Dia-Mel) | 1-gram packet | 3 | 1.0 |
| *Sug'r Like* (Featherweight) | 1 tsp. | 2 | 1.0 |
| *Suprose* (Whitlock) | 1-gram packet | 4 | .9 |
| *Sweet'ner* (Weight Watchers) | 1-gram packet | 3 | 1.0 |
| *Sweet'n-it* (Dia-Mel) | | | |
| Liquid | 5 drops | 0 | .0 |
| *Sweet\* 10* (Pillsbury) | ⅛ tsp. | 0 | .0 |
| **\*SUKIYAKI DINNER** (Chun King) stir fry | ⅙ of pkg. | 100 | 3.0 |
| **SUNDAE**, canned, *Swiss Miss*: | | | |
| Chocolate | 4¼-oz. container | 190 | 28.0 |
| Vanilla | 4¼-oz. container | 180 | 26.0 |
| **SUNFLOWER SEED:** | | | |
| (USDA): | | | |
| In hulls | 4 oz. (weighed in hull) | 343 | 12.2 |
| Hulled | 1 oz. | 159 | 5.6 |
| (Flavor House) dry roasted | 1 oz. | 179 | 4.0 |
| (Frito-Lay's) | 1 oz. | 181 | 4.7 |
| (Planters) dry roasted | 1 oz. | 160 | 5.0 |
| (Planters) unsalted | 1 oz. | 170 | 5.0 |
| **SUNFLOWER SEED FLOUR** (See FLOUR) | | | |
| **SUZY Q** (Hostess): | | | |
| Banana | 2¼-oz. cake | 244 | 38.4 |
| Chocolate | 2½-oz. cake | 240 | 36.5 |
| **SWAMP CABBAGE** (USDA): | | | |
| Raw, whole | 1 lb. (weighed untrimmed) | 107 | 19.8 |

| Food and Description | Measure or Quantity | Calories | Carbo-hydrates (grams) |
|---|---|---|---|
| Boiled, trimmed, drained | 4 oz. | 24 | 4.4 |
| **SWEETBREADS** (USDA): | | | |
| Beef, raw | 1 lb. | 939 | 0. |
| Beef, braised | 4 oz. | 363 | 0. |
| Calf, raw | 1 lb. | 426 | 0. |
| Calf, braised | 4 oz. | 191 | 0. |
| Hog (See **PANCREAS**) | | | |
| Lamb, raw | 1 lb. | 426 | 0. |
| Lamb, braised | 4 oz. | 198 | 0. |
| **SWEET POTATO:** | | | |
| Raw (USDA): | | | |
| All kinds, unpared | 1 lb. (weighed whole) | 419 | 96.6 |
| All kinds, pared | 4 oz. | 129 | 29.8 |
| Firm-fleshed, Jersey types, pared | 4 oz. | 116 | 25.5 |
| Soft-fleshed, Puerto Rico variety, pared | 4 oz. | 133 | 31.0 |
| Baked (USDA) peeled after baking | 3.9-oz. sweet potato (5″ x 2″) | 155 | 35.8 |
| Baked (USDA) peeled after boiling | 5-oz. sweet potato (5″ x 2″) | 168 | 38.7 |
| Candied (USDA) home recipe | 6.2-oz. sweet potato (3½″ x 2¼″) | 294 | 59.8 |
| Canned, regular pack: (USDA): | | | |
| In syrup, solids & liq. | 4 oz. | 129 | 31.2 |
| Vacuum or solids pack | 4 oz. | 118 | 27.1 |
| (King Pharr) | ½ cup | 118 | 22.4 |
| (King Pharr) yam | ½ cup | 114 | 27.0 |

(USDA): United States Department of Agriculture
(HEW/FAO): Health, Education and Welfare/Food and Agriculture Organization
* Prepared as Package Directs

| Food and Description | Measure or Quantity | Calories | Carbo-hydrates (grams) |
|---|---|---|---|
| Canned, dietetic or low calorie, without added sugar & salt (USDA) | 4 oz. | 52 | 12.2 |
| Dehydrated flakes (USDA) dry | ½ cup (2 oz.) | 220 | 52.2 |
| *Dehydrated flakes (USDA) prepared with water | ½ cup (4.4 oz.) | 120 | 28.5 |
| Frozen: | | | |
| (Green Giant) glazed, Southern recipe | ⅓ of 10-oz. pkg. | 120 | 22.7 |
| (Mrs. Paul's): | | | |
| Candied, with apple | ⅓ of 12-oz. pkg. | 162 | 37.1 |
| Candied, yellow | ⅓ of 12-oz. pkg. | 182 | 44.3 |
| **SWEETSOP** (See **SUGAR APPLE**) | | | |
| *SWEET & SOUR DINNER (Chun King) stir fry | ⅕ pkg. | 140 | 10.0 |
| **SWEET & SOUR ORIENTAL,** canned (La Choy): | | | |
| With chicken | ½ of 17-oz. can | 340 | 71.1 |
| With pork | ½ of 17-oz. can | 361 | 69.0 |
| **SWISS STEAK,** frozen (Swanson) | 10-oz. dinner | 350 | 19.0 |
| **SWORDFISH** (USDA): | | | |
| Raw, meat only | 1 lb. | 535 | 0. |
| Broiled, with butter or margarine | 3″ x 3″ x ½″ steak (4.4 oz.) | 218 | 0. |
| Canned, solids & liq. | 4 oz. | 116 | 0. |
| **SYLVANDER WINE** (Louis M. Martini) 12½% alcohol | 3 fl. oz. | 90 | .2 |
| **SYRUP** (See individual listings by kind, such as **PANCAKE & WAFFLE SYRUP**, or by brand name, such as **LOG CABIN**) | | | |

| Food and Description | Measure or Quantity | Calories | Carbo- hydrates (grams) |
|---|---|---|---|

**I**

**TABASCO SAUCE** (See SAUCE, Tabasco)

**TACO:**

| | | | |
|---|---|---|---|
| *(Ortega) | 1 taco | 220 | 13.0 |
| Seasoning mix: | | | |
| *(Durkee) | 1 cup | 641 | 7.5 |
| (French's) | 1¾-oz. pkg. | 50 | 30.0 |
| Shell (Ortega) | 1 shell | 50 | 7.3 |

**TAMALE, canned:**

| | | | |
|---|---|---|---|
| (Derby) beef, with sauce | 1 tamale (2.2 oz.) | 120 | 6.5 |
| (Hormel) beef, *Short Orders* | ½ of 7½-oz. can | 135 | 8.5 |
| (Nalley's): | | | |
| Beef | 4-oz. serving | 134 | 12.5 |
| Chicken | 4-oz. serving | 104 | 12.5 |
| Olive, ripe | 4-oz. serving | 124 | 13.6 |

**TAMALE PIE, canned**

| | | | |
|---|---|---|---|
| (Nalley's) | 4-oz. serving | 113 | 12.5 |

**TAMARIND, fresh (USDA):**

| | | | |
|---|---|---|---|
| Whole | 1 lb. (weighed with pods & seeds) | 520 | 136.1 |
| Flesh only | 4 oz. | 271 | 70.9 |

***TANG*, instant breakfast drink:**

| | | | |
|---|---|---|---|
| Grape | ½ cup (4 oz.) | 64 | 16.0 |
| Grapefruit | ½ cup | 61 | 15.0 |
| Orange | ½ cup | 62 | 15.3 |

(USDA): United States Department of Agriculture
(HEW/FAO): Health, Education and Welfare/Food and Agriculture
                Organization
* Prepared as Package Directs

| Food and Description | Measure or Quantity | Calories | Carbohydrates (grams) |
|---|---|---|---|
| **TANGELO, fresh (USDA):** | | | |
| Whole | 1 lb. (weighed with peel, membrane & seeds) | 104 | 24.6 |
| Juice | ½ cup (4.4 oz.) | 51 | 12.0 |
| **TANGERINE or MANDARIN ORANGE:** | | | |
| Fresh (USDA): | | | |
| Whole | 1 lb. (weighed with peel, membrane & seeds) | 154 | 38.9 |
| Whole | 4.1-oz. tangerine (2⅜" dia.) | 39 | 10.0 |
| Sections (without membranes) | 1 cup (6.8 oz.) | 89 | 22.4 |
| Canned, regular pack (Del Monte) solids & liq. | ¼ of 22-oz. can | 106 | 25.3 |
| Canned, dietetic or low calorie: | | | |
| (Diet Delight) solids & liq. | ½ cup | 56 | 13.4 |
| (Featherweight) water pack, solids & liq. | ½ cup | 35 | 8.0 |
| (Tillie Lewis) *Tasti Diet* | ½ cup | 44 | 11.0 |
| **TANGERINE JUICE:** | | | |
| Fresh (USDA) | ½ cup (4.4 oz.) | 53 | 12.5 |
| Canned, unsweetened (USDA) | ½ cup (4.4 oz.) | 53 | 12.6 |
| Canned, sweetened (USDA) | ½ cup (4.4 oz.) | 62 | 14.9 |
| Frozen: | | | |
| *(USDA) | ½ cup (4.4 oz.) | 57 | 13.4 |
| *(Minute Maid) sweetened | 6 fl. oz. | 85 | 20.8 |
| **TAPIOCA, dry, quick cooking, granulated:** | | | |
| (USDA) | 1 cup (5.4 oz.) | 535 | 131.3 |
| (USDA) | 1 T. (10 grams) | 35 | 8.6 |
| **TARO, raw (USDA):** | | | |
| Tubers, whole | 1 lb. (weighed with skin) | 373 | 90.3 |

| Food and Description | Measure or Quantity | Calories | Carbo-hydrates (grams) |
|---|---|---|---|
| Tubers, skin removed | 4 oz. | 111 | 26.9 |
| Leaves & stems | 1 lb. | 181 | 33.6 |
| **TARRAGON** (French's) | 1 tsp. | 5 | .7 |
| **TAUTUG or BLACKFISH,** raw (USDA): | | | |
| Whole | 1 lb. (weighed whole) | 149 | 0. |
| Meat only | 4 oz. | 101 | 0. |
| **TEA** (See also TEA MIX, ICED): | | | |
| Bag (Lipton) | 1 bag | 0 | 0. |
| Bag (Tender Leaf) | 1 bag | 1 | |
| Bottle (Lipton) | 10 fl. oz. | 140 | 35.0 |
| Canned (Lipton) lemon-flavored | 12 fl. oz. | 130 | 32.0 |
| Canned (Lipton) lemon-flavored, sugar free | 12 fl. oz. | 2 | 0. |
| Instant: | | | |
| (USDA) dry powder, slightly sweetened | 1 tsp. | 1 | .4 |
| *(USDA) beverage, slightly sweetened | 1 cup (8.4 oz.) | 5 | .9 |
| *(Lipton) lemon-flavored | 1 cup (8 fl. oz.) | 4 | 1.0 |
| *(Lipton) 100% tea | 8 fl. oz. | 0 | 0. |
| *Nestea* | 1 tsp. (.6 grams) | 0 | 0. |
| (Tender Leaf) | 1 tsp. | 1 | |
| **TEAM,** cereal | 1 cup (1 oz.) | 110 | 24.0 |
| **TEA MIX, ICED:** Regular: | | | |
| (A&P) *Our Own,* lemon-flavored | 1 tsp. (1.5 grams) | 6 | 1.4 |

(USDA): United States Department of Agriculture
(HEW/FAO): Health, Education and Welfare/Food and Agriculture
              Organization
* Prepared as Package Directs

| Food and Description | Measure or Quantity | Calories | Carbohydrates (grams) |
|---|---|---|---|
| *(A&P) Our Own, lemon-flavored with sugar | 8 fl. oz. | 85 | 21.2 |
| *(Lipton) lemon-flavored | 8 fl. oz. | 60 | 16.0 |
| *Nestea, lemon-flavored | 8 fl. oz. | 20 | .2 |
| *Nestea, lemon-flavored with sugar | 6 fl. oz. | 70 | 17.0 |
| *(Salada) all flavors | 1 cup | 57 | 13.6 |
| *(Wyler's) | 1 cup | 56 | 14.0 |
| Dietetic or low calorie: | | | |
| (Ann Page) | 1 tsp. (1.5 grams) | 6 | 1.4 |
| *(Lipton) lemon-flavored | 8 fl. oz. | 2 | 0. |
| **TEMPTYS** (Tastykake): | | | |
| Chocolate creme | 2-oz. pkg. | 197 | DNA |
| Lemon | 2-oz. pkg. | 272 | DNA |
| **TENDERGREEN** (See MUSTARD SPINACH) | | | |
| **TERIYAKI**, frozen (Stouffer's) beef, with rice & vegetables | ½ of 10-oz. pkg. | 183 | 20.4 |
| **TEQUILA** (See DISTILLED LIQUOR) | | | |
| **TEQUILA SUNRISE COCKTAIL**, canned (Mr. Boston) 12½% alcohol | 3 fl. oz. | 120 | 14.4 |
| **TEXTURED VEGETABLE PROTEIN:** | | | |
| *Breakfast links, Morningstar Farms | .8-oz. link | 62 | .3 |
| *Breakfast patties, Morningstar Farms | 1¼-oz. pattie | 109 | 3.1 |
| *Breakfast strips Morningstar Farms | 4.8-gram strip | 34 | .2 |
| Chili seasoning (Williams) | 4-oz. pkg. | 428 | 47.4 |
| *Grillers, hamburger-like patties, Morningstar Farms | 2¼-oz. pattie | 201 | 4.8 |

| Food and Description | Measure or Quantity | Calories | Carbo-hydrates (grams) |
|---|---|---|---|
| Hamburger seasoning (Williams) | 4-oz. pkg. | 385 | 53.6 |
| Luncheon slices, *Morning-star Farms* | ¾-oz. slice | 25 | 1.4 |
| Meatloaf seasoning (Williams) | 4-oz. pkg. | 393 | 54.2 |
| *Pathmark Plus:* | | | |
| Dry | ⅛ oz. | 28 | 3.0 |
| *Prepared | 4 oz. | 178 | 2.9 |
| Sloppy Joe seasoning (Williams) | 4-oz. pkg. | 382 | 55.8 |
| *Sloppy Joe seasoning (Williams) | 4 oz. | 186 | 9.4 |
| *Spaghetti sauce (Williams) | 4-oz. serving | 118 | 7.6 |
| Taco seasoning (Williams) | 4-oz. pkg. | 378 | 48.7 |
| **THUNDERBIRD WINE** (Gallo): | | | |
| 14% alcohol | 3 fl. oz. | 86 | 8.1 |
| 20% alcohol | 3 fl. oz. | 106 | 7.5 |
| **THURINGER,** sausage: | | | |
| (USDA) | 1 oz. | 87 | .5 |
| (Hormel): | | | |
| Buffet, sliced | 1-oz. serving | 95 | .3 |
| Old smokehouse | 1-oz. serving | 100 | .1 |
| Summer sausage | 1-oz. slice | 76 | .2 |
| (Oscar Mayer): | | | |
| Summer sausage | .8-oz. slice | 97 | .3 |
| Summer sausage, beef | .8-oz. slice | 73 | .5 |
| **THYME,** dried (French's) | 1 tsp. | 5 | 1.0 |
| **TIA MARIA,** liqueur (Hiram Walker) 63 proof | 1 fl. oz. | 92 | 10.0 |
| **TIGER TAILS** (Hostess) | 2.2-oz. piece | 222 | 38.1 |

(USDA): United States Department of Agriculture
(HEW/FAO): Health, Education and Welfare/Food and Agriculture Organization

* Prepared as Package Directs

| Food and Description | Measure or Quantity | Calories | Carbohydrates (grams) |
|---|---|---|---|
| **TILEFISH (USDA):** | | | |
| Raw, whole | 1 lb. (weighed whole) | 183 | 0. |
| Baked, meat only | 4 oz. | 156 | 0. |
| **TOASTER CAKE:** | | | |
| (Nabisco) all varieties | 1.7-oz. piece | 190 | 35.0 |
| (Thomas') fresh or frozen, *Toast-r-Cake:* | | | |
| Blueberry | 1.3-oz. cake | 110 | 17.5 |
| Bran | 1 piece | 112 | 19.6 |
| Corn | 1.3-oz. cake | 116 | 18.3 |
| ***TOASTY O's*, cereal** | 1¼ cups (1 oz.) | 113 | 19.9 |
| **TODDLER BABY FOOD (See BABY FOOD)** | | | |
| ***TOFFEE CRUNCH BAR*** | | | |
| (Sealtest) | 3 fl. oz. | 150 | 12.0 |
| **TOFU (See SOYBEAN CURD)** | | | |
| **TOMATO:** | | | |
| Fresh (USDA): | | | |
| Green: | | | |
| Whole, untrimmed | 1 lb. (weighed with core & stem end) | 99 | 21.1 |
| Trimmed, unpeeled | 4 oz. | 27 | 5.8 |
| Ripe: | | | |
| Whole, eaten with skin | 1 lb. | 100 | 21.3 |
| Whole, peeled | 1 lb. (weighed with skin, stem ends & hard core) | 88 | 18.8 |
| Whole, peeled | 1 med. (2" x 2½", 5.3 oz.) | 33 | 7.0 |
| Whole, peeled | 1 small (1¾" x 2½", 3.9 oz.) | 24 | 5.2 |
| Sliced, peeled | ½ cup (3.2 oz.) | 20 | 4.2 |
| Boiled (USDA) | ½ cup (4.3 oz.) | 31 | 6.7 |

| Food and Description | Measure or Quantity | Calories | Carbohydrates (grams) |
|---|---|---|---|
| Canned, regular pack: | | | |
| (USDA) whole, solids & liq. | ½ cup (4.2 oz.) | 25 | 5.1 |
| (Contadina): | | | |
| Sliced, baby | 4 oz. | 35 | 8.0 |
| Stewed | 4 oz. | 35 | 8.0 |
| Whole, round & pear | 1 cup | 53 | 10.6 |
| (Del Monte): | | | |
| Stewed, solids & liq. | ½ cup (4.2 oz.) | 39 | 8.2 |
| Wedges, solids & liq. | ½ cup (4.1 oz.) | 35 | 7.2 |
| (Hunt's): | | | |
| Stewed | 4 oz. | 30 | 8.0 |
| Whole, peeled | 4 oz. | 25 | 5.0 |
| (Libby's) | | | |
| Stewed | ½ of 16-oz. can | 61 | 12.7 |
| Whole, peeled, solids & liq. | ½ of 16-oz. can | 50 | 9.8 |
| (Stokely-Van Camp): | | | |
| Stewed, solids & liq. | ½ cup (4.2 oz.) | 35 | 7.5 |
| Whole, solids & liq. | ½ cup (4.3 oz.) | 25 | 5.0 |
| Canned, dietetic or low calorie: | | | |
| (USDA) low sodium | 4 oz. | 23 | 4.8 |
| (Diet Delight) whole, peeled | ½ cup (4.3 oz.) | 27 | 5.4 |
| (Featherweight) | ½ cup | 20 | 4.0 |
| (Featherweight) stewed | ½ cup | 35 | 9.0 |
| (Tillie Lewis) *Tasti Diet* | ½ cup (4.3 oz.) | 25 | 6.1 |
| **TOMATO & HOT GREEN CHILI PEPPERS,** canned (Ortega) | 1-oz. serving | 7 | 1.4 |
| **TOMATO JUICE:** | | | |
| Canned, regular pack: | | | |
| (USDA) | ½ cup (4.3 oz.) | 23 | 5.2 |
| (Campbell) | 6-fl.-oz. can | 35 | 8.0 |
| (Del Monte) | 6 fl. oz. | 36 | 7.4 |

(USDA): United States Department of Agriculture
(HEW/FAO): Health, Education and Welfare/Food and Agriculture
                    Organization
* Prepared as Package Directs

| Food and Description | Measure or Quantity | Calories | Carbo-hydrates (grams) |
|---|---|---|---|
| (Libby's) | 6 fl. oz. | 39 | 7.5 |
| (Sacramento) | 5½ fl. oz. | 33 | 7.7 |
| (Stokely-Van Camp) | ½ cup (4.2 oz.) | 23 | 4.5 |
| Canned, dietetic or low calorie: | | | |
| (USDA) | 4 oz. (by wt.) | 22 | 4.9 |
| (Diet Delight) | 6 fl. oz. | 36 | 7.5 |
| (Featherweight) | ½ of 12-oz. can | 35 | 8.0 |
| (Tillie Lewis) *Tasti Diet* | 6 fl. oz. | 35 | 8.0 |
| Concentrate (USDA) canned | 4 oz. (by wt.) | 86 | 19.4 |
| *Concentrate (USDA) canned, diluted with 3 parts water by volume | 4 oz. (by wt.) | 23 | 5.1 |
| *Dehydrated (USDA) | ½ cup (4.3 oz.) | 24 | 5.4 |
| **TOMATO JUICE COCKTAIL:** | | | |
| (USDA) | 4 oz. (by wt.) | 14 | 5.7 |
| (USDA) | 6-oz. can | 139 | 31.6 |
| (Sacramento): | | | |
| Peppy | ½ cup (4.3 oz.) | 28 | 6.6 |
| *Tomato Plus* | 5½-fl.-oz. can | 49 | 9.9 |
| *Snap-E-Tom* | 6 fl. oz. | 38 | 6.8 |
| **TOMATO PASTE, canned:** | | | |
| Regular pack: | | | |
| (USDA) | 6-oz. can | 139 | 31.6 |
| (USDA) | ½ cup (4.6 oz.) | 106 | 24.0 |
| (USDA) | 1 T. (.6 oz.) | 13 | 3.0 |
| (Contadina) | 6-oz. can | 150 | 35.0 |
| (Del Monte) | 6-oz. can | 164 | 33.8 |
| (Hunt's) | 6-oz. can | 140 | 30.0 |
| Dietetic (Featherweight) low sodium | 6-oz. can | 150 | 35.0 |
| **TOMATO, PICKLED,** canned (Claussen) Kosher, green, halves | ¼ of 32-oz. jar | 44 | 8.4 |
| **TOMATO PUREE:** | | | |
| Canned, regular pack: | | | |
| (USDA) | 1 cup (8.8 oz.) | 98 | 22.2 |

| Food and Description | Measure or Quantity | Calories | Carbo-hydrates (grams) |
|---|---|---|---|
| (Contadina) heavy | 1 cup (8.8 oz.) | 110 | 26.4 |
| Canned, dietetic or low calorie (USDA) | 8 oz. (by wt.) | 88 | 20.0 |
| **TOMATO SAUCE:** | | | |
| Canned, regular pack: | | | |
| (Contadina) | 1 cup | 87 | 19.6 |
| (Del Monte) | | | |
| Regular | 1 cup (8 oz.) | 85 | 17.0 |
| With mushroom | 1 cup | 103 | 21.4 |
| With onions | 1 cup | 109 | 23.0 |
| With tomato tidbits | 1 cup | 130 | 5.7 |
| (Hunt's): | | | |
| With bits | 4 oz. | 35 | 8.0 |
| With cheese | 4 oz. | 70 | 10.0 |
| With herbs | 4 oz. | 80 | 12.0 |
| With mushrooms | 4 oz. | 40 | 9.0 |
| With onions | 4 oz. | 45 | 10.0 |
| Plain | 4 oz. | 35 | 8.0 |
| *Prima Salsa:* | | | |
| Regular | 4 oz. | 110 | 20.0 |
| With meat | 4 oz. | 120 | 20.0 |
| With mushrooms | 4 oz. | 110 | 20.0 |
| Special | 4 oz. | 40 | 10.0 |
| (Libby's) | ½ of 8-oz. can | 46 | 9.8 |
| (Stokely-Van Camp) | ½ cup (4.5 oz.) | 35 | 6.5 |
| **TOMATO SOUP:** | | | |
| Canned, regular pack: | | | |
| (USDA) condensed | 8 oz. (by wt.) | 163 | 28.8 |
| *(USDA) condensed, prepared with equal volume water | 1 cup (8.6 oz.) | 88 | 15.7 |
| *(USDA) condensed, prepared with equal volume milk | 1 cup (8.8 oz.) | 172 | 22.5 |
| *(Ann Page) condensed | 1 cup | 73 | 14.1 |

(USDA): United States Department of Agriculture
(HEW/FAO): Health, Education and Welfare/Food and Agriculture Organization
* Prepared as Package Directs

| Food and Description | Measure or Quantity | Calories | Carbo-hydrates (grams) |
|---|---|---|---|
| *(Ann Page) condensed, & rice | 1 cup | 115 | 20.1 |
| *(Campbell) condensed, prepared with equal volume milk | 10-oz. serving | 210 | 27.0 |
| *(Campbell) condensed, prepared with equal volume water | 10-oz. serving | 110 | 20.0 |
| *(Campbell) condensed, bisque | 10-oz. serving | 160 | 29.0 |
| *(Campbell) condensed, & rice, old fashioned | 10-oz. serving | 150 | 29.0 |
| *(Campbell) semi-condensed, Royale, *Soup For One* | 7¾-oz. can | 180 | 33.0 |
| (Progresso) | 1 cup (8 oz.) | 110 | 23.0 |
| Canned, dietetic or low calorie: | | | |
| (Campbell) low sodium | 7¼-oz. can | 130 | 22.0 |
| (Dia-Mel) | 8-oz. serving | 50 | 11.0 |
| (Featherweight) low sodium | 8-oz. can | 120 | 18.0 |
| Mix: | | | |
| *(Lipton) *Cup-a-Soup* | 6 fl. oz. | 70 | 13.0 |
| *(Nestle) *Souptime* | 6 fl. oz. | 70 | 13.0 |
| **TOMCOD, ATLANTIC,** raw (USDA): | | | |
| Whole | 1 lb. (weighed whole) | 136 | 0. |
| Meat only | 4 oz. | 87 | 0. |
| **TOM COLLINS:** | | | |
| Canned (Party Tyme) 10% alcohol | 2 fl. oz. | 58 | 5.9 |
| Mix (Party Tyme) | ½-oz. pkg. | 50 | 13.3 |
| **TONGUE** (USDA): | | | |
| Beef, medium fat, raw, untrimmed | 1 lb. | 714 | 1.4 |
| Beef, medium fat, braised | 4 oz. | 277 | .5 |
| Calf, raw, untrimmed | 1 lb. | 454 | 3.1 |
| Calf, braised | 4 oz. | 181 | 1.1 |

| Food and Description | Measure or Quantity | Calories | Carbo- hydrates (grams) |
|---|---|---|---|
| Hog, raw, untrimmed | 1 lb. | 741 | 1.7 |
| Hog, braised | 4 oz. | 287 | .6 |
| Lamb, raw, untrimmed | 1 lb. | 659 | 1.7 |
| Lamb, braised | 4 oz. | 288 | .6 |
| Sheep, raw, untrimmed | 1 lb. | 877 | 7.9 |
| Sheep, braised | 4 oz. | 366 | 2.7 |

**TONGUE, CANNED**
**(USDA):**

| | | | |
|---|---|---|---|
| Pickled | 1 oz. | 76 | <.1 |
| Potted or deviled | 1 oz. | 82 | .2 |

**TOPPING:**
Sweetened:
Butterscotch:

| | | | |
|---|---|---|---|
| (Kraft) | 1 T. | 57 | 12.4 |
| (Smucker's) | 1 T. | 70 | 16.5 |
| Caramel: | | | |
| (Kraft) | 1 T. | 54 | 12.7 |
| (Smucker's) | 1 T. | 70 | 16.5 |
| Cherry (Smucker's) | 1 T. | 65 | 16.0 |
| Chocolate: | | | |
| (Hershey's) fudge | 1 T. | 49 | 7.3 |
| (Kraft) | 1 oz. | 73 | 18.0 |
| (Kraft) fudge | 1 T. | 68 | 10.9 |
| (Smucker's): | | | |
| Regular | 1 T. | 65 | 13.5 |
| Fudge | 1 T. | 65 | 15.5 |
| Fudge, nut | 1 T. | 70 | 15.5 |
| Milk | 1 T. | 70 | 15.5 |
| Marshmallow (Kraft) | 1 T. | 38 | 9.4 |
| Peanut butter caramel (Smucker's) | 1 T. | 75 | 14.5 |
| Pecan: | | | |
| (Kraft) | 1 oz. | 122 | 13.6 |
| (Smucker's) in syrup | 1 T. | 65 | 14.0 |
| Pineapple (Smucker's) | 1 T. | 65 | 16.0 |
| Strawberry (Smucker's) | 1 T. | 60 | 15.0 |

| Food and Description | Measure or Quantity | Calories | Carbo-hydrates (grams) |
|---|---|---|---|
| Walnuts, in syrup (Smucker's) | 1 T. | 65 | 13.5 |
| Dietetic or low calorie: Chocolate: | | | |
| (Diet Delight) | 1 T. (.6 oz.) | 16 | 3.6 |
| (Tillie Lewis) *Tasti Diet* | 1 T. (.5 oz.) | 17 | 3.9 |
| **TOPPING, WHIPPED:** | | | |
| (USDA) pressurized | 1 cup (2.5 oz.) | 190 | 9.0 |
| (USDA) pressurized | 1 T. (4 grams) | 10 | Tr. |
| *Cool Whip* (Birds Eye) frozen, nondairy | 1 T. (.2 oz.) | 19 | 1.3 |
| *Richwhip*, liquid | 1 T. (¼ oz.) | 20 | 1.2 |
| *Spoon 'N Serve* (Rich's), frozen, nondairy | 1 T. (.14 oz.) | 14 | 1.1 |
| *Whip Topping* (Rich's) aerosol | ½-oz. serving | 20 | 1.2 |
| Dietetic (Featherweight) | 1 T. | 6 | 1.0 |
| **TORTILLA:** | | | |
| (USDA) | .7-oz. tortilla | 42 | 9.7 |
| (Amigos) | 1-oz. tortilla | 111 | 19.7 |
| ***TOTAL***, cereal (General Mills) | 1 cup (1 oz.) | 110 | 23.0 |
| **TOWEL GOURD,** raw (USDA): | | | |
| Unpared | 1 lb. (weighed with skin) | 69 | 15.8 |
| Pared | 4 oz. | 20 | 4.6 |
| **TRIPE:** | | | |
| Beef, commercial (USDA) | 4 oz. | 113 | 0. |
| Beef, pickled (USDA) | 4 oz. | 70 | 0. |
| Canned (Libby's) | ¼ of 24-oz. can | 290 | 1.1 |
| **TRIPLE SEC LIQUEUR:** | | | |
| (Bols) | 1 fl. oz. | 101 | 8.8 |
| (Garnier) | 1 fl. oz. | 83 | 8.5 |
| (Hiram Walker) | 1 fl. oz. | 105 | 9.8 |
| (Leroux) | 1 fl. oz. | 102 | 8.9 |

| Food and Description | Measure or Quantity | Calories | Carbohydrates (grams) |
|---|---|---|---|
| (Mr. Boston) | 1 fl. oz. | 79 | 8.5 |
| **TRIX**, cereal (General Mills) | 1 cup (1 oz.) | 110 | 25.0 |
| **TROUT:** | | | |
| Brook, fresh, whole (USDA) | 1 lb. (weighed whole) | 224 | 0. |
| Brook, fresh, meat only (USDA) | 4 oz. | 115 | 0. |
| Lake (See **LAKE TROUT**) | | | |
| Rainbow (USDA): | | | |
| Fresh, meat with skin | 4 oz. | 221 | 0. |
| Canned | 4 oz. | 237 | 0. |
| **TUNA:** | | | |
| Raw (USDA): | | | |
| Bluefin, meat only | 4 oz. | 164 | 0. |
| Yellowfin, meat only | 4 oz. | 151 | 0. |
| Canned in oil: | | | |
| (USDA) solids & liq. | 6½-oz. can | 530 | 0. |
| (USDA) drained solids | 6½-oz. can | 309 | 0. |
| (Breast O'Chicken) solids & liq. | 6½-oz. can | 427 | 0. |
| (Bumble Bee) drained solids | ½ cup (3 oz.) | 167 | 0. |
| (Carnation) solids & liq. | 6½-oz. can | 427 | 0. |
| (Chicken of the Sea): | | | |
| Chunk, light, solids & liq. | 6½-oz. can | 405 | <1.8 |
| Chunk, light, drained solids | 6½-oz. can | 294 | 0. |
| (Star Kist): | | | |
| Chunk, light, solids & liq. | 6½-oz. can | 427 | 0. |
| Chunk, white, solids & liq. | 6½-oz. can | 467 | 0. |
| Flakes or grated, solids & liq. | 6¼-oz. can | 426 | 0. |

(USDA): United States Department of Agriculture
(HEW/FAO): Health, Education and Welfare/Food and Agriculture Organization

* Prepared as Package Directs

| Food and Description | Measure or Quantity | Calories | Carbo-hydrates (grams) |
|---|---|---|---|
| Solid, light, solids & liq. | 7-oz. can | 459 | 0. |
| Solid, light, in Tonno olive oil, solids & liq. | 7-oz. can | 443 | 0. |
| Solids, white, solids & liq. | 7-oz. can | 503 | 0. |
| Canned in water: | | | |
| (USDA) solids & liq. | 6½-oz. can | 234 | 0. |
| (Breast O'Chicken) | 6½-oz. can | 211 | 0. |
| (Bumble Bee) solids & liq. | ½ cup | 150 | 0. |
| (Carnation) solids & liq. | 6½-oz. can | 211 | 0. |
| (Featherweight) solids & liq., low sodium | 6½-oz. can | 220 | 0. |
| (Star Kist): | | | |
| Chunk, light, solids & liq. | 6½-oz. can | 194 | 0. |
| Chunk, white, solids & liq. | 6½-oz. can | 240 | 0. |
| Solid, light, solids & liq. | 7-oz. can | 235 | 0. |
| Solid, white, imported Albacore, solids & liq. | 7-oz. can | 235 | 0. |
| Solid, white, local Albacore, solids & liq. | 7-oz. can | 334 | 0. |
| *TUNA MIX, Tuna Helper (General Mills): | | | |
| Country dumplings noodles & tuna casserole | ⅕ pkg. | 230 | 31.0 |
| Creamy noodles & tuna casserole | ⅕ pkg. | 280 | 31.0 |
| Noodles & cheese sauce & tuna casserole | ⅕ pkg. | 230 | 28.0 |
| TUNA NOODLES CASSEROLE, frozen (Stouffer's) | ½ of 11½-oz. pkg. | 193 | 18.0 |

| Food and Description | Measure or Quantity | Calories | Carbo-hydrates (grams) |
|---|---|---|---|
| **TUNA & PEAS,** frozen (Green Giant) creamed, *Toast Toppers* | 5-oz. serving | 136 | 9.8 |
| **TUNA PIE,** frozen: | | | |
| (Banquet) | 8-oz. pie | 434 | 42.7 |
| (Morton) | 8-oz. pie | 373 | 36.4 |
| **TUNA SALAD:** | | | |
| Home recipe (USDA) made with tuna, celery, mayonnaise, pickle, onion & egg | 4-oz. serving | 193 | 4.0 |
| Canned (Carnation) *Spreadable* | 1½-oz. serving | 81 | 3.2 |
| **TURBOT, GREENLAND,** raw (USDA): | | | |
| Whole | 1 lb. (weighed whole) | 344 | 0. |
| Meat only | 4 oz. | 166 | 0. |
| **TURBOT MEAL,** frozen (Weight Watchers): | | | |
| 2-compartment meal | 8-oz. meal | 316 | 12.0 |
| 3-compartment meal, stuffed | 16-oz. meal | 420 | 25.9 |
| **TURKEY:** | | | |
| Raw (USDA) ready-to-cook | 1 lb. (weighed with bones) | 722 | 0. |
| Raw (USDA) light meat | 4 oz. | 132 | 0. |
| Raw (USDA) dark meat | 4 oz. | 145 | 0. |
| Raw (USDA) skin only | 4 oz. | 459 | 0. |
| Roasted (USDA): Flesh, skin & giblets | From 13½-lb. raw ready-to-cook turkey | 9678 | 0. |

(USDA): United States Department of Agriculture
(HEW/FAO): Health, Education and Welfare/Food and Agriculture Organization
* Prepared as Package Directs

| Food and Description | Measure or Quantity | Calories | Carbo-hydrates (grams) |
|---|---|---|---|
| Flesh & skin | From 13½-lb. raw ready-to-cook turkey | 7872 | 0. |
| Flesh & skin | 4 oz. | 253 | 0. |
| Meat only: | | | |
| Chopped | 1 cup (5 oz.) | 268 | 0. |
| Diced | 4 oz. | 200 | 0. |
| Light | 4 oz. | 200 | 0. |
| Light | 1 slice (4" x 2" x ¼", 3 oz.) | 75 | 0. |
| Dark | 4 oz. | 230 | 0. |
| Dark | (2½" x 1⅝" x ¼", .7 oz.) | 43 | 0. |
| Skin only | 1 oz. | 128 | 0. |
| Giblets, simmered (USDA) | 2 oz. | 132 | .9 |
| Canned, boned: | 1 slice | | |
| (USDA) | 4 oz. | 229 | 0. |
| (Swanson) chunk meat | ½ of 5-oz. can | 120 | 0. |
| Packaged: | | | |
| (Eckrich) sliced | 1-oz. slice | 47 | 1.3 |
| (Oscar Mayer) breast | .8-oz. slice | 23 | 0. |
| **TURKEY DINNER or ENTREE, frozen:** | | | |
| (USDA) sliced turkey mashed potatoes, peas | 12-oz. dinner | 381 | 43.2 |
| (Banquet): | | | |
| Dinner | 11-oz. dinner | 293 | 27.8 |
| Dinner, *Man Pleaser* | 19-oz. dinner | 620 | 73.8 |
| (Morton): | | | |
| Dinner | 11-oz. dinner | 338 | 34.4 |
| Dinner, King Size | 19-oz. dinner | 583 | 64.8 |
| Dinner, sliced, *Country Table* | 15-oz. dinner | 580 | 81.1 |
| Entree, sliced, *Country Table* | 12¼-oz. entree | 390 | 34.9 |
| (Swanson): | | | |
| Dinner | 11½-oz. dinner | 360 | 45.0 |
| Dinner, *Hungry Man* | 19-oz. dinner | 740 | 80.0 |
| Dinner, 3-course | 16-oz. dinner | 520 | 60.0 |

| Food and Description | Measure or Quantity | Calories | Carbo-hydrates (grams) |
|---|---|---|---|
| Entree, with gravy & dressing | 9¼-oz. entree | 310 | 21.0 |
| Entree, with gravy & dressing & whipped potatoes | 8¾-oz. entree | 260 | 27.0 |
| Entree, *Hungry Man* | 13¼-oz. entree | 380 | 35.0 |
| (Weight Watchers) sliced breast, 3-compartment | 16-oz. meal | 350 | 26.8 |
| **TURKEY GIZZARD** (USDA): | | | |
| Raw | 4 oz. | 178 | 1.2 |
| Simmered | 4 oz. | 222 | 1.2 |
| **TURKEY PIE:** | | | |
| Home recipe (USDA) baked | ⅛ of 9″ pie | 550 | 42.2 |
| Frozen: | | | |
| (USDA) unheated | 8-oz. pie | 447 | 45.6 |
| (Banquet) | 9-oz. pie | 415 | 40.6 |
| (Morton) | 8-oz. pie | 334 | 31.8 |
| (Stouffer's) | 10-oz. pie | 451 | 34.7 |
| (Swanson) | 8-oz. pie | 450 | 40.0 |
| (Swanson) *Hungry Man* | 16-oz. pie | 790 | 60.0 |
| **TURKEY, POTTED** (USDA) | 1 oz. | 70 | 0. |
| **TURKEY SALAD,** canned (Carnation) *Spreadable* | 1½-oz. serving | 86 | 3.0 |
| **TURKEY SOUP,** canned: | | | |
| *(USDA) condensed, prepared with equal volume water | 1 cup (8.8 oz.) | 82 | 8.8 |
| *(Ann Page) & noodle | 1 cup | 129 | 17.8 |
| *(Ann Page) 7 vegetable | 1 cup | 63 | 8.9 |
| (Campbell): | | | |
| *Condensed, & noodle | 10-oz. serving | 80 | 10.0 |
| *Condensed, & vegetable | 10-oz. serving | 90 | 10.0 |

(USDA): United States Department of Agriculture
(HEW/FAO): Health, Education and Welfare/Food and Agriculture Organization
* Prepared as Package Directs

| Food and Description | Measure or Quantity | Calories | Carbo-hydrates (grams) |
|---|---|---|---|
| *Chunky* | 18½-oz. can | 280 | 30.0 |
| Dietetic, low sodium | 7½-oz. can | 130 | 22.0 |
| **TURKEY TETRAZZINI,** frozen: | | | |
| (Stouffer's) | ½ of 12-oz. pkg. | 248 | 16.9 |
| (Weight Watchers) | 13-oz. meal | 401 | 51.0 |
| **TUMERIC** (French's) | 1 tsp. | 7 | 1.3 |
| **TURNIP** (USDA) | | | |
| Fresh, without tops | 1 lb. (weighed with skins) | 117 | 25.7 |
| Fresh, pared, diced | ½ cup (2.4 oz.) | 20 | 4.4 |
| Fresh, pared, slices | ½ cup (2.3 oz.) | 19 | 4.2 |
| Boiled, drained, diced | ½ cup (2.8 oz.) | 18 | 3.8 |
| Boiled, drained, mashed | ½ cup (4 oz.) | 26 | 5.6 |
| **TURNIP GREENS,** leaves & stems: | | | |
| Fresh (USDA) | 1 lb. (weighed untrimmed) | 107 | 19.0 |
| Boiled (USDA) in small amount water, short time, drained | ½ cup (2.5 oz.) | 14 | 2.6 |
| Boiled (USDA) in large amount water, long time, drained | ½ cup (2.5 oz.) | 14 | 2.4 |
| Canned (USDA) solids & liq. | ½ cup (4.1 oz.) | 21 | 3.7 |
| Canned (Stokely-Van Camp) chopped | ½ cup (4.1 oz.) | 23 | 3.5 |
| Frozen: | | | |
| (USDA) boiled, drained | ½ cup (2.9 oz.) | 19 | 3.2 |
| (Birds Eye): | | | |
| Chopped | ⅓ of 10-oz. pkg. | 20 | 3.0 |
| Chopped, with sliced turnip | ⅓ of 10-oz. pkg. | 20 | 3.0 |
| (McKenzie & Seabrook Farms): | | | |
| Chopped | ⅓ of 10-oz. pkg. | 25 | 3.4 |
| Diced | 1-oz. serving | 4 | .8 |

| Food and Description | Measure or Quantity | Calories | Carbo-hydrates (grams) |
|---|---|---|---|
| **TURNOVER** (See individual kinds) | | | |
| **TURTLE, GREEN** (USDA): | | | |
| Raw, in shell | 1 lb. (weighed in shell) | 97 | 0. |
| Raw, meat only | 4 oz. | 101 | 0. |
| Canned | 4 oz. | 120 | 0. |
| *TWINKIE* (Hostess): | | | |
| Regular | 1½-oz. cake | 147 | 26.1 |
| Devil's food | 1½-oz. cake | 150 | 24.7 |

# V

| | | | |
|---|---|---|---|
| **VALPOLICELLA WINE,** Italian red (Antinori) | 3 fl. oz. | 84 | 6.3 |
| *VANDERMINT*, Dutch liqueur (Park Avenue Imports) 60 proof | 1 fl. oz. | 90 | 10.2 |
| **VANILLA EXTRACT** (Virginia Dare) 34% alcohol | 1 tsp. | 10 | Tr. |
| **VANILLA ICE CREAM** (See also individual brand names): | | | |
| (Breyer's): | | | |
| Plain | ¼ pt. | 150 | 16.0 |
| & strawberry | ¼ pt. | 150 | 20.0 |
| (Dean): | | | |
| 10.1% fat | 1 cup (5.3 oz.) | 296 | 33.8 |
| 12% fat | 1 cup (5.6 oz.) | 341 | 34.9 |

(USDA): United States Department of Agriculture
(HEW/FAO): Health, Education and Welfare/Food and Agriculture Organization
* Prepared as Package Directs

| Food and Description | Measure or Quantity | Calories | Carbo-hydrates (grams) |
|---|---|---|---|
| (Meadow Gold) | ¼ pt. | 140 | 16.0 |
| (Sealtest): | | | |
| Cherry | ¼ pt. | 130 | 17.0 |
| Fudge royale | ¼ pt. | 150 | 20.0 |
| *Party Slice* | ¼ pt. | 140 | 16.0 |
| & red raspberry & orange sherbet | ¼ pt. | 130 | 21.0 |
| 10.2% fat | ¼ pt. | 150 | 16.0 |
| (Swift's) sweet cream | ½ cup (2.3 oz.) | 127 | 15.7 |
| **VEAL, medium fat (USDA):** | | | |
| Chuck, raw | 1 lb. (weighed with bone) | 628 | 0. |
| Chuck, braised, lean & fat | 4 oz. | 266 | 0. |
| Flank, raw | 1 lb. (weighed with bone) | 1410 | 0. |
| Flank, stewed, lean & fat | 4 oz. | 442 | 0. |
| Foreshank, raw | 1 lb. (weighed with bone) | 368 | 0. |
| Foreshank, stewed, lean & fat | 4 oz. | 245 | 0. |
| Loin, raw | 1 lb. (weighed with bone) | 681 | 0. |
| Loin, broiled, medium done, chop, lean & fat | 4 oz. | 265 | 0. |
| Plate, raw | 1 lb. (weighed with bone) | 828 | 0. |
| Plate, stewed, lean & fat | 4 oz. | 344 | 0. |
| Rib, raw, lean & fat | 1 lb. (weighed with bone) | 723 | 0. |
| Rib, roasted, medium done, lean & fat | 4 oz. | 305 | 0. |
| Round & rump, raw | 1 lb. (weighed with bone) | 573 | 0. |
| Round & rump, broiled, steak or cutlet, lean & fat | 4 oz. (weighed without bone) | 245 | 0. |
| **VEAL DINNER or ENTREE, frozen:** | | | |
| (Banquet): | | | |
| Buffet, parmigian with tomato sauce | 2-lb. pkg. | 1563 | 119.1 |

| Food and Description | Measure or Quantity | Calories | Carbohydrates (grams) |
|---|---|---|---|
| Cooking bag, parmigian | 5-oz. bag | 387 | 19.5 |
| Dinner, parmigian | 11-oz. dinner | 421 | 42.1 |
| (Green Giant) parmigiana, breaded | 14-oz. pkg. | 621 | 36.6 |
| (Morton) parmigiana | 11-oz. dinner | 272 | 28.1 |
| (Swanson): | | | |
| Parmigiana | 12¼-oz. dinner | 460 | 41.1 |
| Parmigiana, *Hungry Man* | 20½-oz. dinner | 910 | 70.0 |
| **VEGETABLE BOUILLON:** | | | |
| (Herb-Ox) | 1 cube | 6 | .5 |
| (Herb-Ox) | 1 packet | 12 | 2.2 |
| *MBT* | 6-gram packet | 12 | 2.0 |
| **VEGETABLE FAT (See FAT)** | | | |
| **VEGETABLE JUICE COCKTAIL,** | | | |
| Canned: | | | |
| (USDA) | 4 oz. (by wt.) | 19 | 4.1 |
| *V-8* (Campbell): | | | |
| Regular & spicy hot | 6 fl. oz. | 35 | 8.0 |
| Low sodium | 6 fl. oz. | 35 | 8.0 |
| **VEGETABLES, MIXED:** | | | |
| Canned, regular pack: | | | |
| (Chun King) chow mein, solids & liq. | ¼ of 16-oz. can | 20 | 2.0 |
| (Del Monte): | | | |
| solids & liq. | ½ cup (4 oz.) | 38 | 6.9 |
| Drained solids | ½ cup (3.2 oz.) | 41 | 7.4 |
| (La Choy): | | | |
| Chinese style | 1 cup (5.5 oz.) | 24 | 1.6 |
| Chop suey | 1 cup (5.5 oz.) | 36 | 6.9 |
| (Libby's) solids & liq. | ½ cup (4.2 oz.) | 49 | 9.8 |
| (Stokely-Van Camp) solids & liq. | ½ cup (4.3 oz.) | 40 | 8.5 |

(USDA): United States Department of Agriculture
(HEW/FAO): Health, Education and Welfare/Food and Agriculture Organization
* Prepared as Package Directs

| Food and Description | Measure or Quantity | Calories | Carbohydrates (grams) |
|---|---|---|---|
| Canned, dietetic or low calorie (Featherweight) low sodium | ½ cup | 35 | 8.0 |
| Frozen: | | | |
| (USDA) boiled, drained | ½ cup (3.2 oz.) | 58 | 12.2 |
| (Birds Eye): | | | |
| *Americana Recipe:* | | | |
| New England style | ⅓ of 10-oz. pkg. | 69 | 11.7 |
| New Orleans style | ⅓ of 10-oz. pkg. | 69 | 13.8 |
| Pennsylvania Dutch style | ⅓ of 10-oz. pkg. | 44 | 7.3 |
| San Francisco style | ⅓ of 10-oz. pkg. | 42 | 6.4 |
| Wisconsin style | ⅓ of 10-oz. pkg. | 44 | 6.4 |
| Bavarian style beans & spaetzle with seasoned sauce | ⅓ of 10-oz. pkg. | 63 | 10.6 |
| Cantonese style, stir fry | ⅓ of 10-oz. pkg. | 50 | 10.2 |
| Chinese style, with seasoned sauce | ⅓ of 10-oz. pkg. | 28 | 5.2 |
| Chinese style, stir fry | ⅓ of 10-oz. pkg. | 37 | 7.0 |
| (Kounty Kist): | | | |
| Regular | ⅙ of 20-oz. pkg. | 55 | 10.4 |
| California blend | ⅙ of 18-oz. pkg. | 29 | 4.6 |
| (La Choy): | | | |
| Chinese style | ½ of 10-oz. pkg. | 36 | 5.3 |
| Japanese style | ½ of 10-oz. pkg. | 36 | 5.8 |
| (La Sueur): | | | |
| Pea, pea pod & water chestnuts in sauce | ⅓ of 10-oz. pkg. | 72 | 8.9 |
| Pea, onion & carrots in butter sauce | ⅓ of 10-oz. pkg. | 67 | 7.6 |
| (Ore-Ida) stew | ⅛ of 24-oz. pkg. | 60 | 13.0 |

**VEGETABLE OYSTER (See SALISIFY)**

**VEGETABLE SOUP:**
Canned, regular pack:
*(USDA) beef, prepared with equal volume water

| | | | |
|---|---|---|---|
| | 1 cup (8.6 oz.) | 78 | 9.6 |

| Food and Description | Measure or Quantity | Calories | Carbo-hydrates (grams) |
|---|---|---|---|
| *(USDA) with beef broth, prepared with equal volume water | 1 cup (8.8 oz.) | 80 | 13.8 |
| *(USDA) vegetarian, prepared with equal volume water | 1 cup (8.6 oz.) | 78 | 13.2 |
| *(Ann Page) with beef stock | 1 cup | 130 | 20.0 |
| *(Ann Page) vegetarian | 1 cup | 70 | 12.3 |
| (Campbell): | | | |
| Chunky | 10¾-oz. can | 140 | 24.0 |
| Chunky | 19-oz. can | 260 | 42.0 |
| *Condensed | 10-oz. serving | 100 | 16.0 |
| *Condensed, beef | 10-oz. serving | 90 | 10.0 |
| *Condensed, old-fashioned | 10-oz. serving | 90 | 11.0 |
| *Condensed, vegetarian | 10-oz. serving | 90 | 16.0 |
| *Semicondensed, Soup For One, old world | 7¾-oz. can | 120 | 18.0 |
| Canned, dietetic or low calorie: | | | |
| (Campbell) low sodium | 7¼-oz. can | 90 | 14.0 |
| (Campbell) beef, low sodium | 7½-oz. can | 90 | 8.0 |
| *(Dia-Mel) | 8-oz. serving | 60 | 12.0 |
| *(Dia-Mel) & beef | 8-oz. serving | 80 | 11.0 |
| (Featherweight) & beef | 8-oz. can | 180 | 28.0 |
| *Frozen (USDA) with beef, prepared with equal volume water | 8-oz. (by wt.) | 79 | 7.7 |
| Mix: | | | |
| *(Lipton): | | | |
| Alphabet vegetable, Cup-a-Soup | 6 fl. oz. | 40 | 6.0 |
| Vegetable beef | 8 fl. oz. | 60 | 9.0 |
| Vegetable beef, Cup-a-Soup | 6 fl. oz. | 60 | 9.0 |

(USDA): United States Department of Agriculture
(HEW/FAO): Health, Education and Welfare/Food and Agriculture Organization
* Prepared as Package Directs

| Food and Description | Measure or Quantity | Calories | Carbohydrates (grams) |
|---|---|---|---|
| Vegetable beef with shells | 8 fl. oz. | 100 | 18.0 |
| Vegetable, country | 8 fl. oz. | 70 | 13.0 |
| Vegetable, Italian | 8 fl. oz. | 100 | 19.0 |
| Vegetable, Spring, Cup-a-Soup | 6 fl. oz. | 45 | 7.0 |
| *(Nestlé) Souptime cream of | 6 fl. oz. | 80 | 9.0 |

## "VEGETARIAN FOODS":

Canned or dry:

| Food and Description | Measure or Quantity | Calories | Carbohydrates (grams) |
|---|---|---|---|
| Big franks, drained (Loma Linda) | 1.9-oz. frank | 100 | 4.1 |
| Chili (Worthington) | ½ cup (4.9 oz.) | 190 | 20.0 |
| Choplet (Worthington) | 1.6-oz. slice | 50 | 3.0 |
| Cutlet (Worthington) | 2.2-oz. slice | 63 | 2.6 |
| Dinner cuts, drained (Loma Linda) | 1.6-oz. cut | 54 | 1.6 |
| Dinner cuts, no salt added (Loma Linda) | 1.5-oz. cut | 43 | 2.6 |
| FriChik (Worthington) | 1.6-oz. piece | 95 | 1.0 |
| Granburger (Worthington) | 6 T. (1.2 oz.) | 130 | 12.0 |
| Linketts, drained (Loma Linda) | 1.3-oz. link | 74 | 2.2 |
| Little links (Loma Linda) | .8-oz. link | 45 | 1.3 |
| Non-meat balls (Worthington) | .6-oz. meatball | 40 | 2.3 |
| Numete (Worthington) | ½" slice (2.4 oz.) | 160 | 9.0 |
| Nutena (Loma Linda) | ½" slice (2.4 oz.) | 165 | 7.6 |
| Peanuts & soya, canned (USDA) | 4 oz. | 269 | 15.2 |
| Proteena (Loma Linda) | ½" slice (2.6 oz.) | 144 | 6.5 |
| Protose (Worthington) | ½" slice (2.7 oz.) | 190 | 7.0 |
| Redi-burger (Loma Linda) | ½" slice (2.4 oz.) | 132 | 8.8 |
| Sandwich spread (Loma Linda) | 1 T. (.6 oz.) | 25 | 1.8 |
| Sandwich spread (Worthington) | 2½-oz. serving | 120 | 2.0 |
| Saucettes (Worthington) | 1.2-oz. link | 65 | 1.5 |
| Savorex (Loma Linda) | 1 T. (.5 oz.) | 32 | 2.0 |
| Skallops (Worthington) drained | ½ cup | 70 | 3.0 |

| Food and Description | Measure or Quantity | Calories | Carbo-hydrates (grams) |
|---|---|---|---|
| Soyagen, all-purpose powder (Loma Linda) | 1 T. (10 grams) | 48 | 4.7 |
| Soyalac, concentrate, liquid (Loma Linda) | 1 cup (9 oz.) | 177 | 17.0 |
| Soyalac powder (Loma Linda) | 1 oz. | 136 | 12.4 |
| Soyalac, ready-to-use (Loma Linda) | 1 cup (8.5 oz.) | 166 | 15.9 |
| Soyameat (Worthington): | | | |
| Beef-like slices | 1-oz. slice | 55 | 1.5 |
| Chicken-like, diced | ¼ cup (2 oz.) | 120 | 2.0 |
| Chicken-like, sliced | 1.1-oz. slice | 65 | 1.0 |
| Salisbury steak-like slices | 2.3-oz. slice | 160 | 2.0 |
| Soyamel (Worthington) | 1 oz. | 140 | 15.2 |
| Soyamel, low fat (Worthington) | 1 oz. | 110 | 14.0 |
| Stew pac, drained (Loma Linda) | 2-oz. serving | 73 | 5.6 |
| Super links (Worthington) | 1.9-oz. link | 120 | 4.0 |
| Swiss steak & gravy (Loma Linda) | 2¾-oz. steak | 138 | 8.9 |
| Tender bits (Loma Linda) | .6-oz. piece | 23 | 1.1 |
| Tender rounds, drained (Loma Linda) | 1-oz. round | 39 | 2.3 |
| Vegeburger (Loma Linda) | ½ cup (3.8 oz.) | 116 | 4.3 |
| Vegeburger, no salt added (Loma Linda) | ½ cup (3.9 oz.) | 130 | 6.9 |
| Vegelona (Loma Linda) | ½" slice (2.4 oz.) | 102 | 7.0 |
| Vegetable steak (Worthington) | 1.3-oz. piece | 40 | 2.8 |
| Vegetarian burger (Worthington) | ⅓ cup (3.3 oz.) | 130 | 6.0 |
| Veja-Bits (Worthington) | 4.3-oz. serving | 70 | 4.0 |
| Veja-Links (Worthington) | 1.1-oz. link | 70 | 1.5 |
| Vita-Burger (Loma Linda) | 3 T. (.75 oz.) | 70 | 6.4 |

(USDA): United States Department of Agriculture
(HEW/FAO): Health, Education and Welfare/Food and Agriculture Organization
* Prepared as Package Directs

| Food and Description | Measure or Quantity | Calories | Carbo-hydrates (grams) |
|---|---|---|---|
| Wheat protein, nuts or peanuts, canned (USDA) | 4 oz. | 240 | 20.1 |
| Wheat protein, vegetable oil, canned (USDA) | 4 oz. | 214 | 5.9 |
| Wheat soy protein, soy or other vegetable oil canned (USDA) | 4 oz. | 170 | 10.8 |
| Wheat or soy protein (USDA) canned | 4 oz. | 118 | 8.6 |
| Wheat protein (USDA) | 4 oz. | 124 | 10.0 |
| *Worthington 209*, turkey-like flavor | 1.1-oz. slice | 75 | 1.5 |
| Frozen: | | | |
| Beef-like roll (Worthington) | 2½-oz. slice | 140 | 4.0 |
| Beef-like slices (Worthington) | 1-oz. slice | 60 | 2.0 |
| Beef pie (Worthington) | 8-oz. pie | 470 | 51.0 |
| Bologna (Loma Linda) | 1-oz. slice | 77 | 2.8 |
| Bolono (Worthington) | .7-oz. slice | 35 | 1.5 |
| Breakfast sausage (Loma Linda) | 3⅓" slice (3 oz.) | 214 | 4.3 |
| Chicken (Loma Linda) | 1-oz. slice | 57 | 1.5 |
| Chicken, fried (Loma Linda) | 2-oz. piece | 188 | 3.6 |
| Chicken-like pie (Worthington) | 8-oz. pie | 450 | 42.0 |
| Chicken-like roll (Worthington) | 2½-oz. piece | 170 | 2.0 |
| Chicken-like slices (Worthington) | 1-oz. slice | 70 | 1.0 |
| *Chic-Ketts* (Worthington) | ½ cup (3 oz.) | 180 | 6.0 |
| Corned beef-like roll (Worthington) | 2½-oz. piece | 190 | 6.0 |
| Corned beef-like, sliced (Worthington) | .5-oz. slice | 40 | 2.3 |
| Croquettes (Worthington) | 1-oz. croquette | 75 | 5.0 |
| Fillets (Worthington) | 1.7-oz. piece | 108 | 5.0 |
| FriPats (Worthington) | 2.5-oz. piece | 180 | 3.0 |
| Meatballs (Loma Linda) | .8-oz. meatball | 46 | 2.2 |
| Meatless salami (Worthington) | .7-oz. slice | 50 | 1.5 |

| Food and Description | Measure or Quantity | Calories | Carbohydrates (grams) |
|---|---|---|---|
| *Prosage* Links (Worthington) | .8-oz. link | 60 | 1.7 |
| *Prosage* patties (Worthington) | 1.3-oz. pattie | 100 | 3.5 |
| *Prosage* roll (Worthington) | ⅜" slice (1.2 oz.) | 90 | 3.0 |
| Roast beef (Loma Linda) | 1-oz. slice | 65 | 1.3 |
| Salami (Loma Linda) | 1-oz. slice | 65 | 1.7 |
| Sizzle burger (Loma Linda) | 2.5-oz. burger | 210 | 13.3 |
| Smoked beef-like roll (Worthington) | 2½-oz. piece | 170 | 7.0 |
| Smoked beef-like luncheon slice (Worthington) | .3-oz. slice | 22 | 1.0 |
| Smoked turkey-like roll (Worthington) | 2½-oz. piece | 180 | 3.0 |
| Smoked turkey-like slices (Worthington) | .7-oz. slice | 50 | .8 |
| Stakelets (Worthington) | 3-oz. piece | 180 | 8.0 |
| Stripples (Worthington) | .3-oz. strip | 25 | .8 |
| Tuno (Worthington) | 2-oz. serving | 90 | 3.0 |
| Tuno pot pie (Worthington) | 8-oz. pie | 460 | 43.0 |
| Turkey (Loma Linda) | 1-oz. slice | 61 | 1.6 |
| *Wham*, roll (Worthington) | 2½-oz. piece | 140 | 4.0 |
| *Wham*, sliced (Worthington) | .8-oz. slice | 47 | 1.3 |
| **VENISON**, raw, lean meat only (USDA) | 4 oz. | 143 | 0. |
| **VERMOUTH:** Dry: | | | |
| (C&P) 19% alcohol | 3 fl. oz. | 90 | 3.0 |
| (Gallo) 18% alcohol | 3 fl. oz. | 75 | 1.7 |

(USDA): United States Department of Agriculture
(HEW/FAO): Health, Education and Welfare/Food and Agriculture Organization
* Prepared as Package Directs

| Food and Description | Measure or Quantity | Calories | Carbo-hydrates (grams) |
|---|---|---|---|
| (Great Western) 16% alcohol | 3 fl. oz. | 87 | 1.6 |
| (Lejon) 18.5% alcohol | 3 fl. oz. | 99 | 2.2 |
| (Noilly Pratt) 19% alcohol | 3 fl. oz. | 101 | 1.6 |
| (Taylor) 17% alcohol | 3 fl. oz. | 99 | 3.0 |
| Rosso (Gancia) 21% alcohol | 3 fl. oz. | 153 | 6.9 |
| Sweet: | | | |
| (C&P) 16% alcohol | 3 fl. oz. | 120 | 14.4 |
| (Gallo) 18% alcohol | 3 fl. oz. | 118 | 12.3 |
| (Great Western) 16% alcohol | 3 fl. oz. | 132 | 12.4 |
| (Lejon) 18.5% alcohol | 3 fl. oz. | 134 | 11.4 |
| (Noilly Pratt) 16% alcohol | 3 fl. oz. | 128 | 12.1 |
| (Taylor) 17% alcohol | 3 fl. oz. | 132 | 12.3 |
| White (Gancia) 16.8% alcohol | 3 fl. oz. | 132 | 7.8 |
| White (Lejon) 18.5% alcohol | 3 fl. oz. | 101 | 2.6 |
| **VICHYSSOISE SOUP** (Crosse & Blackwell) cream of | ½ of 13-oz. can | 70 | 5.0 |
| **VIENNA SAUSAGE, CANNED:** | | | |
| (USDA) | 1 oz. | 68 | <.1 |
| (Libby's): | | | |
| In barbecue sauce | .7-oz. sausage | 50 | .5 |
| In beef broth | .7-oz. sausage | 45 | .2 |
| **VILLA ANTINORI**, Italian white wine, 12½% alcohol | 3 fl. oz. | 87 | 6.3 |
| **VINEGAR:** | | | |
| Cider: | | | |
| (USDA) | ½ cup (4.2 oz.) | 17 | 7.1 |
| (USDA) | 1 T. (.5 oz.) | 2 | .9 |
| Distilled: | | | |
| (USDA) | ½ cup (4.2 oz.) | 14 | 6.0 |
| (USDA) | 1 T. (.5 oz.) | 2 | .8 |
| Red or white wine (Regina): | | | |
| Champagne | 1 T. (.5 oz.) | <1 | .1 |
| Red, plain or with garlic | 1 T. (.5 oz.) | <1 | .8 |

| Food and Description | Measure or Quantity | Calories | Carbo-hydrates (grams) |
|---|---|---|---|
| **VINESPINACH or BASELLA**, raw (USDA) | 4 oz. | 22 | 3.9 |
| *VIN KAFE* (Lejon) 19.7% alcohol | 3 fl. oz. | 183 | 22.8 |
| **VIN ROSE** (See **ROSE WINE**) | | | |
| **VIRGIN SOUR MIX** (Party Tyme) | ½-oz. pkg. | 50 | 13.3 |
| **VODKA**, unflavored (See **DISTILLED LIQUOR**) | | | |
| **VODKA & TONIC**, canned (Party Tyme) 10% alcohol | 2 fl. oz. | 55 | 5.1 |
| **VOIGNY WINE** (Chanson) 13% alcohol | 3 fl. oz. | 96 | 7.5 |

# W

| Food and Description | Measure or Quantity | Calories | Carbo-hydrates (grams) |
|---|---|---|---|
| **WAFER** (See **COOKIE or CRACKER**) | | | |
| **WAFFLE:** | | | |
| Home recipe (USDA) | 7" waffle (2.6 oz.) | 209 | 28.1 |
| Frozen: | | | |
| (USDA) | 1.6-oz. waffle (8 in 13-oz. pkg.) | 116 | 19.3 |
| (USDA) | .8-oz. waffle (6 in 5-oz. pkg.) | 61 | 10.1 |
| (Aunt Jemima) jumbo | 1¼-oz. waffle | 86 | 13.6 |

(USDA): United States Department of Agriculture
(HEW/FAO): Health, Education and Welfare/Food and Agriculture Organization
* Prepared as Package Directs

| Food and Description | Measure or Quantity | Calories | Carbo-hydrates (grams) |
|---|---|---|---|
| (Downyflake): | | | |
| Blueberry or jumbo | 1 waffle | 85 | 16.0 |
| Regular | 1 waffle | 55 | 10.5 |
| (Eggo): | | | |
| Blueberry | 1.4-oz. waffle | 130 | 18.0 |
| Bran | 2-oz. waffle | 170 | 20.0 |
| Plain | 1.4-oz. waffle | 120 | 17.0 |
| Strawberry | 1.4-oz. waffle | 130 | 18.0 |
| **WAFFLE MIX** (USDA) (See also **PANCAKE & WAFFLE MIX**): | | | |
| Dry, complete mix | 1 oz. | 130 | 18.5 |
| *Prepared with water | 2.6-oz. waffle (½″ x 4½″ x 5½″, 7″ dia.) | 229 | 30.2 |
| Dry, incomplete mix | 1 oz. | 101 | 21.5 |
| *Prepared with egg & milk | 2.6-oz. waffle (7″ dia.) | 206 | 27.2 |
| *Prepared with egg & milk | 7.1-oz. waffle (9″ x 9″ x ⅝″, 1⅛ cup batter) | 550 | 72.4 |
| **WAFFLE SYRUP** (See **SYRUP** and also individual names such as **LOG CABIN**) | | | |
| **WALLBANGER COCKTAIL,** (Mr. Boston) 12½% alcohol | 3 fl. oz. | 102 | 9.6 |
| **WALNUT:** | | | |
| (USDA): | | | |
| Black, in shell, whole | 1 lb. (weighed in shell) | 627 | 14.8 |
| Black, shelled, whole | 4 oz. (weighed whole) | 712 | 16.8 |
| Black, chopped | ½ cup (2.1 oz.) | 377 | 8.9 |
| English or Persian, in shell, whole | 1 lb. (weighed in shell) | 1329 | 32.2 |
| English or Persian, shelled, whole | 4 oz. | 738 | 17.9 |

| Food and Description | Measure or Quantity | Calories | Carbohydrates (grams) |
|---|---|---|---|
| English or Persian, chopped | ½ cup (2.1 oz.) | 391 | 9.5 |
| English or Persian, halves | ½ cup (1.8 oz.) | 326 | 7.9 |
| (Diamond) halves & pieces | 1 cup (3.5 oz.) | 679 | 12.8 |
| (Hammon's) kernels | 4 oz. | 746 | 11.6 |
| **WATER CHESTNUT, CHINESE:** | | | |
| Raw (USDA): | | | |
| Whole | 1 lb. (weighed unpeeled) | 272 | 66.5 |
| Peeled | 4 oz. | 90 | 21.5 |
| Canned: | | | |
| (Chun King) solids & liq. | ½ of 8½-oz. can | 70 | 11.0 |
| (La Choy) drained | 8-oz. can | 65 | 14.6 |
| **WATERCRESS, raw (USDA):** | | | |
| Untrimmed | ½ lb. (weighed untrimmed) | 40 | 6.2 |
| Trimmed | ½ cup (.6 oz.) | 3 | .5 |
| **WATERMELON, fresh (USDA):** | | | |
| Whole | 1 lb. (weighed with rind) | 54 | 13.4 |
| Wedge | 2-lb. wedge (4″ x 8″ measured with rind) | 111 | 27.3 |
| Slice | ½ slice (12.2 oz., ¾″ x 10″) | 41 | 10.2 |
| Diced | 1 cup (5.6 oz.) | 42 | 10.2 |
| **WAX GOURD, raw (USDA):** | | | |
| Whole | 1 lb. (weighed with skin & cavity contents) | 41 | 9.4 |

(USDA): United States Department of Agriculture
(HEW/FAO): Health, Education and Welfare/Food and Agriculture Organization
* Prepared as Package Directs

| Food and Description | Measure or Quantity | Calories | Carbo-hydrates (grams) |
|---|---|---|---|
| Flesh only | 4 oz. | 15 | 3.4 |
| **WEAKFISH (USDA):** | | | |
| Raw, whole | 1 lb. (weighed whole) | 263 | 0. |
| Broiled, meat only | 4 oz. | 236 | 0. |
| **WELSH RAREBIT:** | | | |
| Home recipe (USDA) | 1 cup (8.2 oz.) | 415 | 14.6 |
| Frozen: | | | |
| (Green Giant) with cheddar & swiss cheese, *Toast Topper* | 5-oz. serving | 219 | 11.4 |
| (Stouffer's) | ½ of 10-oz. pkg. | 359 | 16.9 |
| **WESTERN DINNER, frozen:** | | | |
| (Banquet) | 11-oz. dinner | 417 | 32.4 |
| (Morton) *Round-Up* | 11¾-oz. dinner | 426 | 33.5 |
| (Swanson) | 11⅜-oz. dinner | 460 | 41.0 |
| (Swanson) *Hungry Man* | 17¾-oz. dinner | 890 | 77.0 |
| **WEST INDIAN CHERRY (See ACEROLA)** | | | |
| **WHALE MEAT, raw (USDA)** | 4 oz. | 177 | 0. |
| **WHEAT CHEX, cereal (Ralston Purina)** | ⅔ cup (1 oz.) | 110 | 23.0 |
| **WHEATENA, dry** | ¼ cup (1.1 oz.) | 112 | 22.5 |
| **WHEAT FLAKES, cereal:** | | | |
| (USDA) crushed | 1 cup (2.5 oz.) | 248 | 56.4 |
| (Van Brode) | ¾ cup (1 oz.) | 106 | 22.7 |
| **WHEAT GERM, crude, commercial, milled (USDA)** | 1 oz. | 103 | 13.2 |
| **WHEAT GERM CEREAL:** | | | |
| (USDA) | ¼ cup (1 oz.) | 110 | 14.0 |
| (Kretschmer): | | | |
| Regular | ¼ cup (1 oz.) | 110 | 13.0 |
| With sugar & honey | ¼ cup (1 oz.) | 110 | 17.0 |

| Food and Description | Measure or Quantity | Calories | Carbo-hydrates (grams) |
|---|---|---|---|
| **WHEATIES,** cereal (General Mills) | 1 cup (1 oz.) | 110 | 23.0 |
| **WHEAT, ROLLED** (USDA): | | | |
| Uncooked | 1 cup (3.1 oz.) | 296 | 66.3 |
| Cooked | 1 cup (7.7 oz.) | 163 | 36.7 |
| **WHEAT, SHREDDED,** cereal (See **SHREDDED WHEAT**) | | | |
| **WHEAT, WHOLE-GRAIN** (USDA), hard red spring | 1 oz. | 94 | 19.6 |
| **WHEAT, WHOLE-MEAL,** cereal (USDA): | | | |
| Dry | 1 oz. | 96 | 20.5 |
| Cooked | 4 oz. | 51 | 10.7 |
| **WHEY** (USDA): | | | |
| Dry | 1 oz. | 99 | 20.8 |
| Fluid | 1 cup (8.6 oz.) | 63 | 12.4 |
| **WHISKEY or WHISKY** (See **DISTILLED LIQUOR**) | | | |
| **WHISKEY SOUR COCKTAIL:** | | | |
| Canned: | | | |
| (Hiram Walker) | 3 fl. oz. | 177 | 12.0 |
| (Mr. Boston) 12½% alcohol | 3 fl. oz. | 120 | 14.4 |
| (National Distillers) *Duet,* 12½% alcohol | 8-fl.-oz. can | 256 | 17.6 |
| Mix: | | | |
| (Bar-Tender's) | ⅝-oz. serving | 70 | 17.2 |
| (Holland House) dry | .6-oz. pkg. | 69 | 17.0 |
| (Holland House) liquid | 1½ fl. oz. | 82 | 19.6 |
| (Party Tyme) | ½-oz. pkg. | 50 | 13.5 |

(USDA): United States Department of Agriculture
(HEW/FAO): Health, Education and Welfare/Food and Agriculture
           Organization
\* Prepared as Package Directs

| Food and Description | Measure or Quantity | Calories | Carbo- hydrates (grams) |
|---|---|---|---|
| **WHITEFISH, LAKE** (USDA): | | | |
| Raw, whole | 1 lb. (weighed whole) | 330 | 0. |
| Raw, meat only | 4 oz. | 176 | 0. |
| Baked, stuffed, made with bacon, butter, onion, celery & bread crumbs, home recipe | 4 oz. | 244 | 6.6 |
| Smoked | 4 oz. | 176 | 0. |
| **WHITEFISH & PIKE** (See **GEFILTE FISH**) | | | |
| **WIENER** (See **FRANKFURTER**) | | | |
| **WILD BERRY**, fruit drink (Hi-C) | 6 fl. oz. | 88 | 22.0 |
| **WILDBERRY DRINK**, canned (Ann Page) | 1 cup (8.7 oz.) | 124 | 30.9 |
| **WILD RICE**, raw (USDA) | ½ cup (2.9 oz.) | 289 | 61.7 |
| **WINE** (most wines are listed by kind, brand, vineyard, region or grape name): | | | |
| Cooking, Sauterne (Regina) | ¼ cup | 2 | .5 |
| Cooking, sherry (Regina) | ¼ cup | 19 | 4.7 |
| Dessert (USDA) 18.8% alcohol | 3 fl. oz. | 122 | 6.9 |
| Table (USDA) 12.2% alcohol | 3 fl. oz. | 75 | 3.7 |
| *WON TON SOUP, frozen (La Choy) | 1 cup | 92 | 12.3 |
| **WORCESTERSHIRE SAUCE** (See **SAUCE**, Worcester- shire) | | | |
| **WRECKFISH**, raw (USDA) meat only | 4 oz. | 129 | 0. |

| Food and Description | Measure or Quantity | Calories | Carbo-hydrates (grams) |
|---|---|---|---|

**Y**

**YAM (USDA):**
| | | | |
|---|---|---|---|
| Raw, whole | 1 lb. (weighed with skin) | 394 | 90.5 |
| Raw, flesh only | 4 oz. | 115 | 26.3 |
| Canned & frozen (See **SWEET POTATO**) | | | |

**YAM BEAN, raw (USDA):**
| | | | |
|---|---|---|---|
| Unpared tuber | 1 lb. (weighed unpared) | 225 | 52.2 |
| Pared tuber | 4 oz. | 62 | 14.5 |

**YEAST:**
| | | | |
|---|---|---|---|
| Baker's: | | | |
| Compressed (USDA) | 1 oz. | 24 | 3.1 |
| Compressed (Fleischmann's) | ⅗-oz. cake | 19 | 1.9 |
| Dry (USDA) | 1 oz. | 80 | 11.0 |
| Dry (USDA) | 1 pkg. (7 grams) | 20 | 2.7 |
| Dry (Fleischmann's) | ¼ oz. (pkg. or jar) | 24 | 2.9 |
| Brewer's dry, debittered (USDA) | 1 oz. | 80 | 10.9 |
| Brewer's dry, debittered (USDA) | 1 T. (8 grams) | 23 | 3.1 |

**YELLOWTAIL, raw, meat only (USDA)**
| | | | |
|---|---|---|---|
| | 4 oz. | 156 | 0. |

**YOGURT:**
| | | | |
|---|---|---|---|
| Regular: | | | |
| Made from whole milk (USDA) | ½ cup (4.3 oz.) | 76 | 6.0 |
| Made from partially skimmed milk, plain or vanilla (USDA) | 8-oz. container | 61 | 6.3 |

(USDA): United States Department of Agriculture
(HEW/FAO): Health, Education and Welfare/Food and Agriculture Organization
* Prepared as Package Directs

| Food and Description | Measure or Quantity | Calories | Carbo-hydrates (grams) |
|---|---|---|---|
| Plain: | | | |
| (Alta-Dena) *Maya* | 1 container | 210 | 18.0 |
| (Alta-Dena) *Naja* | 1 container | 180 | 20.0 |
| (Breyer's) | 1 cup | 180 | 17.0 |
| (Dannon) | 8-oz. container | 150 | 17.0 |
| (Dean) | 8-oz. container | 143 | 18.4 |
| (Sealtest) *Light'n Lively* | 1 cup | 150 | 18.0 |
| *Viva*, Swiss style | 8-oz. container | 180 | 23.0 |
| *Yoplait* (General Mills) | 6-oz. container | 130 | 14.0 |
| Apple, *Yoplait* (General Mills) | 6-oz. container | 190 | 32.0 |
| Apple crisp (New Country) | 8-oz. container | 240 | 41.4 |
| Apricot: | | | |
| (Breyer's) | 1 cup | 270 | 47.0 |
| (Dannon) | 8-oz. container | 260 | 49.0 |
| (Sealtest) *Light'n Lively* | 1 cup | 250 | 48.0 |
| Apricot crunch (New Country) | 8-oz. container | 251 | 42.5 |
| Banana: | | | |
| (Breyer's) | 1 cup | 270 | 47.0 |
| (Dannon) | 8-oz. container | 260 | 49.0 |
| Blueberry: | | | |
| (Breyer's) | 1 cup | 270 | 47.0 |
| (Dannon) | 8-oz. container | 260 | 49.0 |
| (Dean) | 8-oz. container | 259 | 50.6 |
| (Sealtest) *Light'n Lively* | 1 cup | 250 | 49.0 |
| (Sweet 'N Low) | 8-oz. container | 150 | 28.0 |
| *Yoplait* (General Mills) | 6-oz. container | 190 | 32.0 |
| Blueberry ripple (New Country) | 8-oz. container | 240 | 43.0 |
| Boysenberry (Dannon) | 8-oz. container | 260 | 49.0 |
| Cherry: | | | |
| (Breyer's) black | 1 cup | 270 | 47.0 |
| (Dannon) | 8-oz. container | 260 | 49.0 |
| (Dean) | 8-oz. container | 245 | 47.9 |
| (Sealtest) *Light'n Lively* | 1 cup | 240 | 45.0 |
| (Sweet 'N Low) | 8-oz. container | 150 | 28.0 |
| *Yoplait* (General Mills) | 6-oz. container | 190 | 32.0 |

| Food and Description | Measure or Quantity | Calories | Carbo-hydrates (grams) |
|---|---|---|---|
| Cherry supreme (New Country) | 8-oz. container | 240 | 44.0 |
| Coffee (Dannon) | 8-oz. container | 200 | 32.0 |
| Date walnut (New Country) | 8-oz. container | 257 | 42.6 |
| Dutch apple (Dannon) | 8-oz. container | 260 | 49.0 |
| Flavored (Alta-Dena) *Maya* | 1 container | 280 | 39.0 |
| Flavored (Alta-Dena) *Naja* | 1 container | 250 | 40.0 |
| French vanilla ripple (New Country) | 8-oz. container | 240 | 42.0 |
| Fruit crunch (New Country) | 8-oz. container | 240 | 42.0 |
| Grape (Breyer's) | 1 cup | 270 | 47.0 |
| Hawaiian salad (New Country) | 8-oz. container | 250 | 42.0 |
| Honey (Dannon) | 8-oz. container | 260 | 49.0 |
| Honey'n berries (New Country) | 8-oz. container | 240 | 43.0 |
| Lemon: | | | |
| (Breyer's) | 1 cup | 230 | 32.0 |
| (Dannon) | 8-oz. container | 200 | 32.0 |
| (Sealtest) *Light'n Lively* | 8-oz. container | 250 | 47.0 |
| (Sweet 'N Low) | 8-oz. container | 150 | 28.0 |
| *Yoplait* (General Mills) | 6-oz. container | 190 | 32.0 |
| Lemon ripple (New Country) | 8-oz. container | 240 | 43.0 |
| Mandarin orange (Sealtest) *Light'n Lively* | 1 cup | 240 | 46.0 |
| Orange: | | | |
| (Dean) | 8-oz. container | 311 | 62.9 |
| *Yoplait* (General Mills) | 6-oz. container | 190 | 32.0 |
| Orange-pineapple (Breyer's) | 1 cup | 270 | 47.0 |

(USDA): United States Department of Agriculture
(HEW/FAO): Health, Education and Welfare/Food and Agriculture
                    Organization
* Prepared as Package Directs

| Food and Description | Measure or Quantity | Calories | Carbo-hydrates (grams) |
|---|---|---|---|
| Orange supreme (New Country) | 8-oz. container | 240 | 43.0 |
| Peach: | | | |
| (Breyer's) | 1 cup | 270 | 47.0 |
| (Dannon) | 8-oz. container | 260 | 49.0 |
| (Dean) | 8-oz. container | 259 | 49.1 |
| (Sweet 'N Low) | 8-oz. container | 150 | 28.0 |
| Peach melba (Sealtest) *Light'n Lively* | 1 cup | 250 | 48.0 |
| Peaches'n Cream (New Country) | 8-oz. container | 240 | 43.0 |
| Pineapple: | | | |
| (Breyer's) | 1 cup | 270 | 47.0 |
| (Dean) | 8-oz. container | 265 | 48.7 |
| (Sealtest) *Light'n Lively* | 1 cup | 250 | 50.0 |
| Pineapple-orange (Dannon) | 8-oz. container | 260 | 49.0 |
| Raspberry: | | | |
| (Breyer's) | 1 cup | 270 | 47.0 |
| (Dannon) red | 8-oz. container | 260 | 49.0 |
| (Sealtest) *Light'n Lively*, red | 1 cup | 230 | 43.0 |
| (Sweet 'N Low) | 8-oz. container | 150 | 28.0 |
| *Yoplait* (General Mills) | 6-oz. container | 190 | 32.0 |
| Raspberry ripple (New Country) | 8-oz. container | 240 | 43.0 |
| Strawberry: | | | |
| (Breyer's) | 1 cup | 270 | 47.0 |
| (Dannon) | 8-oz. container | 260 | 49.0 |
| (Dean) | 8-oz. container | 256 | 46.8 |
| (Sealtest) *Light'n Lively* | 1 cup | 250 | 47.0 |
| (Sweet 'N Low) | 8-oz. container | 150 | 28.0 |
| *Viva*, Swiss style | 8-oz. container | 250 | 47.0 |
| *Yoplait* (General Mills) | 6-oz. container | 190 | 32.0 |
| Strawberry supreme (New Country) | 8-oz. container | 240 | 43.0 |
| Vanilla: | | | |
| (Breakstone) | 8-oz. container | 195 | 29.5 |
| (Breyer's) | 1 cup | 230 | 32.0 |
| (Dannon) | 8-oz. container | 200 | 32.0 |

| Food and Description | Measure or Quantity | Calories | Carbo-hydrates (grams) |
|---|---|---|---|
| **Frozen (Dannon):** | | | |
| **Banana:** | | | |
| *Danny-in-a-Cup* | 8-oz. cup | 210 | 42.0 |
| *Danny-Yo* | 3½-oz. serving | 110 | 21.0 |
| Blueberry, *Danny Parfait* | ¼ of 16-oz. container | 160 | 35.0 |
| **Boysenberry:** | | | |
| *Danny-On-A-Stick*, carob coated | 2½-fl.-oz. bar | 135 | 13.0 |
| *Danny-Yo* | 3½-oz. serving | 110 | 21.0 |
| Cherry, *Danny-in-a-Cup* | 8-oz. cup | 210 | 42.0 |
| Chocolate, *Danny-Yo* | 3½-oz. serving | 110 | 21.0 |
| Lemon, *Danny-in-a-Cup* | 8-oz. cup | 180 | 20.0 |
| **Peach:** | | | |
| *Danny-in-a-Cup* | 8-oz. cup | 210 | 42.0 |
| *Danny Parfait* | ¼ of 16-oz. container | 160 | 35.0 |
| **Piña Colada:** | | | |
| *Danny-in-a-Cup* | 8-oz. cup | 210 | 42.0 |
| *Danny-On-A-Stick* | 2½-fl.-oz. bar | 65 | 13.0 |
| Pineapple-orange, *Danny Parfait* | ¼ of 16-oz. container | 160 | 35.0 |
| **Raspberry, red:** | | | |
| *Danny-in-a-Cup* | 8-oz. cup | 210 | 42.0 |
| *Danny Parfait* | ¼ of 16-oz. container | 160 | 35.0 |
| *Danny-On-A-Stick*, chocolate coated | 2½-fl.-oz. bar | 135 | 13.0 |
| **Strawberry:** | | | |
| *Danny-in-a-Cup* | 8-oz. cup | 210 | 42.0 |
| *Danny Flip*, with strawberry topping | 5-fl.-oz. serving | 175 | 37.0 |
| *Danny Parfait* | ¼ of 16-oz. container | 160 | 35.0 |
| *Danny-On-A-Stick* | 2½ fl. oz. bar | 65 | 13.0 |
| *Danny-On-A-Stick*, chocolate-coated | 2½-fl.-oz. bar | 135 | 13.0 |

(USDA): United States Department of Agriculture
(HEW/FAO): Health, Education and Welfare/Food and Agriculture
          Organization
\* Prepared as Package Directs

| Food and Description | Measure or Quantity | Calories | Carbo-hydrates (grams) |
|---|---|---|---|
| *Danny-Yo* Vanilla: | 3½-oz. serving | 110 | 21.0 |
| *Danny-in-a-Cup* | 8-oz. cup | 180 | 20.0 |
| *Danny Flip*, with red raspberry topping | 5-fl.-oz. serving | 175 | 37.0 |
| *Danny-On-A-Stick* | 2½-fl.-oz. bar | 65 | 13.0 |
| *Danny-On-A-Stick*, carob coated | 2½-fl.-oz. bar | 135 | 13.0 |
| *Danny Yo* Vanilla-strawberry, | 3½-oz. serving | 110 | 21.0 |
| *Danny Sampler* | 3-fl.-oz. serving | 70 | 14.0 |
| **YOGURT CHIFFON PIE,** frozen (Sara Lee) *Light'n Luscious:* | | | |
| Blueberry | ⅛ of pie | 120 | 20.4 |
| Cherry | ⅛ of pie | 121 | 21.1 |
| Strawberry | ⅛ of pie | 118 | 19.4 |

# Z

| | | | |
|---|---|---|---|
| **ZINFANDEL WINE:** | | | |
| (Inglenook) Estate, 12% alcohol | 3 fl. oz. | 58 | .3 |
| (Inglenook) vintage, 12% alcohol | 3 fl. oz. | 59 | .3 |
| (Italian Swiss Colony) 13% alcohol | 3 fl. oz. | 61 | .9 |
| (Louis M. Martini) 12½% alcohol | 3 fl. oz. | 90 | .2 |
| **ZITI,** frozen (Ronzoni) baked | 4½-oz. serving | 130 | 19.0 |
| **ZUCCHINI (See SQUASH, SUMMER)** | | | |
| **ZWEIBACK:** | | | |
| (USDA) | 1 oz. | 120 | 21.1 |
| (Gerber) | .2-oz. piece | 30 | 5.2 |
| (Nabisco) | .3-oz. piece | 30 | 5.0 |

# Bibliography

Dawson, Elsie H., Gilpin, Gladys L., and Fulton, Lois H. *Average weight of a measured cup of various foods.* U.S.D.A. ARS 61–6, February 1969. 19 pp.

Leung, W. T. W., Busson, F., and Jardin, C. *Food composition table for use in Africa.* U.S. Department of Health, Education and Welfare and Food and Agriculture Organization of the United Nations. 1968. 306 pp.

Leung, W. T. W., Butrum, R. V., and Chang, F. H. *Food composition table or use in East Asia.* U.S. Department of Health, Education and Welfare and Food and Agriculture Organization of the United Nations. December 1972. 334 pp.

Merrill, A. L. and Watt, B. K., *Energy value of foods—basis and derivation.* U.S.D.A. Handb. 74, 105 pp. 1955.

Pecot, Rebecca K., Jaeger, Carol M., and Watt, Bernice K., *Proximate composition of beef from carcass to cooked meat: Method of derivation and tables of values.* U.S.D.A. Home Economics Research Report 31, 32 pp. 1965.

Pecot, Rebecca K. and Watt, Bernice K., *Food yields: Summarized by different stages of preparation.* U.S.D.A. Handb. 102, 93 pp. 1956.

U.S.D.A. Nutritive value of foods. Home and Garden Bul. 72, 36 pp. 1964 and revised edition, 1970. 41 pp.

U.S.D.A. Unpubl. Data 1969.

Watt, Bernice K., Merrill, Annabel L., et. al., *Composition of foods: Raw, processed, prepared.* U.S.D.A. Agriculture Handb. 8, 190 pp. 1963.